C0-GGZ-398

SERVING THE SERIOUSLY MENTALLY ILL: PUBLIC–ACADEMIC LINKAGES IN SERVICES, RESEARCH, AND TRAINING

PAUL WOHLFORD

HECTOR F. MYERS

JOANNE E. CALLAN

EDITORS

AMERICAN PSYCHOLOGICAL ASSOCIATION
WASHINGTON, DC

Barry University Library
Miami, Fla. 33161

Copyright © 1993 by the American Psychological Association. All rights reserved. Except as permitted under the United States Copyright Act of 1976, no part of this publication may be reproduced or distributed in any form or by any means, or stored in a database or retrieval system, without the prior written permission of the publisher.

(Copyright is not claimed for foreword and chapters 1, 2, 7, 20, and 26, which are in the public domain.)

Published by the
American Psychological Association
750 First Street, NE
Washington, DC 20002

Copies may be ordered from
APA Order Department
P.O. Box 2710
Hyattsville, MD 20784

In the UK and Europe, copies may be ordered from
American Psychological Association
3 Henrietta Street
Covent Garden, London
WC2E 8LU England

This book was typeset in Century Schoolbook by Innodata Corp., Hanover, MD

Printer: Victor Graphics, Inc., Baltimore, MD
Cover designer: Sans Serif Graphics, Arlington, VA
Technical/production editor: Paula R. Bronstein
Copy Editor: Diane Stuart

Library of Congress Cataloging-in-Publication Data
Serving the seriously mentally ill: public-academic linkages in services, research, and training/Paul E. Wohlford, Joanne E. Callan, and Hector F. Myers, editors.
p. cm.
Includes bibliographical references.
ISBN 1-55798-216-3 (acid-free paper)
1. Clinical psychologists—Training of. 2. Clinical psychology—Study and teaching. 3. Mentally ill—Services for. 4. Mental health services. I. Wohlford, Paul, 1938- II. Callan, Joanne E. III. Myers, Hector F.
RC467.7.S47 1993
362.2—dc20 93-32056
CIP

British Library Cataloging-in-Publication Data
A CIP record is available from the British Library.

Printed in the United States of America
First edition

RC
467.7
.S47
1993

This book is dedicated to Louis D. Cohen, Norman Garmezy, Eliot H. Rodnick, Stanley F. Schneider, Milton Shore, and Sam Silverstein, who, through their commitment to excellence and innovation in training for psychological services, continue to be role models for many.

This book is also dedicated to the memory of Thomas O. Hilliard and Saleem Shah whose work for the underserved must be carried forward by others.

Contents

Foreword ix
Bernard S. Arons and Frederick K. Goodwin

Preface xi
Raymond D. Fowler

Acknowledgments xiii

Introduction

1. Public–Academic Linkages 3
Paul Wohlford, Joanne E. Callan, and Hector F. Myers

Part I Efforts to Improve Clinical Training for Psychological Services to Targeted Groups

2. Seriously Emotionally Disturbed Children, Adolescents, and Their Families 19
Paul Wohlford and Phyllis R. Magrab

3. Seriously Mentally Ill Adults 27
Dale L. Johnson

4. Psychological Services for Older Adults 33
Linda Teri

5. Ethnic Minorities With Mental Disorders 43
Hector F. Myers

6. Clients With Substance Abuse and Comorbid Diagnoses 51
Holly A. Hills, Robert A. Zucker, and Steven L. Seitz

Part II Public Mental Health Service Responsibilities for the Mentally Ill

7. The Role of the State in Public–Academic Linkages for Clinical Training — 63
James P. Stratoudakis, Henry Tomes, Paul Wohlford, and James Stockdill

8. The Community Support Program and Psychology: Trends and Opportunities — 69
Andrea K. Blanch

9. Public–Academic Collaboration in Training Child Mental Health Professionals — 77
Lenore B. Behar

10. The Human Resource Development Program: Improving Community-Based Mental Health Services — 85
Susan E. Salasin, Thomas E. Backer, and Frank D. McGuirk

11. The Role of Community Mental Health Centers in Public–Academic Linkages — 95
David S. Hargrove

12. Consumer Impact on Mental Health Services, Clinical Training, and Public–Academic Linkages: Some Personal Reflections — 99
Frederick J. Frese

Part III: Models of Effective Public–Academic Collaboration

13. State Mental Health Systems and Universities: A Conceptual Model for Collaborative Service — 105
King E. Davis

14. The North Carolina Children and Youth Demonstration Project: Increasing Professionals' Understanding of Service Systems — 115
Lenore B. Behar, Tom Bainbridge, and Richard Munger

15. Initiatives in Ohio With Seriously Emotionally Disturbed Children and Adolescents — 131
W. Rodney Hammond and Betty Yung

16. The Cincinnati Consortium: Training for Services to Seriously Mentally Disabled Adults and Their Families — 137
David T. Hellkamp

17. Developing the Maryland Training Consortium on Serious Mental Illness 143
Robert D. Coursey, Stanley E. Weinstein, and Lee E. Deckelnick

18. Creating a Competent Workforce in Vermont: Promoting Public–Academic Linkages and Human Resource Development 157
Annamarie T. Cioffari, John D. Burchard, Paul J. Carling, and Rodney E. Copeland

19. The Colorado Postdoctoral Training Consortium: An Innovative Postdoctoral Program in Public Psychology 165
Carl N. Zimet and Courtenay Harding

Part IV: Ensuring Quality and Competence in Training for Mental Health Services

20. Using Research and Evaluation to Develop a Competent Workforce for Mental Health Services 175
Paul Wohlford and Ronald W. Manderscheid

21. Assessing the Competencies of Clinical Psychologists 185
Lee Sechrest and Anne Scott

22. The Role of the State in Ensuring Quality in Health Care Service Delivery and Its Linkage With the Private and Public Sectors 195
Judy E. Hall

23. Improving the Clinical Training of Psychologists: A Role for Accreditation? 207
Paul D. Nelson

24. Clinical Training and Research for Children's Services 213
Robert M. Friedman

25. Public Mental Health Systems and Research: Can This Relationship Survive? 219
Michael F. Hogan

Conclusion

26. Current Progress and Future Directions 227
Paul Wohlford, Hector F. Myers, and Joanne E. Callan

Appendixes

A.	Policy Recommendations From the National Conference on Implementing Public–Academic Linkages for Clinical Training in Psychology	245
B.	National Conference on Implementing Public–Academic Linkages for Clinical Training in Psychology, Participants List	257
C.	State Mental Health Planning	263
D.	Public–Academic Linkages in Clinical Training Programs in Psychology Supported by CMHS/NIMH, 1988–1993	271

Foreword

Our nation faces an extraordinary public health challenge: to improve the care provided to the millions of people with serious and disabling mental disorders. These are individuals who suffer from conditions that devastate their lives and often the lives of those around them. Efforts to deinstitutionalize seriously mentally ill individuals have resulted in their being discharged from state psychiatric hospitals and returned to communities, often without adequate treatment and psychosocial rehabilitation programs. Other priority populations also presently underserved by the public mental health system include children and adolescents with serious emotional disturbances, elderly and ethnic minorities with mental disorders, persons with mental disorders living in rural areas, and individuals with dual disorders (e.g., with a mental illness and with substance abuse).

The mission of a mental health delivery system is inexorably tied to human resources, its most valued asset. As the focus shifts from state hospitals to innovative community programs, the most urgent issue in mental health human resources development today is to improve training of the core mental health professionals, including clinical psychologists, and thereby instill in them appropriate values, roles, and skills. Community treatment will not be successful if the available personnel, professional organizations, and academic programs are not receptive to changes in the delivery of services to seriously impaired persons. Methods must be found to recruit new staff to work with these clients, especially in community settings, to redeploy staff from mental hospitals into the community, and, within the community, to move staff from practitioners' offices into the client's natural environment.

If staff and training needs are to be addressed, it is clear that enhanced collaboration among academic training programs and state and local mental health agencies is needed. As a major step in this direction, the Georgetown University Child Development Center and the National Institute of Mental Health (NIMH) cosponsored the National Conference on Implementing Public–Academic Linkages for Clinical Training in Psychology, in December 1990. Consistent with the concepts that the conference was promoting, the participants represented a wide spectrum of consumer, family, and advocacy mental health organizations; public mental health or substance abuse organizations at the federal, state, and local levels; academic and internship training programs in psychology; and graduate students. Of particular significance in this age of specialization and compartmentalization is the fact that support and funding for this conference came from five different federal programs and cut across divisional and agency boundaries. Funding sources included two major divisions within NIMH, the Division of Clinical Research and the Division of Applied and Services Research, as well as the Office of Substance Abuse Prevention, demonstrating collaboration between services and clinical training and also between mental health and substance abuse prevention.

It is to be hoped that efforts to implement the recommendations of these conferences will be facilitated by the recent major reorganization of NIMH. The Alcohol, Drug Abuse, and Mental Health Administration Reorganization Act of 1992 mandated the creation of a national Center for Mental Health Services (CMHS) within a new agency, the Substance Abuse and Mental Health Services Administration (SAMSHA). The Center now has major responsibility for improving mental health services, as well as for conducting related clinical training, information collection, and evaluation activities. This book, the Center's first published project on human resources or workforce development, continues NIMH's tradition of policy development for improving mental health services.

When Congress created the new CMHS with service and clinical training functions that were separate from NIMH and its research functions, concerns were expressed that mental health research would be split from mental health services. Thus, Congress explicitly mandated collaboration between the two agencies so that research-based knowledge about mental disorders and treatment is transferred from NIMH to CMHS to improve mental health services. This reorganization has created certain structures to help facilitate the knowledge translation and transfer.

A major challenge in clinical training is to minimize discrepancies between the state of science, the state of clinical training, and the typical state of practice. To address these systems problems, the latest and soundest scientific knowledge about effective mental health services should be translated into ongoing education and training curricula for use in both the preservice training of new service providers and the continuing education of current service providers. In short, our aim is to translate the latest scientific knowledge into practice via training. By strengthening and extending linkages between public service agencies and academic training programs, we hope to close the gaps between the latest science-based knowledge, what is taught, and the actual practice of providing services to persons with mental illness.

BERNARD S. ARONS, MD
Acting Director
Center for Mental Health Services
Substance Abuse and Mental Health Services Administration

FREDERICK K. GOODWIN, MD
Director
National Institute of Mental Health
National Institute of Health

Preface

The National Institute of Mental Health (NIMH) is to be commended for its leadership over the years in giving focus to the many needs of this country's seriously mentally ill and also for its attention to the training of mental health professionals. Its past support of clinical training for psychologists, initiated in 1948, was a major force in establishing outstanding doctoral and internship programs across the United States. More recently, its commitment to relating the clinical training of psychologists to the mental health needs of the nation's most underserved populations has provided direction in the midst of reduced resources.

This volume draws on the thinking of more than 100 representatives of public service and academic organizations, mostly psychologists, who participated in the 1990 National Conference on Implementing Public–Academic Linkages for Clinical Training in Psychology, cosponsored by NIMH and Georgetown University. It presents recommendations developed in the conference to advance the clinical training of psychologists and, especially, to meet the mental health needs of the major underserved populations. In highlighting what can be done by psychologists to respond to the needs of such underserved groups through linkages between public and academic agencies, this volume holds promise for more efficient, effective, and relevant clinical training.

With 114,000 members and affiliates, the American Psychological Association (APA) is the largest scientific and professional association of psychologists in the world. APA's commitment to promoting the conduct of relevant research and the training of psychologists who can deliver services responsive to our country's compelling mental health needs is congruent with the Conference recommendations.

Just as APA has enjoyed a collaborative association with NIMH for more than 4 decades in supporting the clinical training of psychologists, it encourages collaboration among all agencies and institutions similarly committed. Indeed, APA looks to the gains that can be realized in research, training, and service through such linkages.

Raymond D. Fowler
Chief Executive Officer
American Psychological Association

Acknowledgments

This book grew out of the issues discussed at the National Conference on Implementing Public–Academic Linkages for Clinical Training in Psychology held in Washington, D.C. on December 10–12, 1990. The conference was cosponsored by the National Institute of Mental Health (NIMH) and Georgetown University through an interagency agreement with the Bureau of Maternal and Child Health and Resources Development. Special thanks go to Alan I. Leshner, who was the Acting Director of NIMH when this conference was held, for his support and encouragement.

The cosponsors of the Conference included the Education and Training Branch of the Division of Clinical Research, NIMH; the Systems Development and Community Support Branch and the Child and Family Support Branch of the Division of Applied and Services Research, NIMH; and the Office of Substance Abuse Prevention, Alcohol, Drug Abuse, and Mental Health Administration. The Conference was conducted by the Georgetown University Child Development Center, directed by Phyllis R. Magrab, and coordinated by Ellen Kagan. Much of the manuscript was prepared by Rebecca Levine and Ernest Fields.

Introduction

CHAPTER

1

Public–Academic Linkages

Paul Wohlford
Center for Mental Health Services

Joanne E. Callan
American Psychological Association

Hector F. Myers
University of California, Los Angeles

Although new federal and state policies have directed resources to the seriously mentally ill over the last decade, the education of key mental health professionals has generally not stayed in step. University training programs have continued to produce graduates trained to serve clients who have less serious problems. On this score, professional psychology is as indictable as the other mental health professions. Over 3,000 psychologists are working in state mental hospitals (Manderscheid & Barrett, 1987), approximately 2,100 PhDs and 2,800 MA psychologists are working in Community Mental Health Centers (CMHCs; National Council of CMHCs, 1987). Unfortunately, very few of these psychologists have been trained to be expert in treating the seriously mentally ill.

According to Johnson, (1990; this volume) and to Sechrest and Pion (1990), many psychology faculties continue to instill outmoded ideas for the care of these patients, or provide no ideas or relevant experience whatsoever. Sechrest and Pion found that "it is quite possible for students in clinical psychology to go all through their training without any contact with persons who are seriously mentally ill" (1990, p. 29). They concluded, "Over time, clinical psychology has . . . largely abandoned work with the seriously mentally ill" (1990, p. 29). This abandonment by clinical psychology as a field is ironic because individual clinical psychologists have contributed to many of the most powerful systems presently available for assessing and treating or managing systems of care for the seriously mentally ill (Johnson, 1990). Mechanisms are needed to bridge the increasing gap between professional psychology training programs and the needs of the public sector, in order to better serve the seriously mentally ill.

A growing sense of concern over this situation has led to a renewed interest in clinical training in psychology from mental health policymakers at national, state, and local levels; from consumers of mental health services and their family members; and from psychologists themselves. Indeed, a similar renewal of interest in clinical training has occurred in all mental health disciplines. This renewed interest has embraced all related mental health functions including research and administration, and, especially, services. More specifically,

The opinions expressed in this chapter are those of the authors and do not necessarily reflect the official policy or position of the Center for Mental Health Services, the American Psychological Association, or the University of California at Los Angeles.

the interface between public mental health services and clinical training in psychology has been of central interest, and it is this interface that constitutes the theme of the present volume, as reflected in its title: *Serving the Seriously Mentally Ill: Public–Academic Linkages in Services, Research, and Training.*

Seriously mentally ill is intended to be a general term for underserved priority populations, including children, the elderly, and adults, as discussed below.

Several different sets of forces have converged, giving rise to the emphasis on public–academic linkages for services and training. The illumination of these goals is one focus of the introduction, and major themes running throughout the volume reflect them. The goals include improving the quality of care for unserved or underserved groups of mentally ill; instituting more collaborative relationships, service-driven training, and consumer-driven services; ensuring competence of psychologists (and other service providers); laying strong foundations in science; translating and transferring knowledge from research to services via training; and increasing incentives for the development and implementation of the best clinical service-training-research models. An additional set of issues has very recently catapulted itself to the foreground: How mental health services will be included under national health care reform, what constitutes quality public mental health services, and the role of competent personnel in delivering these services.

This book has two main purposes: The first is to consolidate and facilitate the implementation of recommendations from recent training conferences that have focused on the underserved priority populations of seriously mentally ill adults, children and adolescents with serious emotional disturbances, and elderly and ethnic minorities with mental disorders. The second purpose is to suggest and promote ways of expanding the collaboration referred to as "public–academic linkages for clinical training." The chapters that follow contain a wealth of ideas as to how this can be done.

In this chapter, we will first discuss the background of issues and conferences that led up to the 1990 National Conference on Implementing Public–Academic Linkages for Clinical Training in Psychology (Linkages Conference). Then we will describe the Linkages Conference itself. Finally, we present an overview of the chapters in this volume.

Background

Until October 1, 1992, the National Institute of Mental Health (NIMH) Education and Training Branch[1] was responsible for clinical training of mental health professionals who are concerned with treatment of the priority populations mentioned above. In 1987, NIMH invited discussion of a plan to improve clinical training for providing services to such populations. It had become clear not only that economic issues must be considered, but also that many other important factors had to be reconciled; and, further, that a good, consensus-based policy resolution would require a long process. Because additional funds were made available by Congress for NIMH clinical training in 1988 (for the first time in seven years), it was possible to plan for systematic program improvement, including the scheduling of several conferences designed to discuss factors affecting training and to make policy recommendations.

In 1987, two NIMH-sponsored interdisciplinary conferences layed the foundation for subsequent training activities, and the proceedings were published in the report, *Interdisciplinary Collaboration Between State Mental Health and Higher Education* (Davis and Sanchez, 1987). The purpose of these conferences was to explore ways to increase collaboration between university-based mental health professional education and training programs and the array of state and local mental health programs serving the public sector. This basic concept of collaboration has been refined to become public–academic linkages for services and training. Another objective of these conferences was to identify barriers that often frustrate efforts to initiate, support, and maintain collaboration between state mental health programs and higher education. The major barriers identified were (a) lack of information, (b) lack of shared goals and purposes, (c) lack of motivation, (d) lack of faculty knowledge and skills regarding state services and clients, and most important, (e) lack of comprehensive state and academic planning.

[1] Since October 1, 1992, when Public Law 102-321, the ADAMHA Reorganization Act, went into effect, the responsibility for mental health clinical training was transferred to the new Center for Mental Health Services (CMHS), part of the new Substance Abuse and Mental Health Services Administration (SAMHSA), within the Department of Health and Human Services (DHHS). Specifically, clinical training is the responsibility of the Human Resources Planning and Development Branch in CMHS's Division of State and Community Systems Development.

In summary, these conferences found that the academic preparation of mental health professionals in all disciplines, including psychology, was perceived by the public mental health community as increasingly irrelevant to the mental health service needs of the public sector. Public mental health service programs, by the same token, were perceived by training program directors as unstable and shifting in direction and priority. These issues were reaffirmed in three 1988 conferences and in subsequent meetings on clinical training, and indeed are just as important now as they were in 1987.

The 1988 National Conferences on Clinical Training in Psychology

In 1988, in order to focus clinical training in psychology on services to priority populations, the following three national conferences were held:

- Training Psychologists to Work with the Seriously Mentally Ill, April 6–8, 1988, University of Houston (Johnson, 1990).
- Clinical Training in Psychology: Improving Psychological Services for Children and Adolescents With Severe Mental Disorders, May 18–20, 1988, Georgetown University (Magrab and Wohlford, 1990).
- Improving Training and Psychological Services for Ethnic Minorities, June 8–10, 1988, University of California, Los Angeles (Myers, Wohlford, Guzman, & Echemendia, 1991).

The purpose of each of these conferences was to improve clinical training and services for a specific priority population by focusing on more effective collaboration across service programs and training programs, as shown schematically in Figure 1. Note that under service programs the priority population to receive services (seriously mentally ill adults, etc.) appears separated from the state and local mental health agencies. This separation serves to underscore the view that quality service programs and training should be guided by consumer needs.

At each of the three 1988 conferences, 40 to 60 national leaders intensively examined training issues and recommended policy directions. Each conference was both large enough to be representative of the nation's best programs (many of which had been supported by NIMH) and focused enough to allow in-depth discussion. Each conference agenda covered a matrix of training issues, focusing primarily on what constitutes the best training models to provide the skills and experiences necessary for professionals to serve the needs of a specific population. In addition, each agenda considered level of training (e.g., masters, predoctoral academic, predoctoral internship, and postdoctoral fellowship), type of setting and client (e.g., dual diagnosis, homeless), and type of support mechanism (e.g., student stipend, faculty support, faculty development, curriculum development). Each conference was charged with making specific sets of recommendations to the following institutions:

- NIMH for funding priorities, clinical training policies, and administrative procedures.
- American Psychological Association (APA) boards and committees for improving the quality of training in given areas.
- Other institutions, including state and local mental health agencies.

The three components of psychology training programs distinguished in Figure 1 are academic programs and faculty; students and trainees; and practicum, internship, and postdoctoral training programs. The latter component is sometimes conducted in a state or local mental health agency, thus creating a partial bridge between psychology training programs and services programs (noted in Figure 1 by dotted brackets). Because this relationship between academic programs and internship programs may be tenuous or, in some instances, nonexistent, such bridging is unreliable at best. Sometimes the students or trainees, themselves, are the chief bridge between the academic programs and the service programs. Therefore, at a minimum, several actions are needed: (a) improve academic internship program communications and relations, (b) strengthen and extend direct relations between academic programs and service programs, (c) directly acquaint students with all aspects of service programs from the local agencies to state policy making, and (d) involve training programs with primary consumers and their families. In summary, a major purpose of the 1988 conferences on clinical training in psychology was to enhance collaboration across clinical service and training programs, that is, to make the clinical training program more service-driven.

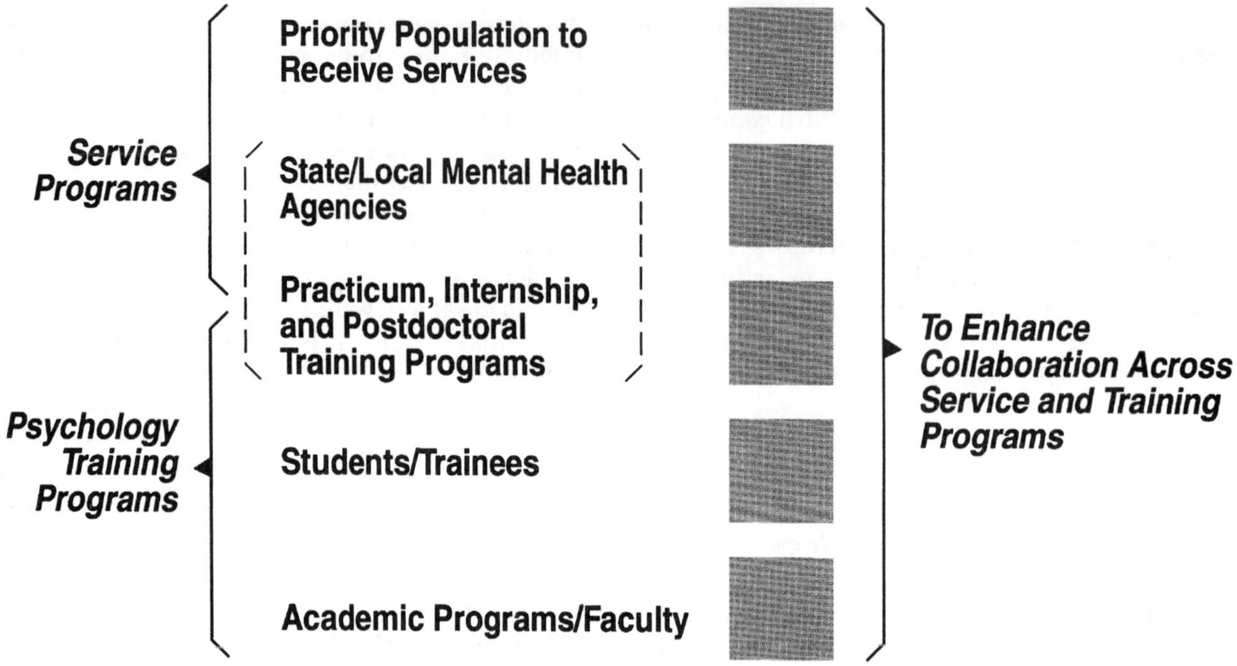

Figure 1. A major purpose of the 1988 national conferences on clinical training in psychology was to enhance collaboration across services and training programs. Note: Practicum, internship, and postdoctoral training programs are sometimes conducted in state or local mental health agencies.

In August, 1988, at the APA Annual Convention in Atlanta, the steering committees of the three conferences discussed implementation of their recommendations regarding funding priorities and general policies. There was agreement on general as well as specific recommendations across the three conferences, although some topics were discussed in only one conference. The most salient recommendation that emerged independently from each of the three conferences was that *more young psychologists should be recruited for careers in public service to the priority populations.* The conferees also concurred on other policy recommendations, such as adding ethnic minorities as another NIMH clinical training priority population and recognizing the importance of institutional faculty development, curriculum development, and continuing education. It is interesting to note that the conferees at each of the three conferences displayed qualities observable both in the conference process and in the outcome, such as cooperation, helping, and sharing rather than competitiveness and secretiveness. These qualities were reflected by the endorsement, at all three conferences, of sharing new curricular models and materials through such means as faculty development activities or some new type of national curriculum clearinghouse. Perhaps this cooperative spirit was due to a general recognition that psychologists in the public service sector constitute a special subset of the whole profession, a recognition that led also to the uniting of participants in the three conferences for the explicit purpose of helping one another implement all recommendations.

Implementation of recommendations from the three 1988 conferences involved four steps:

1. Working with appropriate offices of the APA to ensure the implementation of policy recommendations to NIMH. (This step has been achieved to some extent; the 1989, 1990, 1991, and 1992 NIMH clinical training announcements reflect input from the three conferences. Several changes in NIMH clinical training announcements, two of which are very significant, resulted from conference input: The 1990 announcement highlighted and for the first time required public–academic linkages for clinical training, and the 1991 announcements included ethnic minorities with mental disorders as a primary priority population.)

2. Seeking a broader base for implementing recommendations by APA boards and committees through the dissemination of published conference proceedings and public discussions at the 1989 APA Annual Convention. (The latter was accom-

plished when conference recommendations were presented at three separate symposia).

3. Publishing books based on each of the three conferences. These were published by APA (Johnson, 1990; Magrab & Wohlford, 1990; Myers, Wohlford, Guzman, & Echemendia, 1991) and distributed to the training program directors of APA-accredited doctoral programs and internship programs, and to the key leadership of APA divisions, boards and committees.

4. Establishing a structure or committee, with representation from all three conferences to oversee the implementation of the recommendations. (In December, 1990, NIMH and Georgetown University sponsored a conference on public–academic linkages for clinical training in psychology to support this effort.)

Multidisciplinary National Conferences on Clinical Training

The recommendations from the three 1988 conferences on clinical training in psychology contributed to four corresponding multidisciplinary clinical training conferences held between 1988 and 1990:

- National Forum for Educating Mental Health Professionals to Work with the Seriously Mentally Ill and Their Families, September 14–16, 1988, National Alliance for the Mentally Ill (National Institute of Mental Health, 1990).
- Clinical Training for Services to the Long-Term Seriously Mentally Ill: A Multidisciplinary Review and Assessment, September 22–24, 1989, University of Cincinnati (Paulson and Paulson, 1991).
- National Conference on Multidisciplinary Clinical Training for Services for Seriously Emotionally Disturbed Children and Adolescents, September 6–8, 1989, Georgetown University (Kagan, Magrab, & Wohlford, 1992).
- National Conference on Multidisciplinary Clinical Training and Services for Seriously Mentally Ill Ethnic Minorities, October 31–November 2, 1990, Howard University (Gary & Weaver, 1991).

The focus on service-driven training from earlier conferences, and as described above, led to a multidisciplinary focus and cooperation. Figure 2 shows how the focus on collaboration across service and training in psychology was expanded to reflect a multidisciplinary perspective.

Psychology has taken the lead on NIMH multidisciplinary clinical training programs. Seven out of 10 multidisciplinary programs funded in 1991 by NIMH involve psychology. Usually a psychologist serves as the training program director. All seven of these psychology programs are internship or postdoctoral training programs; none are doctoral programs. It may be that at this early stage in the development of such collaborative initiatives, it is easier for disciplines to collaborate in actual service settings in which these internships are located than it is to bridge the gap between a department of psychology within a university and some other entity, such as a school of nursing.

The 1990 National Conference on Implementing Public–Academic Linkages for Clinical Training in Psychology

Recommendations from the three 1988 conferences on clinical training in psychology and the subsequent follow-up meetings, provide important guidelines for future development and expansion of training relevant to the treatment of the seriously mentally ill in the United States. These recommendations are pertinent to federal and state agencies that are responsible for service delivery and that employ psychologists to provide services, and to those institutions and individuals who train current and future psychologists.

Nevertheless, implementation of the recommendations has presented a serious challenge. In response to this challenge and to the extent that the recommendations are similar, it would be possible to have common advocacy from a broad constituency, thereby increasing the likelihood of implementing them. By strengthening public–academic linkages, the conceptual and strategic aspects of the various conference recommendations could be promoted, and thus, service-driven clinical training could be enhanced.

In December, 1990, NIMH and Georgetown University sponsored a fourth conference in the series on training in psychology, the National Conference on Implementing Public–Academic Linkages for Clinical Training in Psychology (or Linkages Conference). The two major purposes of the Linkages Conference as presented in this volume are sum-

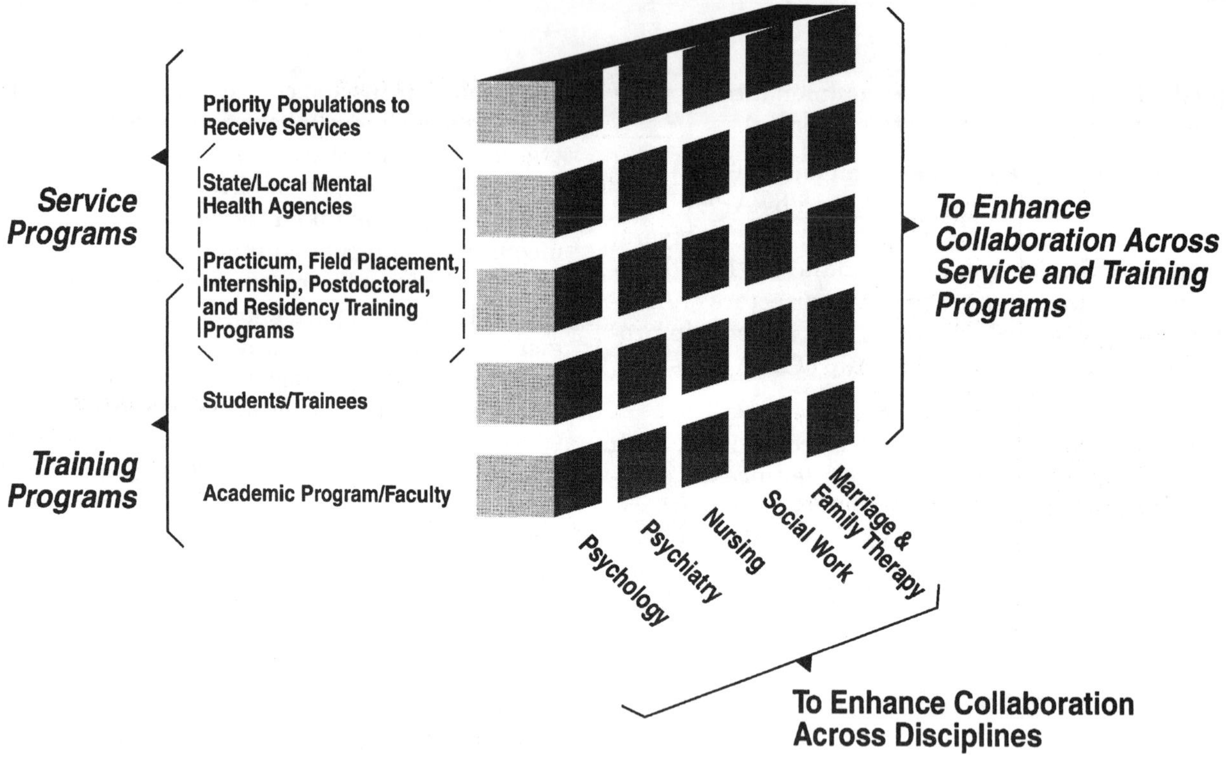

Figure 2. Major purposes of the 1988–1990 multidisciplinary national conferences on clinical training were to enhance collaboration across service and training programs and across disciplines. Note: Practicum, internship, and postdoctoral training programs are sometimes conducted in state or local mental health agencies.

marized in Figure 3. They are (a) to promote collaboration across priority populations by integrating previous recommendations into one coherent, feasible plan for clinical training in psychology; and (b) to enhance collaboration across service programs and training programs by strengthening public–academic linkages in support of clinical training in psychology.

The Linkages Conference included 105 participants, all leaders in services and training, and focused on the identified priority populations: adults with serious mental illnesses; children, elderly,[2] and minorities with mental disorders; individuals with mental disorders living in rural areas; and individuals with dual diagnoses (e.g., mental disorders and substance abuse).[3] See Appendix B of this volume for a list of conference participants. Representatives from universities, state and local public (including private nonprofit) mental health service systems, national organizations such as APA and NIMH, and consumers met in plenary sessions and work groups. The purpose of these sessions was to develop specific implementation recommendations regarding services for priority populations, academic issues, internship and postdoctoral training, faculty development, curriculum development, and research and continuing education and inservice training. Expert presentations as well as workgroup discussions highlighted unique contributions that psychologists, through their science base, can make to the public mental health system. Noted in particular were psychologists' skills in developing specific psychosocial and other interventions, as well as those in program evaluation.

The conference's first purpose, to promote collaboration across priority populations by integ-

[2] A fourth area, aging, was the focus of an April, 1992, clinical training conference sponsored by NIMH and APA, and is summarized by Teri in Chapter 4 of this volume. Although this conference had not yet occurred at the time of the Linkages Conference, recommendations were available from the 1981 "Older Boulder" Conference (Santos & VandenBos, 1982) and from the 1990 Training Committee of APA Division 20 (Division on Adult Development and Aging; Zarit et al., 1990). Because planners of the Linkages Conference did not want to exclude the area of aging, these recommendations, although provisional, were considered.

[3] Clinical training conferences on dual diagnosis (e.g., mental disorder and substance abuse) and on rural services and training are proposed for the near future.

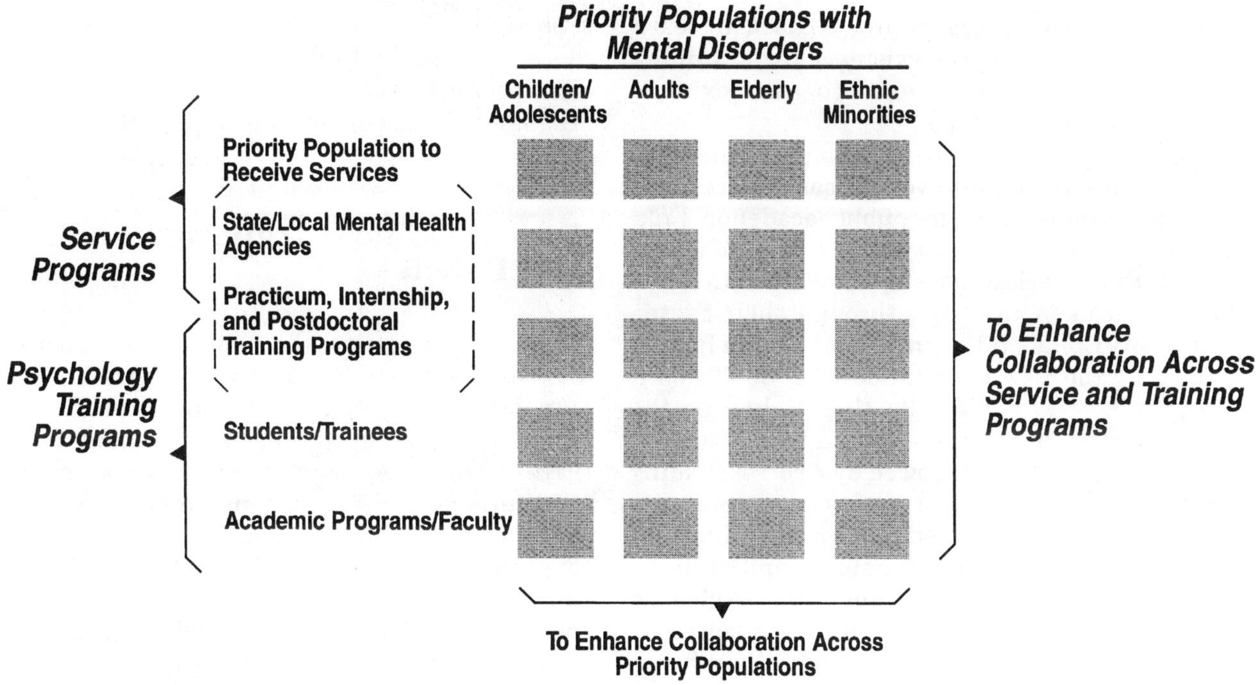

Figure 3. Major purposes of the 1990 National Conference on Implementing Public–Academic Linkages for Clinical Training in Psychology were to enhance collaboration across service and training programs and across priority populations.

rating recommendations from earlier conferences on NIMH priority populations, was accomplished in two ways. First, prior to the Linkages Conference, recommendations from the previous four conferences were consolidated into a single document, referred to as the *Consolidated Recommendations,* and made available as a working draft to conference participants.[4] Second, conference participants convened in work groups and developed a new set of recommendations, which are presented in Appendix A as policy recommendations. Work groups were formed to take advantage of geographic connections, and each included academic training program directors, internship directors, public service representatives, and advocates for all priority populations including Community Support Program (CSP) and Child and Adolescent Service System Program (CASSP) directors. As work groups produced recommendations, their interactions generated observable synergy in that individuals representing training and services made connections with their counterparts from same and nearby states, often for the first time.

The second main purpose of the Linkages Conference was to advance public–academic linkages for clinical training in psychology from the 1990 high water mark to the next higher level of collaboration. In the 1980s, NIMH clinical training announcements encouraged clinical training in the public sector and encouraged collaboration between academic training programs and the public sector. An informal survey of the 1989 clinical training grantees revealed that although all training was done in public or private, nonprofit facilities, successful collaboration was quite mixed. Some programs did a good job, but others did not. Among problems contributing to these mixed outcomes were rather loosely stated announcement guidelines and the lack of a mechanism to ensure accountability.

Guided by specific recommendations from the earlier conferences on clinical training, the 1990 NIMH clinical training announcement made public–academic linkages for clinical training a major review criterion. Application instructions provided a state-by-state list of names and phone numbers of CSP, CASSP, and other state program contacts. After this information was issued, both training program directors and state directors

[4] The policy recommendations described in Appendix A are similar in some ways to the *Consolidated Recommendations* on which they were based in part. However, the latter set of recommendations is longer and more detailed. It is available from the Georgetown University CASSP TA Center, 2233 Wisconsin Avenue, NW, Washington, DC 20007.

were frequently surprised and pleased to learn about their counterparts' existence (e.g., "I didn't know these resources . . . and programs existed" was a frequent response).

The central theme of the Linkages Conference and this book—to improve clinical services and clinical training through public–academic linkages—is too important to restrict to psychology. In fact, the American Psychiatric Association has moved ahead in this area through their State–University Collaboration in Mental Health Project funded by the Pew Foundation in 1989 (Talbott, 1991; Talbott & Rabinowitz, 1986). Just as the psychology training conferences on each of the priority populations was followed by a corresponding multidisciplinary training conference to enhance collaboration, as discussed earlier (see Figures 1 and 2), so, too, it was important to expand the focus of the Linkages Conference from just psychology (Figure 3) to a more multidisciplinary perspective. The solution was a future multidisciplinary conference on public–academic linkages to enhance collaboration across service and training programs, across priority populations, and across all disciplines (see Figure 4). Strategically, the most likely way to implement Linkages Conference recommendations in psychology is to expand the focus to enhance collaboration across all disciplines. In February, 1993, such a multidisciplinary conference was held, "Building a Competent Mental Health Workforce for the 21st Century" (CMHS, 1993a). It is discussed in Chapter 26.

Recent Clinical Training Funding and Policies

In several instances, the newfound collaboration at the Linkages Conference generated state-supported stipends for the training programs. It was particularly gratifying to learn about this positive outcome because in many cases, excellent institutional clinical training programs could not be funded by NIMH. In 1990, only 14% of approved applications were funded; in 1991, 26% were funded; in 1992, 22% were funded; and in 1993, no new applications were accepted, and for the first time, even committed continuation grants will be cut.

As documented recently (Wohlford, 1990, pp. 20–21), NIMH's clinical training budget grew from $1 million in 1948 to a high point of $93 million in 1969. Then, it plateaued and slightly declined to $70 million in 1980, before plummeting to about $31 million in 1982, and then tapering downward

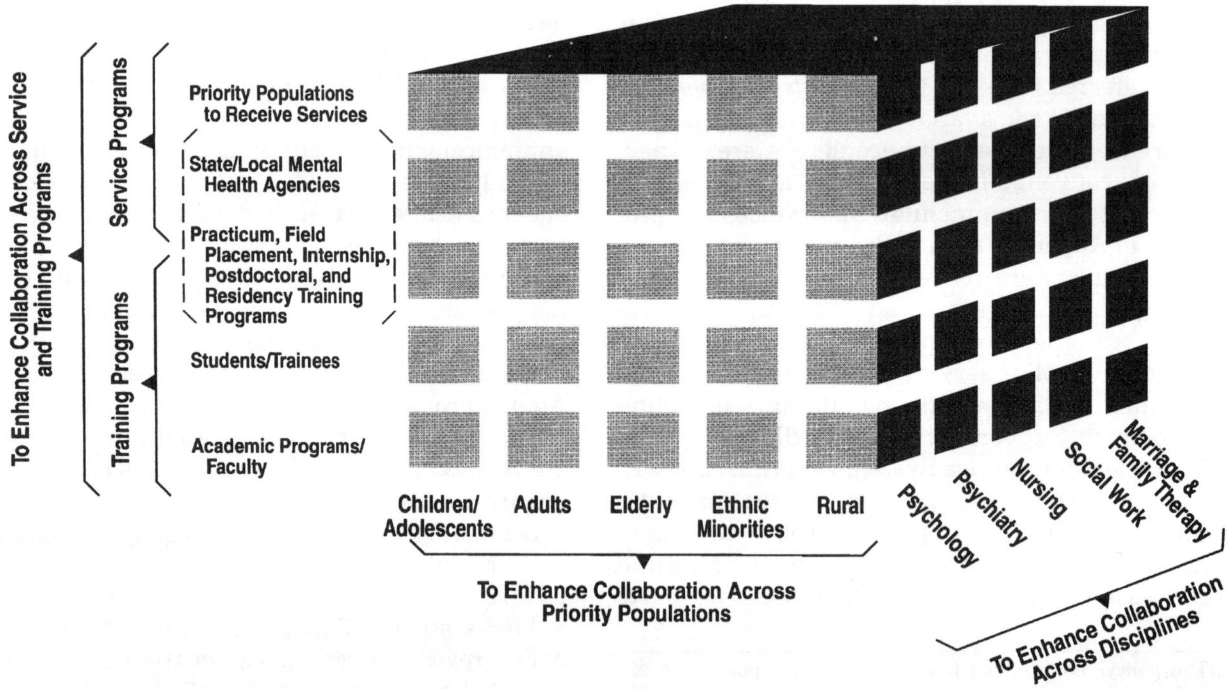

Figure 4. Major purposes of a future multidisciplinary national conference on public–academic linkages for clinical training are to enhance collaboration across service and training programs, across disciplines, and across priority populations.

to $15 million in 1987. Its 1988 increase to $16.8 million was the first increase in seven years, and it fluctuated during the five year period from 1987 to 1992, shifting between $10.8 million and $16.8 million (up, down, up, up, down).

During the period from 1981 to 1992, in spite of the Reagan and Bush Administrations' consistent attempts to eliminate NIMH's clinical training budget, Congress repeatedly saved the program, but added the requirements of payback service and training for service to priority populations (Wohlford, 1990, 1991). In 1993, however, Congress slashed the clinical training budget—now in the new CMHS of the newly created Substance Abuse and Mental Health Services Administration (SAMHSA)—by 73%, to about $3 million, citing no specific problems, only a general budgetary concern. Congress also mandated a detailed evaluation of the clinical training payback service requirement. The report of this evaluation is discussed in Chapter 20.

Congress has not yet, however, required a more general evaluation of clinical training with respect to the service needs of the priority population: Have clinical training programs failed or succeeded in training sufficient numbers of providers with the latest skills to provide quality services to the priority populations? This is a complex question; a satisfactory analysis must consider the strategic timing and relative impact of federal support. When NIMH clinical training supported one fourth to one third of all mental health trainees two or three decades ago, the impact of NIMH policies was very pervasive. During this period, these policies were quite laissez faire, focusing upon the priorities of the leadership of the disciplines. However, in the last decade, when the funding of clinical training plummeted, only 1% or 2% of these trainees have received mental health training support; thus the impact of these policies has also fallen off dramatically. Ironically, this decrease in policy impact came in the early 1980s precisely when the policies began to clearly focus on service to the seriously mentally ill priority populations. The new programs supported since 1981 have increasingly changed their curricula in keeping with the new policies, and their graduates have found public sector employment working with the priority populations (CMHS, 1993b). Unfortunately since this new policy direction was taken, 98% to 99% of the trainees have not been supported or trained in such programs. Therefore, it is understandable that public sector employers must frequently hire new providers who lack appropriate skills.

In summary, in the last decade there has been significant interest in developing more effective linkages between the public mental health service sector and the academic institutions that train psychologists. The impetus for this has come from the realization that most psychologists are ill-equipped to serve the populations of greatest need within the public sector, that is, the seriously mentally ill adults, seriously emotionally disturbed children and adolescents, elderly and ethnic minorities with mental disorders, and mentally ill in rural areas. The series of national conferences sponsored by CMHS/NIMH brought together representatives from the various interest groups and galvanized this interest into a more coherent movement for change.

Overview of the Structure of the Book

Part I: Efforts to Improve Clinical Training for Psychological Services to Targeted Groups

A detailed discussion of the issues addressed in each of the conferences and the follow-up activities noted in the previous discussion are provided in the chapters in Part I of this book. They describe the service needs and training issues specific to each of the five priority populations, including a discussion on improving clinical training for service delivery to the dually diagnosed. The challenges in training psychologists to meet the service needs of seriously emotionally disturbed children and adolescents and their families are discussed by Wohlford and Magrab in chapter 2. Although approximately 15% of the 7.5 million children and youth under age 18 have serious emotional disturbances, only about 10%–15% of them receive adequate treatment or services (National Advisory Mental Health Council, 1990). Wohlford and Magrab (chapter 2) point to the urgent need for practitioners to respond to these needs. They emphasize the particularly urgent need of minority youth and adolescents. Johnson discusses training for providing services to seriously mentally ill adults in chapter 3. Pointing to specific training needs and deficits, he suggests that postdoctoral training opportunities preparing psychologists to work with the seriously mentally ill adult be developed. He also encourages predoctoral programs to include a greater emphasis, through coursework and applied experiences, on the acquisition of skills relevant to the seriously mentally ill.

In chapter 4, Teri discusses the need for training more psychologists equipped to address the mental health needs of the growing population of the elderly. She notes that although, at the present time, approximately 12% of the U.S. population is over the age of 65, this number will increase 150% by the year 2000. She emphasizes the psychological needs of the older adult, pointing out that the complete range of disturbances seen in younger groups are complicated by other problems peculiar to aging (e.g., physical health and special losses). Given these increasing demands, she stresses the critical need for more comprehensive and relevant training for all clinical psychology students and the need for more psychologists with special competencies for working with older adults.

In chapter 5, Myers discusses the unique issues and problems in training for service to racial and ethnic minorities with mental disorders. He reviews the rationale for increasing the number of trained ethnic minority psychologists, as well as for training all psychologists for competencies in service and research with the increasingly diverse population of the United States.

Although the conference on improving clinical training for psychological services to the dually diagnosed (individuals with both mental disorders and substance abuse) is yet to be held, Hills, Zucker, and Seitz discuss consumer as well as clinical training needs for this population in chapter 6.

Part II: Public Mental Health Service Responsibilities for the Mentally Ill

Part II of this book considers the responsibilities of the states to meet the needs of underserved populations, along with the latest mental health service programs that have been developed in response to those needs. Over the last decade, these responsibilities have been defined by several important changes. First, in 1982, a block grant program shifted responsibility for the CMHCs from the federal government to the states. This was accompanied by a number of other changes in the mental health block grants to the states, the net effect of which was to reduce total funding for mental health services and to give the states more freedom to expend federal monies as they saw fit. Perhaps as a result of this greater freedom, states were uneven in their adoption of modern community-based rehabilitation programs for the seriously mentally ill. In response to this unevenness, in 1986 Congress enacted Public Law 99-660, which required each state to have an acceptable state mental health plan for the period of 1990–92. Chapter 7, by Stratoudakis et al., provides an overview of state and local governments' complex and changing responsibilities toward the seriously mentally ill and describes aspects of the program planning process mandated by PL 99-660. The authors also discuss the need for university training to better prepare mental health professionals for work in the public mental health service, and they make recommendations for improved public–academic linkages.

Three of the chapters in Part II describe programs funded by CMHS/NIMH to support the provision of mental health services in the public sector. In chapter 8, Blanch describes the remarkable success of the Community Support Program (CSP), a program that, since the late 1970s, has successfully demonstrated the provision of services to seriously mentally ill adults, based on community-centered psychosocial rehabilitation and case management approaches. In 1989, CSP programs were operating in almost 50 states, with 113 funded grants totaling $14.8 million; in 1993, $16.2 million is available for CSP.

The success of this program in addressing the comprehensive service needs of seriously mentally ill adults prompted NIMH, in 1984, to launch a parallel program for seriously emotionally disturbed children and adolescents, called the Child and Adolescent Service System Program (CASSP). Many experts have high expectations for CASSP's potential to address fragmentation and other complex problems in children's services. In 1989, the CASSP program for seriously emotionally disturbed children also was operating in almost 50 states and had 51 funded grants totaling $9 million. In 1993, $8.2 million is available for CASSP, a large part of whose program is conducted through joining funding with other federal agencies. In chapter 9, Behar describes historical trends in child mental health that resulted in CASSP, cites subsequent developments, and calls for public–academic collaboration in the training of child mental health professionals.

Since the late 1970s, NIMH has sponsored the state Human Resource Development (HRD) program in all 50 states to help states develop and manage their mental health personnel more effectively. The program provides special grants exclusively to the states or to consortia of states. Out of NIMH's 1989 clinical training budget of $12.8 million, the NIMH state HRD budget was $3.1

million, funding 29 grants to state HRD offices; in 1992, HRD grants totalled about $2.5 million. Salasin, Backer, and McGuirk describe this program in chapter 10.

In chapter 11, Hargrove argues that CMHCs should become key players in the formulation of plans to foster collaboration between the public sector and academia. He notes that with the shift of services from the community to states under the block grant program, CMHCs—the cornerstone of direct services since the mid-1960s—have been effectively excluded from the discussion and planning process.

In the last chapter of this section, chapter 12, Frese compellingly articulates the position of the consumer, advocating improved training to meet the needs of the seriously mentally ill and increased consumer participation in the development of public–academic collaboration.

Part III: Models of Effective Public–Academic Collaboration

The creation of effective collaborative working relationships between public sector mental health systems and universities to ensure the readiness of clinical psychologists and other mental health professionals to meet the needs of seriously mental ill persons is an idea whose time has come. However, achieving such radical system change requires significant change in the conceptualization of how mental health services should be provided, how mental health disciplines should interact, how institutional boundaries should be redefined, and how clinical training should be redefined. Complementary changes in the structural arrangements of mental health care delivery systems and in university training programs will also be required in order to implement the new ideas that emerge from the new conceptual models of training and service delivery.

Part III of this book presents a conceptual model of public–academic linkages for training and services and six examples of how such linkages may actually work. Chapter 13, by Davis, provides a conceptual model of the principles and guidelines to be considered in developing collaborative arrangements between public sector providers and academic institutions. This chapter underscores the following principles: that successful collaborations require a commitment to ensuring that all parties win, that creativity and flexibility in formulating arrangements are essential in order to overcome artificial institutional boundaries of ideology and territory, and that such arrangements must be of co-equals who respect and value each others' expertise and contributions to the common goals.

These principles are brought to life in the examples of public–academic sector collaborations provided in the next six chapters. These chapters describe programs in several states that are different in approach, scope of effort, and in stage of development. Several chapters include the active and meaningful participation of former patients and their families in all aspects of the program, from program design and development to shared roles in teaching and the provision of direct services. For instance, chapter 14 by Munger, Behar, and Bainbridge describes innovative children and adolescent programs in North Carolina, and chapter 15 by Hammond and Yung describes similar programs in Ohio. In chapter 16, Hellkamp describes innovative programs that target seriously mentally ill adults and their families in Cincinnati; and chapter 17, by Coursey, Weinstein, and Deckelnick describes the Maryland Consortium for the seriously mentally ill. In chapter 18, Ciofarri et al., discuss the effort in Vermont to build a competent public sector workforce using public–academic linkages as part of the human resource development efforts. Finally, Zimet and Harding describe in chapter 19 the development of a postdoctoral training consortium in Colorado to train psychologists for public sector service.

Each chapter provides the program's rationale and brief history of its development, as well as details about its perspective, membership, and current status. It is hoped that these examples will encourage other university programs, state and local mental health agencies, and associations to begin exploring ways to forge similar collaborative service and training efforts.

Part IV: Ensuring Quality and Competence in Training for Mental Health Services

Major challenges in fostering effective public–academic sector linkages for clinical training in psychology will be to improve the competencies of service providers and to encourage more public agency-based clinical research and research training. These are challenges as well as opportunities because both academic institutions and public sector mental health settings can benefit from such dialogue and collaboration.

The chapters in Part IV of this book articulate ways in which community–clinical service, training and research objectives can be met through effective collaborations. In chapter 20, Wohlford and Manderscheid first consider mental health service needs, that is, the prevalence and treatment of mental illness and lack of availability of providers. Next, they discuss the improvement of the mental health workforce in the context of a framework within which to organize research and evaluation in order to improve (a) mental health services, (b) training programs, and (c) competencies of individual service providers. Finally, they consider the process of knowledge translation and transfer whereby the latest research findings in mental health are conveyed to training faculty and to service providers.

In chapter 21, Sechrest and Scott make a strong case for the need to develop and implement a comprehensive system of competencies assessment research to ensure the preparation and continuing competency of clinical psychologists who serve the seriously mentally ill. This effort has implications for the profession, and it ensures that those providing clinical services and conducting services research in the public sector are qualified to do so. These authors describe several methods by which such assessments can be conducted.

In chapter 22, Hall discusses the need to include quality assurance, state licensing and continuing education strategies in the training and re-training of psychologists for service to the seriously mentally ill. In the final analysis, unless these priority skills are evaluated as part of licensing requirements, the public mental health sector will continue to exert limited influence on the training of psychologists for service in the public sector. In chapter 23, Nelson, who is the Director of APA's Program Consultation and Accreditation Office, discusses the role of the APA Accreditation process in improving the clinical training of psychologists. He considers the importance of addressing national mental health concerns, saying that teaching and research alone are no longer sufficient, that service to the community is increasingly recognized as a faculty responsibility. He suggests a public health model that would not only integrate academic experience with field experience but would include greater exposure to interdisciplinary research and practice at advanced levels of education.

In chapter 24, Friedman argues for a comprehensive, systems approach to services research. He favors considering the effectiveness of interventions, not simply in terms of either individual or group outcomes, but also the impact of such outcomes on the entire system of care provided in the community. This approach is being implemented as a collaborative effort between the university and the public mental health service system to children in Florida.

Finally, in chapter 25, Hogan argues for states to conduct services research despite the complexities of state bureaucracies and the competing agendas of service versus research. Descriptions of several such efforts funded by NIMH public–academic liaison (PAL) research grants are provided. Although PAL grants for research are not to be confused with public–academic linkages projects for clinical training, mental health research plays an integral role in the improvement of mental health services as articulated in the model offered in the concluding chapter 26.

Together, these chapters in Part IV make compelling arguments for professional psychology to adopt the public health model. A first step would be to explore innovative ways for substantial collaboration between academic clinical training programs and the public mental health authorities to occur, then to address the myriad of questions that arise in the provision of effective mental health care.

Part V: Recommendations and Future Directions

The struggle to improve the quality of mental health services provided to the priority populations of seriously mentally ill adults, children, ethnic minorities, aged, dually diagnosed, and those in rural areas, requires restructuring both the mental health service delivery systems and the training of mental health providers. Direct collaboration between the public sector and academic programs offers a unique opportunity for meeting this objective in ways that are mutually beneficial to these institutions and to consumers, as recommended by the Linkages Conference, presented in Appendix A. In chapter 26, Wohlford, Callan, and Myers review the current progress on these initiatives and identify future trends in the training of psychologists. The jewel in this crown will be the development of models of clinical training that are driven by the service needs of consumers, that effectively link public mental health service agencies and academic institutions, and that train psychologists to be effective members of multidisciplinary service and research teams. In developing these models, however, continual attention must be paid to the integrity and standards of each discipline (e.g., recognizing the scientific base of psychology and respecting its professional identity and independence), ensuring the effective participation of all stakeholders in decision making, and striving for mutually beneficial outcomes.

The editors hope that this volume will serve as a catalyst for those interested in changing the way mental health services are delivered in the public sector to priority populations, the way the science of psychology is used to improve the quality of services provided, and the way psychologists are trained to be effective members of multidisciplinary service delivery and services research teams. It is our firm belief that these goals can best be accomplished by fostering effective public–academic linkages for service, research, and training.

References

Center for Mental Health Services. (1993a, February). *National conference on building a competent mental health workforce for the 21st century,* Washington, DC.

Center for Mental Health Services. (1993b, June). *Report to the United States Congress: Evaluation of the mental health clinical training payback requirement.* Rockville, MD: Department of Health and Human Services.

Davis, M., & Sanchez, A. M. (Eds). (1987). *Interdisciplinary collaboration between state mental health and higher education.* Boulder, CO: Western Interstate Commission on Higher Education.

Gary, L. E., & Weaver, G. D. (Eds). (1991). *A multidisciplinary national conference on clinical training for services to mentally ill ethnic minorities.* Washington, DC: Howard University, Institute for Urban Affairs and Research.

Johnson, D. L. (Ed.). (1990). *Service needs of the seriously mentally ill: Training implications for psychology.* Washington, DC: American Psychological Association.

Kagan, E., Magrab, P. R., & Wohlford, P. (Eds.). (1992). *Clinical training for services to children and adolescents with serious emotional disturbance: Multidisciplinary approaches.* Washington, DC: Georgetown University, Child Development Center.

Magrab, P. R., & Wohlford, P. (Eds.). (1990). *Improving psychological services for children and adolescents with severe mental disorders: Clinical training in psychology.* Washington, DC: American Psychological Association.

Manderschied, R. W., & Barrett, S. A. (1987). *Mental health, United States,* 1987 (DHHS Publication No. ADM 87-1518). Washington, DC: U.S. Government Printing Office.

Myers, H. F., Wohlford, P., Guzman, L. P., & Echemendia, R. J. (Eds.). (1991). *Ethnic minority perspectives on clinical training and services in psychology.* Washington, DC: American Psychological Association.

National Advisory Mental Health Council. (1990). *National plan for research on child and adolescent mental disorders.* DHHS Publication No. ADM 90-1683. Washington, DC: U.S. Government Printing Office.

National Council of Community Mental Health Centers. (1987). *1987 CMHC salary survey.* Rockville, MD: National Council of CMHCs.

National Institute of Mental Health. (1990). *Clinical training in serious mental illness* (DHHS Publication No. ADM 90-1679). Washington, DC: U.S. Government Printing Office.

Paulson, R., & Paulson, P. (1991). *Clinical training for services to the long-term seriously mentally ill: A multidisciplinary review and assessment.* Cincinnati, OH: University of Cincinnati School of Social Work.

Santos, J. F., & VandenBos, G. R. (1982). *Psychology and the older adult: Challenges for training in the 1980s.* Washington, DC: American Psychological Association.

Sechrest, L. & Pion, G. (1990). Developing cross-discipline measures of clinical competencies in diagnosis, treatment, and case management. In D. L. Johnson (Ed.), *Service needs of the seriously mentally ill: Training implications for psychology* (pp. 29–32). Washington, DC: American Psychological Association.

Talbott, J. A. (1991). The Pew Project: A national effort to improve state–university collaboration. *Hospital and Community Psychiatry, 42,* 70.

Talbott, J. A., & Rabinowitz, C. B. (Eds.). (1986). *Working together: State–university collaboration in mental health.* Washington, DC: American Psychiatric Press.

Wohlford, P. (1990). National responsibilities to improve training for psychological services for children, youth, and families in the 1990s. In P. R. Magrab & P. Wohlford (Eds.), *Improving psychological services for children and adolescents with severe mental disorders: Clinical training in psychology* (pp. 11–34). Washington, DC: American Psychological Association.

Wohlford, P. (1991). Trends in NIMH support for clinical training for ethnic minorities. In H. F. Myers, P. Wohlford, L. P. Guzman, & R. J. Echemendia (Eds.). (1991). *Ethnic minority perspectives on clinical training and services in psychology* (pp. 13–21). Washington, DC: American Psychological Association.

Zarit, J. M., Zarit, S. H., Frazer, D. W., Hartman-Stein, P., Knight, R., & Teri, L. (1990). Training in clinical geropsychology: Report of the Division 20 Education Subcommittee on Clinical Practice and Training. *Adult Development and Aging News, 18,* 3–6.

PART I

Efforts to Improve Clinical Training for Psychological Services to Targeted Groups

CHAPTER

2

Seriously Emotionally Disturbed Children, Adolescents, and Their Families

Paul Wohlford
Center for Mental Health Services

Phyllis R. Magrab
Georgetown University

The 1986 Office of Technology Assessment (OTA) study as well as many other earlier studies (e.g., President's Commission on Mental Health, 1978) have noted that millions of children and adolescents with severe mental disorders do not receive adequate services because there is a shortage of trained personnel. Of all children and youth under age 18, 7.5 million have emotional disorders, and half of these children have serious emotional disturbances that impair their present functioning and future potential (National Advisory Mental Health Council [NAMHC], 1990). Just a small proportion of these children, 1.5 million, receive mental health treatment in organized settings (NAMHC, 1990). In particular, minority children and adolescents are frequently underserved. The need to train professionals to serve these children and adolescents is a paramount concern for this decade.

To address this need, in May, 1988, a National Conference on Clinical Training in Psychology on improving services for seriously emotionally disturbed children was conducted by Georgetown University Child Development Center, and supported by the National Institute of Mental Health's (NIMH) Education and Training Branch and the Children and Adolescent Service System Program (CASSP), to make recommendations about improving psychological services for children and adolescents with severe mental disorders, or serious emotional disturbances. Gathered for the conference were 56 leaders in the field of professional child psychology representing such areas as clinical child psychology, pediatric psychology, school psychology, and applied developmental psychology; state CASSP directors; NIMH staff; and a number of graduate students. They represented a cross section of relevant divisions, boards, and committees of the American Psychological Association and related organizations. The following discussion summarizes the conclusions of that conference (which are fully presented in Magrab and Wohlford, 1990) as updated in two subsequent conferences, the 1989 National Conference on Multidisciplinary Clinical Training for Services for Seriously Emotionally Disturbed Children and Adolescents (Kagan, Magrab, &

The opinions expressed in this article are those of the authors and do not necessarily reflect the opinions, official policies, or position of the Center for Mental Health Services (CMHS) or of Georgetown University.

Wohlford, 1992) and the Linkages Conference that is reported in this volume.

Professional Child Psychology

Before examining needed services and training in child psychology, it is important to understand how the field of professional child psychology relates to the overall field of professional psychology. Professional child psychology should be recognized as a specialty within clinical psychology; nevertheless, it is a broad field that itself includes several very different subspecialties, from school psychology to pediatric psychology. Lambert (1990) recommended a sensible nomenclature to describe the field:

Psychology; within it is nested:
  Professional Psychology; within it is nested:
    Professional Child Psychology;
      within it are nested:
      Clinical Child Psychology,
      Pediatric Psychology,
      School Psychology, and perhaps others, such as *Applied Developmental Psychology.*
(cited in Wohlford, 1990, p. 14)

The historical development of clinical psychology serving children and the first recognition of clinical child psychology, per se, was traced by Ross (1959) and updated in 1974 by Williams and Gordon who traced training issues in clinical child psychology as a specialty. The more recent works (Tuma, 1985; Fischer, 1978; Routh, 1977) trace the development of particular psychology training programs for children's services over the last 15 years, and identify training facilities and graduate programs in clinical child psychology and pediatric psychology. These serve as beginning efforts to define the field.

It has not been sufficiently recognized that providing services to children and families requires special skills that go beyond work with adults. It must continuously be reaffirmed that children's mental disorders of childhood and the corresponding assessment procedures and treatment methods for children are often quite different from those used with adults. Within each subspecialty of professional child psychology (clinical child, pediatrics, and school), functional tasks of evaluation, treatment, consultation, and research, as well as different levels of expertise in rendering these services can be specified. After a functional analysis is completed, what constitutes competence for each function can be determined, and standards can be established on the basis of competent performance for each of these functions.

Training for Competence

Professional competence to render quality service to children, youth, and families goes hand in hand with training to attain that competence and with standard-setting or credentialing to confirm that such competence has been attained or maintained. But how should professionals be trained for work with children's services that are comprehensive, multidimensional, and multidisciplinary? Shore (1990) summarized the following critical training issues:

1. What generic training is needed?

2. What are the boundary issues among clinical psychology, school psychology, and applied developmental psychology, all of which are delivering psychological services?

3. What different roles are there, and do they require different kinds of training at different levels?

4. What different models are there? For example, should a multidimensional comprehensive set of services be administered by one individual, or should a person be primarily a facilitator coordinating a multiple number of services?

5. What different standards are there for the different tasks?

6. How do we train for new types of research in service delivery, which is so broad and highly complex?

7. Considering the vast expanse of this model of service delivery, how can we avoid becoming dilettantes who dabble and have merely superficial knowledge of the wealth of information and choices?

Indeed, one of the questions is whether there is so much to learn that there is a danger that we may not know anything well. (p. 50)

Service Needs and Clinical Training

It is essential that training be responsive to service delivery needs. Issues related to service delivery include the need for comprehensive services, multidimensional services, services in different settings, different roles for service providers, multidisciplinary services; and the coordination of service elements. The overarching issue of this conference was how psychologists should be trained to provide services based on these aspects of service delivery. Psychological services to children, youth, and families embrace different functions in different settings and may involve different types and levels of expertise.

Array of Services

In considering training for service needs, one must take into account a system of care for severely emotionally disturbed children and youth. The optimum array of services is composed of both residential and nonresidential services. Nonresidential services include prevention, early identification and intervention, assessment, outpatient treatment, home-based services, day treatment, and emergency services. Residential services include therapeutic foster care, therapeutic group care, therapeutic camp services, independent living services, crisis residential services, inpatient services, and hospitalization. Clinical child psychologists should be exposed to these various options and understand their utility.

A systems approach should be used to improve services for seriously emotionally disturbed children and, simultaneously, to improve clinical training to providers. There are a number of important underlying principles in the delivery of these services that must frame both services and training.

Guiding Principles for the System of Care

1. Emotionally disturbed children should have access to a comprehensive array of services that address the child's physical, emotional, social and educational needs.

2. Emotionally disturbed children should receive individualized services in accordance with the unique needs and potentials of each child, and guided by an individualized service plan.

3. Emotionally disturbed children should receive services within the least restrictive, most normative environment that is clinically appropriate.

4. The families and surrogate families of emotionally disturbed children should be full participants in all aspects of the planning and delivery of services.

5. Emotionally disturbed children should receive services that are integrated, with linkages between child-caring agencies and programs and mechanisms for planning, developing and coordinating services.

6. Emotionally disturbed children should be provided with case management or similar mechanisms to ensure that multiple services are delivered in a coordinated and therapeutic manner, and that they can move through the system of services in accordance with their changing needs.

7. Early identification and intervention for children with emotional problems should be promoted by the system of care in order to enhance the likelihood of positive outcomes.

8. Emotionally disturbed children should be ensured smooth transitions to the adult service system as they reach maturity.

9. The rights of emotionally disturbed children should be protected, and effective advocacy efforts for emotionally disturbed children and youth should be promoted.

10. Emotionally disturbed children should receive services without regard to race, religion, national origin, sex, physical disability, or other characteristics, and services should be sensitive and responsive to cultural differences and special needs. (Stroul and Friedman, 1986, p. vii)

Education and Training for Services to Seriously Emotionally Disturbed Children and Adolescents

The training of psychologists who are capable of delivering clinical services to children with serious emotional disturbances depends on at least four factors: (a) translation of relevant knowledge into the curriculum, (b) the faculty who are entrusted to transmit that knowledge, (c) the characteristics and motivation of the student expected to assimilate that knowledge and its clinical application, and (d) society's needs. This is the challenge in dealing with the seriously emotionally disturbed child.

In 1985, the Hilton Head Conference on Training Clinical Child Psychologists (Tuma, 1985) made substantial progress in articulating the complex issues in the training of clinical child psychologists. Although the mechanisms to implement the conference's recommendations were somewhat unclear, the conference was the kickoff of other meetings that resulted in publication of *Guidelines for Clinical Child Psychology Internship Training* (Elbert, Abidin, Finch, Sigman, & Walker, 1988) and *Guidelines for Postdoctoral Training in Clinical Child Psychology* (Ollendick, Drotar, Friedman, & Hodges, 1988). The Hilton Head Conference apparently used the 1983 APA Division 37 (Child, Youth, and Family Services) guidelines, *Guidelines for Training Psychologists to Work with Children, Youth, and Families* (Roberts, Erickson, & Tuma, 1985), for the academic component of training. Erickson summarized the academic component in *Standards for Training Clinical Child Psychologists in University Doctoral Programs* (1990). The report of the 1988 Georgetown Conference brought together a complete set of guidelines covering academic training, predoctoral internship, and postdoctoral training (Magrab & Wohlford, 1990). This represents a significant advance in the field of professional child psychology.

The content of these initial guidelines is excellent; however, as a set they are rather uneven, lack conciseness, and do not reflect the latest principles of a system of care cited above. Therefore, after reviewing the progress of implementation of the recommendations of the 1990 Linkages Conference as reported in this volume, 12 specific task groups were organized to work on critical issues. One of these is the Task Group on Refining Clinical Training Guidelines for Psychologists for Services to Children and Adolescents with Mental Disorders, co-chaired by Michael C. Roberts and Robert M. Friedman. The new guidelines are expected to be available in 1994.

Clinical child psychology and pediatric psychology are on the threshold of gaining recognition as specialties in professional psychology, aided by structures and processes recommended by the recent APA Task Force on Accreditation Criteria (American Psychological Association [APA], 1988). After many years of discussion and debate, culminating in the 1987 Salt Lake Conference on Graduate Education in Psychology (Bickman, 1987), the 1987 Gainesville Conference on Internship Training in Psychology (Belar et al., 1989), and the 1990 Gainesville National Conference on Scientist–Practitioner Education and Training for the Professional Practice of Psychology (Belar & Perry, 1990), it is clear that graduate training in clinical psychology intends to:

1. Proceed sequentially from broadly based didactic and experiential courses that make up a scientific core and a professional core in the first years of education and training.

2. Focus increasingly on area or field proficiencies in the middle years of education and training.

3. Retain the predoctoral internship as a period of general professional role acquisition.

4. Relegate specialty training primarily to a postdoctoral year (or years).

Recommendations to Improve Clinical Training for Services to Seriously Emotionally Disturbed Children and Adolescents

Just as constructive innovation should occur at each level, stage, or setting to improve services to seriously emotionally disturbed children, so, too, public–academic collaboration should occur at each level, stage, or setting to improve the clinical training of the next generation of psychologists providing services for seriously emotionally disturbed children. This includes, but is not limited to

- faculty development and curriculum development;
- clinical research, as well as clinical competencies and administrative skills;
- academic training at all levels from undergraduate (where interest in helping seriously emotionally disturbed children may first arise) to graduate school (master's and doctoral coursework and research);
- practica, predoctoral internships, and postdoctoral fellowships; and
- retraining and continuing education.

States and the federal government, in collaboration with universities, should develop incentives (e.g., financial support) for faculty and students to become involved in working and training in these settings. Faculty would be offered opportunities either to practice or to conduct research, or both, in public settings with emphasis on the needs of seriously mentally ill persons.

Additionally, predoctoral psychology internships and practicum sites should be developed to involve publicly supported psychology staff members in training partnerships with university faculty members. This could result in the development of meaningful internships in public settings that prepare students for work with seriously emotionally disturbed children. An obstacle to such development in the field of psychology is the uneven level of, and sometimes poor communication between, doctoral training programs and internship programs. It would be particularly helpful if a new clinical training grant program was started that would require both state mental health authorities and psychology training programs (including both doctoral and internship programs) to be cosponsors, with incentives for states to gradually assume some level of financial responsibility, possibly over a three to six year period.

As expanded training efforts begin in professional psychology, it is essential that the human resource needs are understood. The best available estimates of the current number of mental health service providers, including those serving both adults and children, are in the OTA report (OTA, 1986). The OTA report stated, "There are approximately 3,000 child psychiatrists, 5,000 clinical psychologists, 7,000 child and family-oriented social workers, and 1,000 child/family-oriented mental health nurses. . . . Estimates of the numbers of professionals needed have consistently been much higher" (OTA, 1986, p. 141). However, the OTA report does not specify exactly how many professionals are needed to work with children. There is a great need for a careful, data-based study to more precisely determine the number of child mental health professionals needed. A study of future mental health personnel shortages should estimate the number of personnel needed to provide mental health services to the general population, and also should estimate the number of specialized personnel needed to provide direct services and preventive services to children. Also, the impact of drug and alcohol abuse services and AIDS-related services must be included in the mental health personnel equation. Finally, new demands for mental health services may be awakened by national health care reform, as discussed by Wohlford and Manderschied in chapter 20 of this volume. The total number of available mental health professionals and paraprofessionals undoubtedly will be reduced by these new demands.

One potentially useful source of data related to human resource needs may be found in the 50 States Comprehensive Mental Health Plans under PL 99-660, which should include a separate section addressing mental health services for children and adolescents (see Appendix C). These state plans may serve as the foundation of a national data-based management system of child mental health services, which does not yet exist. Such a national data-based management system should be created for management, fiscal, and program accountability. This system would provide a foundation for planning for children's services and, specifically, for estimating the number of personnel who are necessary to provide these services.

In considering the training necessary for serving children with serious emotional disturbances, funding concerns cannot be ignored. Over the three years from 1986–1989, although the overall NIMH clinical training budget was reduced by 36%, from $20 million to $12.8 million, the institutional training grants suffered a relatively larger 59% cut, from $10 million to 4.1 million. In this period, child training grants were cut in number from 77 to 31, a decrease of 60%, and were reduced in amount from $3.3 million to $2.1 million, a decrease of 37%. If both faculty scholar and clinical training grants for children are considered, the reduction was much less, from $3.3 million to $3 million, a decrease of 9%. Although reductions in the overall program were occurring during this period, the proportion of training grants for services for children actually increased from one third of the 1986 awards (77 of 220) to one half of the 1989 awards (43 of 87).

In summary, the long-term solution to upgrade and expand professional child psychology training programs will require action at every level.

The APA and related organizations should upgrade the standards for training, accreditation, and credentialing for children's services. In particular, professional child psychology should be recognized as another specialty, with subspecialties of clinical child psychology, pediatric psychology, school psychology, and so on.

The Center for Mental Health Services (CMHS)[1] and other federal agencies should do the following:

- Assess the expected shortages of mental health personnel for comprehensive services to

[1] PL 102-321, the ADAMHA Reorganization Act, went into effect October 1, 1992. It transferred responsibility for mental health services and clinical training from NIMH to the new CMHS. CMHS is part of the new Substance Abuse and Mental Health Services Administration (SAMHSA) within the Department of Health and Human Services.

children, youth, and their families now and in the years 1995, 2000, 2010, and 2020.

• Determine clinical competencies needed to provide services to children.

• Increase its support for clinical training for children's services.

In promoting clinical training policy for improving services to children, CMHS should restore credibility, integrity, and confidence in the clinical training grants process by seeking to:

• Attract more students in clinical child psychology and related areas to careers in the public service sector that provide services to children, adolescents, and families. Specifically, trainee stipends should be continued, with payback to ensure that trainees begin their careers in the public sector. There should be special incentives for minority students. Special federal–state incentives should be created to draw students who are already experienced in state and community programs.

• Strengthen linkages between state and community service settings and academic and internship training programs; the CASSP model should be used to stimulate stronger linkages through new, creative, flexible funding.

• Stimulate truly interdisciplinary (not just multidisciplinary) training in which professionals from a variety of backgrounds and at different levels may network together, and in which an interactive team may contribute to a child's and a family's functioning.

• Recognize that high quality clinical training for providing services to children with serious emotional disturbances should not be narrowly confined, but it should also include training for providing services to the less seriously emotionally disturbed; training should also cover prevention programs. High quality clinical training must address both issues of breadth (e.g., child in the family, school, medical setting, etc.) and issues of depth (e.g., specialized expert training in child neuropsychology, etc.).

• Encourage academic and internship faculty to develop their skills and curricula in the latest community-based services and clinical services research; create academic–state exchange programs; create special incentives for minority faculty.

Training for Child Mental Health Services in the 21st Century

Child advocates have made tremendous strides in securing the 1991 Comprehensive Child Mental Health Services program that complements the CASSP program. The Clinton administration seems particularly aware of children's issues and preventive approaches, as seen with its immediate action on children's immunization. Most importantly, health care reform may include mental health services, and if so, children's mental health services may also be included. In addition, if health care reform utilizes Total Quality Management (TQM) to help contain costs, feedback from consumers or family members will be critical to the process.

However, future prospects are not all positive. First, the advocates of children's mental health services have sometimes neglected the fact that the quality of these services is only as good as the quality of the provider. For example, paradoxically, the House of Representatives Appropriations Committee recommended an increase from $5 million to $40 million for children's mental health services from 1992 to 1994, and, at the same time, a decrease from $11 million to zero for clinical training. The children's advocates and Congress need to understand a central theme of the recent conferences: quality clinical services are based on quality clinical training, and vice versa.

Second, national health care reform, in order to contain costs, emphasizes generic and primary health providers as opposed to specialists. Thus, it may be necessary to repeat the battles that child mental health professionals have waged for decades within general mental health; children's mental disorders and corresponding services are often quite different from adult disorders and services. There is a ray of hope in the fact that health care reform appears to embrace TQM concepts. Chapter 26 discusses the need for consumer-assisted reform of mental health services and training. A critical part of this reform will be consumer involvement in establishing standards of care and in defining clinical competencies of providers. Finally, as part of the strategy to implement recommendations from the recent conferences, Lenore Behar is cochairing a task group to address clinical competencies and standards of care for children's mental health services.

References

Belar, C. D., Bieliauskas, L. A., Larsen, K. G., Mensh, I. N., Poey, K., & Roelke, H. J. (1989). The National

Conference on Internship Training in Psychology. *American Psychologist, 44,* 60–65.

Belar, C. D., & Perry, N. W. (1990, January). *Resolutions of the National Conference on Scientist–Practitioner Education and Training for the Professional Practice of Psychology.* Gainesville: University of Florida, Department of Clinical and Health Psychology.

Bickman, L. (Ed.). (1987). Proceedings of the National Conference on Graduate Education in Psychology, University of Utah, Salt Lake City, June 13–19, 1987 [special issue]. *American Psychologist, 42,* 1041–1085.

Elbert, J. C., Abidin, R. R., Finch, A. J., Jr., Sigman, M. D., & Walker, C. E. (1988). Guidelines for clinical child psychology internship training. *Journal of Clinical Child Psychology, 17,* 280–287.

Erickson, M. T. (1990). Standards for training clinical child psychologists in university doctoral programs. In P. R. Magrab & P. Wohlford (Eds.), *Improving psychological services for children and adolescents with severe mental disorders: Clinical training in psychology* (pp. 75–78). Washington, DC: American Psychological Association.

Fischer, C. T. (1978). Graduate programs in clinical child psychology and related fields. *Journal of Clinical Child Psychology, 7,* 87–88.

Kagan, E., Magrab, P. R., & Wohlford, P. (Eds.). (1992). *Clinical training for services to children and adolescents with serious emotional disturbances: Multidisciplinary approaches.* Washington, DC: Georgetown University Child Development Center.

Lambert, N. M. (1990). School psychology as a specialty within a group of specialties in professional child psychology: Education and training issues. In P. R. Magrab & P. Wohlford (Eds.), *Improving psychological services for children and adolescents with severe mental disorders: Clinical training in psychology* (pp. 111–116). Washington, DC: American Psychological Association.

Magrab, P. R., & Wohlford, P. (Eds.), (1990). *Improving psychological services for children and adolescents with severe mental disorders: Clinical training in psychology.* Washington, DC: American Psychological Association.

National Advisory Mental Health Council. (1990). *National plan for research on child and adolescent mental disorders* (DHHS Publication No. ADM 90-1683). Washington, DC: U.S. Government Printing Office.

Office of Technology Assessment. (1986). *Children's mental health: Problems and services—A background paper* (Report No. OTA-BP-H-33). Washington, DC: U.S. Government Printing Office.

Ollendick, T. H., Drotar, D., Friedman, M., & Hodges, K. (1988). Guidelines for postdoctoral training in clinical child psychology. *Journal of Clinical Child Psychology, 17,* 288–289.

President's Commission on Mental Health. (1978). *Report to the President from the President's Commission on Mental Health:* (Catalog No. PR 39.8:M52/R29/V.1). Vol. I Washington, DC: U.S. Government Printing Office.

Reich, J. (1988). *Proposed scope of accreditation for education and training in professional psychology* (Report No. 4, Section B). Washington, DC: American Psychological Association, Task Force on Review of the Scope and Criteria of Accreditation.

Roberts, M. C., Erickson, M. T., & Tuma, J. M. (1985). Guidelines for training psychologists to work with children, youth, & families. *Journal of Clinical Child Psychology, 14,* 70–79.

Ross, A. O. (1959). *The practice of clinical child psychology.* New York: Grune & Stratton.

Routh, D. K. (1977). What is a clinical child psychologist? *The Clinical Psychologist, 30,* 23–25.

Shore, M. F. (1990). Background and recent history of psychology's role in improving psychological services for children. In P. R. Magrab & P. Wohlford (Eds.), *Improving psychological services for children and adolescents with severe mental disorders: Clinical training in psychology* (pp. 49–50). Washington, DC: American Psychological Association.

Stroul, B. A., & Friedman, R. M. (1986). *A system of care for seriously emotionally disturbed children and youth.* Washington, DC: CASSP Technical Assistance Center.

Tuma, J. M. (Ed.). (1985). *Proceedings: Conference on Training Clinical Child Psychologists.* Washington, DC: Section on Clinical Child Psychology, Division of Clinical Psychology, American Psychological Association.

Williams, G. J., & Gordon, S. (Eds.). (1974). *Clinical child psychology: Current practices and future perspectives.* New York: Behavioral Publications.

Wohlford, P. (1990). National responsibilities to improve training for psychological services for children, youth, and families in the 1990s. In P. R. Magrab & P. Wohlford (Eds.). *Improving psychological services for children and adolescents with severe mental disorders: Clinical training in psychology.* Washington, DC: American Psychological Association.

CHAPTER

3

Seriously Mentally Ill Adults

Dale L. Johnson
University of Houston

In February, 1988, NIMH brought together in Houston a group of 40 psychologists and other mental health professionals to develop recommendations for training psychologists to work with people who have serious mental illnesses (SMI). Recommendations were developed and published, along with supporting papers, in the conference proceedings (Johnson, 1990). In making the recommendations, participants in the conference agreed that present training practices were not effective in producing professionals who could best treat people with serious mental illnesses. Faculty and students seemed to be unaware of the extensive intervention technology that has been developed over the past 2 decades that could be applied to improve the quality of life of seriously mentally ill people. The recommendations also noted the urgency of correcting existing training deficiencies. The conference participants stipulated that all clinical students should be exposed to the field of work with people with serious mental illnesses; that most students should also have experience in actually working with this population in practicum and internship settings; and that provision should be made for some students, through 2-year internships or postdoctoral training, to develop expert skills in the area. The proceedings have been available since 1990, and the recommendations have been distributed to National Institute of Mental Health (NIMH), the American Psychological Association (APA), and directors of clinical psychology training programs. It is therefore appropriate to review progress that has been made in bringing the recommendations to fruition.

This chapter also reviews the results of a survey conducted of Directors of Clinical Psychology (DCPs) about their practices with regard to training students to work with the SMI population.

Actions Since the Houston Conference

The recommendations from the conference follow, with comments on progress that has been made toward their attainment.

1. Faculty and students need to become more aware of the body of knowledge that now exists and continues to develop in the SMI area. NIMH should facilitate this process by assembling the relevant knowledge and informing faculty and students about it through periodically updated bibliographies and computerized information systems. Information about model programs and model curricula should be included.

Progress: Most importantly, a new journal, *Innovations and Research: Clinical Services, Community Support and Rehabilitation,* has been launched, which is edited and published jointly by the Boston University Psychiatric Rehabilitation group and the National Alliance for the Mentally Ill. William Anthony and Harriet Lefley are the co-editors. Funding to offset start-up costs was provided by NIMH. The journal presents abstracts of the rehabilitation and treatment literature (150 journals now contribute) and each issue includes several review articles.

2. Because it is vital that all graduate students in clinical and counseling psychology have some exposure to the SMI area and because this will occur only if faculty members are knowledgeable and interested, it is recommended that faculty development be promoted by NIMH by providing resources for sabbaticals or summer conference training in appropriate settings.

Progress: One relevant activity stands out even though it was not directed to psychology faculty per se. The APA Practice Directorate has worked with several state psychological associations in developing training sessions. To our knowledge, these have been carried out in California, Massachusetts, Ohio, North Carolina, Pennsylvania, and Texas. These activities show that postdoctoral continuing education can be provided to large numbers of psychologists. It is essential that these be continued to reach psychologists in more states and that additional means be developed to reach academic psychologists.

Academic psychologists do attend and participate in special-topic conferences, as may be seen by the high levels of participation in the Sutherland Conferences sponsored by the Hogg Foundation for Mental Health in Texas (e.g., Bonjean, Coleman, & Iscoe, 1989). The Sutherland Conferences are successful, in part, because presentations tend to be of high quality, invitations to attend are seen as an indication of prestige, and expenses are paid. Whether they have a measurable impact on attitudes or knowledge of participants has never been assessed, but presumably they do have an impact. Key features of these conferences are worth noting: quality presentations, prestige, and expenses paid. It is essential for progress in training professionals for work with the seriously mentally ill that conferences based on the Sutherland model, or on other types, be held to reach a large number of academic clinical psychologists.

The special-topic conference is one way to provide new information to academicians and practitioners, but the Houston conference on training for work with people with serious mental illnesses urged the development of more extensive and intensive training opportunities such as sabbatical periods spent in highly specialized training–research–treatment facilities.

The American Psychological Association can take a leading role in this, but because psychologists have moved to the American Psychological Society, its clinical division, the American Association of Applied and Preventive Psychology, should also be called on for action in this area.

3. In order to develop high levels of expert knowledge in the small group of students who wish to specialize in the SMI area, it is recommended that NIMH provide graduate stipends for students in programs that offer specialized training. These stipends should have appropriate pay-back requirements.

Progress: This has been stalled owing to continued low levels of funds available to the NIMH Clinical Training Program. The Reagan and Bush administrations tried to eliminate the clinical training budget and only through the support of members of Congress have funds been available at all. Recently, two events of importance have occurred. First, the board of the National Alliance for the Mentally Ill has developed policy in support of clinical training directed specifically at training in the area of serious mental illness, including seriously emotionally disturbed children, and has accelerated advocacy for training. Second, the proposed move of NIMH to the National Institutes of Health (NIH) includes provisions that may actually result in greater funding opportunities for clinical training if the proposed changes do occur.

There is no evidence that states have expanded clinical training budgets.

4. It is further recommended that the development of expert-knowledge-level students be fostered by NIMH through the provision of support for 2-year internship programs (1 year predoctoral and 1 year postdoctoral), also with pay-back requirements.

Progress: The 2-year internship concept was supported by the APA-sponsored conference on internship training (Belar, Bieliauskas, Larsen, & Mensh, 1987), but because funds from NIMH or the states are lacking, there has been little action.

5. NIMH should develop regional training–research–treatment facilities to provide training sites for faculty and students in state-of-the-art methods for the treatment and rehabilitation of people with serious mental illnesses.

Progress: The recommendation stemmed, in part, from the success of such facilities as were created for mental retardation in the 1960s (National Institute of Child Health and Human Development, 1986). Nothing comparable was ever done in the SMI area, and it appears that there has been no action on this highly important recommendation. The schizophrenia research centers funded by NIMH approximate the recommendations but differ because funding is on a short-term basis only and because clinical training is treated as incidental to their primary mission of carrying out research. Assurance of long-term funding is essential for the development of such a complex entity, and a new focus on clinical training should be added.

6. In order to extend training activities as widely as possible, NIMH should promote collaboration of state and local agencies (public and nonprofit) with universities in the training of students to serve seriously mentally ill people. It is recommended that NIMH take the lead in funding the training of doctoral-level students and that states take responsibility for funding training of masters-level psychologists, but that collaborative efforts be encouraged at all levels.

Progress: There is evidence in many parts of the country that the NIMH public–academic linkage initiative has been effective in promoting collaborative research projects, but little has been done on training. The Cincinnati project linking the University of Cincinnati and Xavier University with public agencies has been a leader in this effort. A consortium of university and community agencies in Denver has been formed to develop postdoctoral training opportunities. A similar action, but with an emphasis on research, is underway in the Houston–Galveston area. Both of these efforts are promising but not yet fully functioning.

7. It is also recommended that NIMH encourage the involvement of consumers and their families in training of all kinds.

Progress: The survey of directors of clinical psychology training programs, to be discussed below, indicated that only a small proportion (17%) of clinical psychology training programs have included consumers and families in any way.

8. Minorities make up a substantial part of the SMI population, and NIMH should encourage the recruitment of minority students and faculty to work with this group.

Progress: Although most, if not all, clinical training programs actively recruit minority students for all of their training programs, the commonly heard remark is that the pool of available candidates is remarkably small. There is no available evidence on the results of recruiting within programs that place emphasis on people with serious mental illnesses.

9. It is recommended that standing committees instead of ad hoc committees be formed to review training grant applications. These committees should be interdisciplinary and should be made up of experts capable of reviewing applications for training to work with specific priority populations. Equitable funding for each discipline is also recommended.

Progress: This has not been done.

Survey of Directors of Clinical Psychology

Participants at the Houston conference noted that there was not much information available about what clinical training programs were actually doing to train students in the area of serious mental illness. Without knowing what kind of training practices exist at the present time, it is difficult to develop plans to improve training. This survey apparently was the first of its kind.

A one-page questionnaire was mailed to 165 directors of clinical psychology (DCPs) along with a copy of the proceedings of the Houston conference on training. A stamped and addressed envelope was included for return of the survey. DCPs were told to regard serious mental illness as schizophrenia, bipolar disorder, or major depression.

Responses were received from 114 DCPs, a 69% return. Respondees did not differ from nonrespondees in terms of representing public or private universities, schools in the United States or Canada, or geographic location. Fewer professional schools responded (45%) than academic programs (70%).

The mean total number of department of psychology faculty respondees was 28, with a mean clinical faculty of 9. Of the latter, a mean of 3 had a major research and teaching interest in serious mental illness, and a mean of 5 had some experience or special training in the area.

Nearly all (96%) DCPs reported that some material on SMI was included in their training programs. It was obvious, however, from an examination of reported courses taught in this area, that in most instances the only relevant course was one on psychopathology. Respondees (71%) said they offered special courses or seminars on SMI, but in the listings of these courses, only 42% reported courses with titles such as "Seminar on Schizophrenia" or "The Homeless Mentally Ill," which would suggest a special focus. Most of the courses listed (e.g., "Psychological Interventions") seemed to have a more general orientation but might, of course, have included material on serious mental illness.

The issue of specialized versus generic training at the predoctoral level was addressed with a series of questions. Some DCPs have said that they do not provide special tracks in their programs to allow students to develop some degree of special knowledge or skills. Nevertheless, 65% said they preferred to offer special tracks, and 64% were providing special track training. Only 31% preferred generic training.

Although special tracks were available in a majority of programs, these typically were not in the serious mental illness area. Only 8% of DCPs said they offered a special track on serious mental illness. In response to the question of whether DCPs would encourage a student especially interested in people with serious mental illnesses to apply to their program, 26% said they would not.

The number of schools with special courses and seminars on serious mental illness is not large. The survey results suggested that the number might be as few as 13 (11%) and would include the following in approximate order of programmatic strength in the field: University of Houston, University of Maryland at College Park, University of Nebraska, University of California—Los Angeles, University of Wisconsin, University of Minnesota, Howard University, University of Cincinnati, University of Connecticut, University of Pittsburgh, University of Virginia—Charlottesville, Virginia, and Rutgers Graduate School of Applied and Professional Psychology.

The survey reinforces the impressions held by the Houston conference participants that few clinical training programs were available to provide the kind of training needed to improve the quality of care available to people with serious mental illnesses. The survey also revealed that there is interest and that a number of schools have potential for vast improvement. The problems of funding, and other problems noted in the section above on recommendations for training, continue to retard development in this field.

What Needs to Be Done

A beginning has been made, but there is much yet to be done. Few of the recommendations made by participants in the Houston conference have been addressed, let alone realized. In order to improve training for work in the SMI area, the following are essential:

1. There must be an increase in training funds from federal and state sources to recruit students and to direct faculty attention to the area. Payback requirements should be maintained in order to maximize employment in this priority area.

2. Work needs to be done to develop model curriculum materials in order to demonstrate that special predoctoral training programs can be activated. At present, many educators are unclear about what contents might appropriately be included in training.

3. APA accreditation guidelines should mention the need for experience in this area. Existing guidelines call attention to the need for inclusion of minorities and for gender parity, which is an addition brought about by the civil rights movement. As this movement has been expanded to include people with serious mental illness and because people with serious mental illnesses are recognized nationally and in each state as a priority service population who remain underserved, the guidelines need to take this into account. The objection that DCPs would "bristle" at the addition of another requirement is a weak argument against the proposal. Many objected to the inclusion of minority and gender guidelines when first presented, but these are widely accepted now. There is precedent for this requirement: Psychologists in the United Kingdom are required by licensing standards to have experience in working with people with patients who have serious mental illnesses.

4. Specialty certification should be developed to ensure that there is a core of practitioners in this complex field who have special skills and can provide high-quality care. Certification has been developed for other areas, such as addictive disorders, but not yet for the field of serious mental illness. As the Houston conference showed, this is an area with special service requirements, and it may be time to recognize exemplary practitioners in this area and provide a way for others to join their ranks.

5. A stronger case must be made for better clinical training. It is apparent from the recent hiring practices of public and private agencies that quality of care is often being sacrificed for economic reasons. For example, in many hospitals and community mental health centers, doctoral-level psychologists have been replaced with psychologists with masters degrees. There is an unfortunate tendency, apparent in these human resource patterns, to give people with serious mental illnesses the least and poorest care.

Furthermore, because training programs have placed little emphasis on serious mental illness, psychologists at both degree levels too often lack exposure to, experience with, or expert knowledge about this client population and cannot be expected to be able to provide state-of-the-art services. With better, more appropriate training, both masters- and doctoral-level psychologists can provide better services. First, we need more experts on services—the kind of experts that would emerge from postdoctoral training in specialized centers. They would create service settings and set standards for performance. Second, doctoral-level psychologists could carry out key service practices and also provide supervision for masters-level psychologists. At present, with rare exceptions, we lack this blend of talents, experiences, and training in most service settings. Masters-level psychologists now provide services to people with serious mental illnesses in hospital and community settings, but there is little evidence that masters training programs have given much attention to the question of whether their training is appropriate for working with people who have serious mental illnesses.

Members of advocacy groups such as the National Alliance for the Mentally Ill, Depressive and Manic Depressive Association, and the National Mental Health Association need to see that services can be improved through the inclusion of better trained personnel, and they need to direct their advocacy efforts toward improved funding for clinical training. Unfortunately, these advocates do not seem convinced yet, and the idea that services are merely "common sense" is still prevalent. In order to test whether specialized training does result in changes in types of services offered, and perhaps whether services are better, we have initiated a study to follow the graduates of clinical training programs that have had a strong emphasis on serious mental illness. Students who have participated in these programs are expected to be providing high-quality services in the field of serious mental illness. If that proves to be the case, the argument for increasing the force of our advocacy for quality services will be strengthened.

References

Belar, C. D., Bieliauskas, L. A., Larsen, K. G., Mensh, I. N. (Eds.). (1987). *Proceeding: National Conference on Internship Training in Psychology.* Gainesville, FL: Association of Psychology Internship Centers.

Bonjean, C. M., Coleman, M. T., & Iscoe, I. (Eds.). (1989). Community care of the chronically mentally ill. *Proceedings of the Sixth Robert Lee Sutherland Seminar in Mental Health.* Austin, TX: Hogg Foundation for Mental Health.

Johnson, D. L. (Ed.). (1990). *Service needs of the seriously mentally ill: Training implications for psychology.* Washington, DC: American Psychological Association.

National Institute of Child Health and Human Development. (1986). *Centers of excellence: The Mental Retardation Research Centers* (NIH Publication No. 86-2882). Washington, DC: U.S. Government Printing Office.

CHAPTER

4

Psychological Services for Older Adults

Linda Teri
University of Washington

Introduction

Currently, 12% of the U.S. population, approximately 25 million people, is over the age of 65. By the year 2000, it is estimated that this number will increase 150%, with the heaviest growth among the "oldest old," those age 85 and over (Fisher, 1980). Older adults experience the complete range of psychological disorders seen in younger age groups, such as depression and anxiety disorders, alcohol and substance abuse, and paranoia and schizophrenia. Mental disorders with serious symptoms are seen in 15–25% of the general population over the age of 65; in medical and institutional settings such as nursing homes, this figure is dramatically higher, generally estimated at 70–90% of nursing home residents (Burns, 1991; Cohen, 1991). Suicide is among the top 10 causes of death among the elderly, with older White men at greatest risk of all age groups (Blazer, Bachar, & Manton, 1986). Other disorders also increase with age. The prevalence of dementia, for example, increases with age, affecting at least 20% of those over age 85, with estimates ranging up to 47% in some studies (Evans et al., 1989; Mortimer, 1983). Dementing brain disorders, such as Alzheimer's disease, constitute the most common form of mental disturbance in older adults, seriously affecting the cognitive and behavioral function of 4–10% of people over 65 and mildly impairing another 5–10% (Evans et al., 1989). The psychological changes associated with physical illnesses are also a major issue within the elderly population. For example, 80% of those over 65 suffer from at least one chronic ailment, and most must cope with multiple physical conditions, both acute and chronic. These include visual and hearing loss, cardiovascular problems, and metabolic changes, as well as the effects of taking many different medications to treat or control these conditions (Collins, 1988; Salzman & Neevis-Olesen, 1992; U.S. Senate Special Committee on Aging, 1986). In addition, older individuals are exposed to many environmental and psychosocial stressors, including retirement, bereavement, changes in living situation, and changes in interpersonal relationships. Many of the mental and emotional problems of older adults are associated with the physical frailty of advanced old age or with the emotional and lifestyle adjustment to living with increased physical restrictions.

Disorders among our nation's elderly have far-reaching effects in addition to the direct effect on the older individual. Most older adults reside in their own homes or with family members (Brody, 1989). Indeed, over 7.6 million Americans are involved in caring for an older disabled adult; most of these are close family members (Stone, Cafferata, & Sangl, 1987). Thus, the dementias and other major mental disorders influence not only

Preparation of this manuscript was supported, in part, by NIMH grant MH19332. Correspondence concerning this article should be addressed to Linda Teri, Ph.D., University of Washington, Department of Psychiatry and Behavioral Sciences, RP-10, Seattle, Washington 98195.

Barry University Library
Miami, Fla. 33161

the affected elder but also the spouse or other family members providing care. Consequently, the numbers of individuals affected may be doubled and, in some cases, trebled and quadrupled, if one takes into account the impact of the older adult's disability on the careprovider and his or her immediate family.

The impact of various emotional disorders on health-care utilization in younger adults has been well documented (Katon, et al., 1990). The comparable impact of emotional disorders on the health-care utilization of older adults is unknown but is likely to be staggering. Currently, 35% of our total national health-care expenditures go to those age 65 and over; 25–40% of all prescription, hospital, and physician office visit costs go to this segment; and 50% of all Medicaid expenditures support older adults in long-term care settings (Rice & Feldman, 1983). Those with psychological disorders are very likely accounting for a disproportionate percentage of these costs, even though they are not receiving the care they need.

In summary, a number of factors combine to make the mental health needs of older adults an issue of central importance. These include the sheer numbers of older adults affected; the growing proportion of individuals and families affected; the emotional, functional, and social disability incurred by these problems; and the impact on our social service and health-care delivery systems. Thus, the need for well-trained professionals providing relevant, accessible psychological services cannot be overstated. This mandate is even more acute given the recent (and successful) effort to have Medicare expand its coverage to include psychologists and the renewed emphasis on behavioral and psychosocial intervention in long-term care settings because of the Omnibus Budget Reconciliation Act of 1987.

Unfortunately, however, a recent report by the Education Subcommittee on Clinical Practice and Training of the American Psychological Association's Division 20 (Aging) concluded that "little progress has been made" in training psychologists to work in aging since a decade ago (Zarit, et al., 1990), and federal support for research and training in aging no longer meets pre-1980 levels (Maddox, 1987). Mental health clinics continue to represent the smallest segment of the care provided (6% of their caseload is over 65, which has resulted in a mere 2% increase in the past decade), and the one major site for mentally impaired elders is the site least equipped to meet their needs—the nursing home (Gatz & Smyer, 1992).

In response to these human resource issues, in April, 1992, the National Institute of Mental Health (NIMH) collaborated with the American Psychological Association and the Retirement Research Foundation to sponsor a National Conference on Clinical Training in Psychology: Improving Psychological Services for Older Adults (Knight, Teri, Santos, & Wohlford, 1993). On considering the needs of the elderly and the current context of geropsychological training and service provision, the conference participants, who are experts in clinical psychology, aging, and clinical geropsychology, made a series of recommendations that follow in the appendix to this chapter. These recommendations are targeted to three groups seen as critical to the continued development of quality psychological services to older adults: the American Psychological Association, NIMH, and Congress. The recommendations are provided in their entirety because they offer a comprehensive approach to improving psychological services for older adults.

Areas of Responsibility

In addition to these recommendations, and in concert with them, other areas of responsibility and growth can be identified that would enhance the provision of effective psychological services to older adults. These areas include research, service, and teaching.

Research

The continued development of a knowledge base regarding effective intervention with older adults is needed. This includes the systematic investigation, evaluation, and improvement of intervention strategies. Various models of psychotherapy exist, yet few have been systematically applied or studied with older adults. Well-controlled clinical trials on theoretically sound interventions concerning clinically relevant problems and populations are desperately needed. Research and clinical knowledge concerning the interplay between emotional and physical health is needed. Gerontological and clinical theories need to be integrated in order to fully understand the psychological disorders of late life. Applied clinical research conducted in "natural" environments, such as the older adult's home, community center, medical center, congregate care setting, and nursing home, need to be

Barry University Library
Miami, Fla. 33161

developed and studied. Research needs to focus on the efficacy of various therapeutic interventions, on the characteristics of both the therapeutic approach and the older individual that impact the effectiveness of different strategies (including physical and cognitive status, ethnic background, type of symptoms, and expectations of both the client and the therapist), and on the external variables such as accessibility and cost, which are also likely to impact the conduct of psychotherapy with older adults. Special needs of minority and economically and culturally diverse populations need to be recognized and addressed. Brief, goal-oriented, structured intervention strategies are in demand and need to be evaluated.

Measurement development and refinement need to address the possible uniqueness of older adults. Normative samples must include adequate representation of the "oldest old," and rigorous methodological design and psychometric analyses need to be incorporated in the development of new measures.

Clinical Service

The application of this knowledge base to clinical populations is needed now. Obviously, application cannot await final empirical support; however, a strong (and growing) body of literature already provides directions for clinical services. These include (but are not limited to) a diversity of approaches such as psychodynamic, interpersonal, behavioral, cognitive–behavioral therapies, and reminiscence therapies, and have been reviewed recently elsewhere (Gatz & Popkin, 1985; Smyer, Zarit, & Qualls, 1989; Teri, Curtis, Gallagher-Thompson, & Thompson, in press, Zarit, 1990).

Psychologists must be encouraged to study and work with issues relevant to older adults (Lewinsohn, Teri, & Hautzinger, 1984; Storandt, 1983). Although this may be stating the obvious, it is critical that professionals learn to view working with older adults as a challenge rather than as a hopeless or futile effort. Considering that the average life span of an individual born in 1980 is 74 years and that a given individual can live beyond 100 (World Almanac Book of Facts, 1991) and be a "young-old," active, community-residing adult or a frail, institutionalized "old-old" individual, an appreciation of the diversity and complexity of aging is essential.

On-site interventions in natural environments, such as those described earlier (the older adult's home, community center, medical center, congregate care setting, or nursing home), need to be conducted. Significant agreement exists that older adults do not routinely access services as they now exist. New ways to make services accessible and relevant to older adults must be explored.

The special needs of minority and economically and culturally diverse populations need to be recognized and addressed. In chapter 7 of this volume, Stratoudakis, Tomes, Wohlford, and Stockdill discuss how states can ready themselves for providing services to the seriously mentally ill. Many of the same issues apply to the older adult. State mental health agencies are often inadequately staffed with psychologists. So-called multidisciplinary teams frequently lack even a consulting psychologist and rely on non-mental health nonprofessionals to provide much-needed service. Individuals, institutions, and states need to identify the aged as an underserved population and identify ways to increase appropriate utilization of psychological services by the elderly.

Training

In order to meet the unmet needs identified above, psychologists must be trained in this knowledge base and its application. They also must be trained in the critical skills to advance it. The recommendations of the National Conference on Clinical Training in Psychology: Improving Psychological Services for Older Adults (Appendix of this chapter) details the training and funding needs as they now exist. Both training and funding in clinical geropsychology need to be available at the undergraduate and graduate, internship and postdoctoral, and continuing professional levels. Exposure to and training in clinical geropsychology must be offered at each of these levels from introductory undergraduate courses to more specialized advanced graduate, postgraduate, and continuing education courses. Curriculum development needs to be advanced, the existing body of knowledge built on and extended. Training in the evaluation and conduct of clinical research is critical. Psychologists must be familiar with the array of models and their specific application to older adults. If specializing in geriatrics, they must be expert in one or more of these models.

Psychologists need to be trained to function in the array of environments in which psychological services will be provided. These include private practice models, interdisciplinary teams, medical centers, long-term care facilities, community agencies, and so forth. Psychologists working with older adults need to appreciate the diversity of services that older adults need and to identify the unique contribution they can make in addressing those needs.

In summary, the frequent gap between the service needs of older adults and current psychological research, training, and practice must be bridged. This is simplistic and grandiose at the same time. It is simplistic because it forms the core of any integrated approach to clinical training; it is grandiose because it will necessitate widespread changes in our funding, training, and service provision systems. In the current financial and political climate in the United States, it is difficult to recommend increases in funding and programs; however, our population of older adults needs these increases. They may well make the difference between living long and living well.

References

Blazer, D. G., Bachar, J. R., & Manton, K. G. (1986). Suicide in late life: Review and commentary. *Journal of the American Geriatrics Society, 34,* 519–525.

Brody, E. M. (1989). The family at risk. In E. Light & B. Lebowitz (Eds.), *Alzheimer's disease: Treatment and family stress. Directions for research* (pp. 2–49). Rockville, MD: National Institute of Mental Health.

Burns, B. (1991). Mental health services research on the hospitalized and institutionalized CMI elderly. In E. Light & B. Lebowitz (Eds.), *The elderly with chronic mental illness (p. 209).* New York: Springer.

Cohen, C. (1991). The chronic mentally ill elderly: Service research issues. In E. Light & B. Lebowitz (Eds.), *The elderly with chronic mental illness (p. 194).* New York: Springer.

Collins, J. G. (1988). Prevalence of selected chronic conditions, United States, 1983–85. *NCHS Advancedata, 165,* 1–16.

Evans, I. A., Funkenstein, H., Albert, M. S., Scherr, P., Cook, N. R., Chown, M. J., Hebert, L. E., Hennekens, C. H., & Taylor, J. O. (1989). Prevalence of Alzheimer's disease in a community population of older persons—Higher than previously reported. *Journal of the American Medical Association, 262,* 2551–2556.

Fisher, C. R. (1980). Differences by age groups in health care spending. *Health Care Financing Review, 1,* 65–90.

Gatz, M., & Popkin, S. J. (1985). Psychological interventions with older adults. In J. E. Birren & K. W. Schaie (Eds.), *Handbook of the psychology of aging (pp. 755–785).* New York: Van Nostrand Reinhold.

Gatz, M., & Smyer, M. A. (1992). The mental health system and older adults in the 1990s. *American Psychologist, 47,* 741–751.

Katon, W., Von Korff, M., Lin, E., Lipscomb, P., Russo, J., Wagner, E., & Polk, E. (1990). Distressed high utilizers of medical care. *General Hospital Psychiatry, 12,* 355–362.

Knight, B., Teri, L., Santos, J. F., & Wohlford, P. (1993). *Applying geropsychology for older adults: Implications for training and practice.* Unpublished manuscript.

Lewinsohn, P. M., Teri, L., & Hautzinger, M. (1984). Training clinical psychologists for work with older adults: A working model. *Professional Practice: Research and Practice, 15,* 187–202.

Maddox, G. L. (Ed.). (1987). *The encyclopedia of aging.* New York: Springer.

Mortimer, J. A. (1983). Alzheimer's disease and senile dementia: Prevalence and incidence. In B. Reisberg (Ed.), *Alzheimer's disease: The standard reference* (pp. 141–148). New York: Free Press.

Rice, D. R., & Feldman, J. J. (1983). Living longer in the United States: Demographic changes and health needs of the elderly. *Milbank Memorial Fund Quarterly,* 362–396.

Salzman, C., & Neevis-Olesen, J. (1992). Psychopharmacologic treatment. In H. E. Birren, R. B. Sloane, & G. D. Cohen (Eds.), *Handbook of mental health and aging* (2nd ed., pp. 721–762). San Diego, CA: Academic Press.

Smyer, M. A., Zarit, S. H., & Qualls, S. H. (1989). Psychological intervention with the aging individual. In W. Schaie & S. Willis (Eds.), *Handbook of the psychology of aging* (3rd ed.). San Diego, CA: Academic Press.

Stone, R., Cafferata, G. L., & Sangl, J. (1987). Caregivers of the frail elderly: A national profile. *The Gerontologist, 27,* 616–626.

Storandt, M. (1983). Psychology's response to the graying of America. *American Psychologist, 38,* 323–326.

Teri, L., Curtis, J., Gallagher-Thompson, D., & Thompson, L. W. (in press). Cognitive–behavior therapy with depressed older adults. In L. S. Schneider, C. F., Reynolds, B. D., Lebowitz, & A. Friedhoff (Eds.), Diagnosis and treatment of depression in late life. Washington, DC: American Psychiatric Press.

U.S. Senate Special Committee on Aging. (1986). *The health status and health care needs of older Americans* (Serial No. 99–L). Washington, DC: U.S. Government Printing Office.

World Almanac Book of Facts. (1991). *World almanac book of facts.* New York: Author.

Zarit, J. M., Zarit, S. H., Frazer, D. W., Hartman-Stein, P., Knight, R., & Teri, L. (1990). Training in clinical geropsychology: Report of the Division 20 Education Subcommittee on Clinical Practice and Training. *Adult Development and Aging News, 18,* 3–6.

Zarit, S. H. (1990). Interventions with frail elders and their families: Are they effective and why? In M. P. Stephens, J. H. Crowther, S. E. Hoboll, & D. L. Tennebaum (Eds.), *Stress and coping in later life families* (pp. 241–265). Washington, DC: Hemisphere.

APPENDIX

Recommendations From the National Conference on Clinical Training in Psychology: Improving Psychological Services for Older Adults[1]

Introduction

Older adults experience the complete range of psychological disorders seen in younger groups such as depression and anxiety disorders, alcohol and substance abuse, paranoia, and schizophrenia.

- Mental disorders with serious symptoms are seen in 15–25% of the general population over the age of 65. In medical and institutional settings this figure is dramatically higher, generally estimated at 70%.

- Suicide is among the top 10 causes of death among older adults.

- Dementing brain disorders, such as Alzheimer's disease, constitute the most common form of mental disturbance in older adults, seriously affecting the cognitive and behavioral function of 4–10% of people over 65 and mildly impairing another 5–10%. The prevalence of dementia increases with age, affecting at least 20% of those over age 85, with estimates ranging up to 47% in some studies.

- The psychological changes associated with physical illness are a major issue. Eighty percent of those over 65 suffer from at least one chronic ailment; most cope with multiple physical conditions. In addition, older individuals are exposed to many environmental and psychosocial stressors, including retirement, bereavement, changes in living situation, and interpersonal relationship changes. These problems of late life not only affect the older adult but also the spouse or other family members providing care for that individual.

The psychological needs of older people are not adequately met by the health, mental health, or social service systems in the United States. The older adults, for example, are defined as a priority, underserved population by the National Institute of Mental Health. Many older people lack appropriate access to psychological services.

- Although Congress enacted changes to Medicare legislation to allow psychologists to be directly reimbursed as independent mental health service providers to the older adult, Medicare-eligible population, this intent has largely been thwarted by delays in implementing the federal regulations and reimbursement policies required to allow this change to occur. Thus, older adults are deprived of needed mental health services.

Psychologists have expertise that can aid older adults in coping with psychological and health-related problems and enhance the ability of our current health-care system to provide effective, cost-efficient care. Clinical geropsychological services include assessment and intervention in a variety of therapeutic settings for a variety of issues including, but not limited to, serious emotional disorders such as depression and anxiety; alcohol and substance abuse; emotional and behavioral aspects of brain disorders such as Alzheimer's disease and other dementing disorders; guardianship and competency issues; and difficulties in coping with normative life transitions and stresses related to aging such as bereavement, chronic illness, health-care decisions, and retirement.

- Clinical geropsychologists have been most involved in providing testing, evaluation, and diagnostic and therapeutic services within settings where older adults receive health and mental health care, such as hospitals, outpatient clinics, community health centers, private health-care organizations and consulting offices, and nursing homes.

[1] This report was prepared by a collaborative effort of professionals in clinical psychology, gerontology, counseling psychology, and clinical geropsychology, following a 3-day "National Conference on Clinical Training in Psychology: Improving Psychological Services for Older Adults" funded by the American Psychological Association, the National Institute of Mental Health (#91 MH333135-OID), and the Retirement Research Foundation. The authors gratefully acknowledge the contribution of ideas by all those who attended but take full responsibility for any errors contained herein. Those wishing to refer to this conference or its recommendations are asked to use the following citation: Teri, L., Storandt, M., Gatz, M., Smyer, M., and Stricker, G. Recommendations from *A National Conference on Clinical Training in Psychology: Improving Psychological Services for Older Adults.* Unpublished manuscript, 1992. Those wishing additional information or another copy of the recommendations may contact Linda Teri, Ph.D., University of Washington, Department of Psychiatry and Behavioral Sciences, RP-10, Seattle, WA 98195.

• Clinical geropsychologists also have long-standing involvement in forensic issues affecting the elderly population, such as in legal competency determinations and procedures for ensuring that patients are allowed to give informed consent regarding their care, an objective that has been legislatively codified by Congress in the Patient Self-Determination Act.

• Neuropsychological evaluation is an essential element in diagnosing dementing disorders and formulating appropriate care plans for the cognitively impaired.

• Clinical geropsychologists also provide multiple forms of individual, group, and family psychotherapy; behavior therapy; cognitive training; support groups; and other forms of care. In addition, they play a major role in counseling older adults about life transitions, preparing for and adapting to new life roles, and devising prevention efforts to maintain healthy functioning in old age.

• Psychologists have made prominent contributions to improving systems of service delivery and enhancing the quality of life enjoyed by older adults through planned modifications of the physical and social environments in which they reside. In many care settings, psychologists also have a major role in consultation to and on-the-job training of other staff members. In addition, because of their research skills, psychologists are major contributors to efforts to enhance the quality of care based on empirical evaluation of care outcomes.

• Clinical geropsychologists' professional approach is characteristically one of collaborating in a multidisciplinary effort with allied health professions such as medicine, psychiatry, social work, nursing, and marriage and family therapy to ensure accessibility to appropriate services and to deliver the optimum quality of care to the elderly population in need.

There is an acute shortage of well-trained clinical geropsychologists—psychologists appropriately prepared to deliver these much-needed, high-quality services to older adults. In response to these needs, in April, 1992, a National Conference on Clinical Training in Psychology: Improving Psychological Services for Older Adults, cosponsored by the American Psychological Association, NIMH, and the Research Retirement Foundation, was held in Washington, D.C. On considering the needs of the older adult and the current context of clinical geropsychological training and service provision, the experts in clinical psychology, aging, and clinical geropsychology who gathered at this nationwide conference agreed on the series of principles and recommendations that follow.

Background

As a framework within which the following recommendations were developed, the following assumptions are made:

1. The problems and prospects of aging require that psychological services be provided in a variety of settings and through a variety of service delivery mechanisms.

2. The expansion of psychological services to older adults is taking place in the context of an ongoing national debate and various congressional proposals on national health-care reform.

3. The best approaches to expanding knowledge about the aging process and improving psychological services to older adults require that psychologists who work with the older adults receive a combination of training in both clinical and research skills.

4. Quality clinical training must be provided in collaboration with excellent programs of service delivery to older adults.

Because of the graying of our nation and the importance of meeting the mental health needs of those who are aging in our country today—and in the future—the need for concerted action on these recommendations cannot be emphasized enough.

Recommendations to the American Psychological Association (APA)

Public policy and services. Psychologists have expertise that can aid older adults in coping with psychological and health-related problems and enhance the ability of our current health-care system to provide effective, cost-efficient care. Clinical geropsychological services include assessment and intervention in a variety of therapeutic settings for a variety of issues including, but not limited to, serious emotional disorders, such as depression and anxiety and alcohol and substance abuse; emotional and behavior sequelae of neurological diseases, such as Alzheimer's disease and other dementing disorders; guardianship and competency issues; and aiding older adults in coping with aging, such as bereavement, chronic illness, health-care decisions, and retirement.

1. This conference endorses the recent Board of Directors recommendation to implement an interdirectorate initiative within the APA central office for the purpose of coordinating activities in the area of clinical geropsychology. This initiative should be established without delay and with appropriate funding from APA.

2. Once established, this interdirectorate initiative should implement the remainder of the recommendations from this conference. Action on these recommendations should be developed and implemented in collaboration with the task groups identified.

3. An on-going work group in clinical geropsychology should be established to operate in an advisory capacity to the interdirectorate initiative. This work group should include, but not be limited to, members of the current conference steering committee and attendees.

4. APA should monitor and influence policies related to access, delivery, and reimbursement of mental health services for older adults, and develop coalitions of cross-disciplinary and cross-divisional groups to advocate for necessary policy changes.

5. APA should aggressively lobby Congress and the Health Care Financing Administration to reexamine and appropriately adjust reimbursement patterns to clinical geropsychologists providing services to older adults.

6. Given the inadequate amount of support for training at all levels and in all areas of clinical geropsychology, APA should aggressively lobby with Congress and federal agencies to develop services, training, and research initiatives in areas of relevance to clinical geropsychology and to assure that funds are provided for pre- and postdoctoral clinical training and research training and research support mechanisms designed to expand the development of a cadre of future clinical geropsychological researchers.

7. APA should aggressively lobby with Congress and federal agencies to develop greater funding for faculty development of both new and existing faculty in clinical geropsychology.

Professional competencies: Training and research. Students moving through the educational system and professionals already in the field will be working with a much older population than has been true in the past. It is imperative to provide them with the knowledge and skills they will need to be effective clinicians, academicians, and researchers to deal with the full spectrum of older adults from mental health to severe mental illness.

To meet the varying needs of the aging population, education and training should occur across a continuum of levels of preparedness in clinical geropsychology. The conference participants strongly support the integration of clinical geropsychological issues in all levels of training and acknowledge the valuable roles to be played by psychologists trained to different degrees of competence in clinical geropsychology, ranging from minimal exposure to specific experience to specialized expertise. For trainees and practicing professionals, the mechanisms for obtaining this training and the demands for different levels of competence will vary. However, the necessity of educating both trainees and current practitioners cannot be overstated.

At each training level, there must exist a sensitivity to the provision of services to culturally diverse minority elderly populations. Community/state and hospital/academic linkages should be strengthened. Collaborative partnerships are needed that focus on service, teaching, training, and research. Training must incorporate theory, research, and practice in clinical geropsychology across three levels of competencies: exposure, experience, and expertise.

8. *Exposure* to aging issues and lifespan development should be available to all students. As part of the accreditation criteria concerning human diversity, APA should require all professional training programs to expose students to aging. The psychology of aging must include positive mental health as well as psychopathology and be integrated with other areas of psychology such that aging issues are included in basic courses.

9. *Experience* must be available to develop skills in minimum core competency areas of clinical geropsychology. These content areas include normal adult development, psychopathology, assessment and treatment, pharmacology, psychology/medical interface, and so forth. Training in these areas should be provided through didactic and supervised clinical experiences and provide opportunities through the range of settings in which the older adult receives care.

10. APA internship accreditation standards should require internship training programs to provide experiences in working with older adults. Each internship should provide some exposure to issues of normal aging as well as to pathological aging; each internship should also provide a recognition of the ongoing contribution of research and its scholarly context, and the need for the practitioner to contribute to that context.

11. APA should support the development of more extensive and varied continuing education opportunities in clinical geropsychology for professionals currently in the field. A full range of training opportunities should be provided to enable them to receive exposure, experience, and expertise. Both brief and time-extended opportunities need to be developed.

12. *Expertise* requires postdoctoral training that is designed to develop specialization in the substantive area of clinical geropsychology and in the range of multidisciplinary approaches for older adults.

13. APA should aid professionals seeking to specialize in clinical geropsychology via an integrated effort to support such specialization, including the formulation of requirements for a specialty in clinical geropsychology.

14. APA should develop criteria to define the expertise necessary for working with older adults and their families, and for evaluating competencies at both the generalist and specialist levels.

15. APA should support further development and dissemination of appropriate curricula and materials for clinical geropsychological training at all levels. This includes undergraduate, graduate, internship, postdoctoral, continuing education, new, and experienced professionals in the field. Current underdeveloped areas include (but are not limited to) use of psychotherapeutic techniques with older adults, psychopharmacology, medical–psychological interface, and so forth.

16. APA should encourage psychologists to use existing funding mechanisms to secure support for faculty development in clinical geropsychology and academic psychology and in internship, postdoctoral training, and clinical settings. APA should assist in disseminating appropriate information on such mechanisms to its members.

17. APA should encourage psychologists to exploit existing research support mechanisms to conduct research in understudied aspects of clinical geropsychology.

Recommendations to the National Center for Mental Health Services (CMHS)[2]

1. CMHS should conduct a systematic study to assess the numbers and kinds of trained mental health personnel including, but not limited to, psychologists, needed to render quality services to older adults with serious mental disorders in the years 2000 and 2020.

2. CMHS should evaluate the impact and effectiveness of both current clinical training programs and the proposed new clinical training initiatives on service delivery systems, client outcomes, and students.

3. Given the inadequate amount of support for training at all levels and in all areas of clinical geropsychology, CMHS should significantly increase the number of individual and institutional pre- and postdoctoral training grants.

4. CMHS should provide training funds with realistic criteria (e.g., adequate stipends for students and reasonable coverage for faculty time).

5. To strengthen public–academic linkages for clinical training in clinical geropsychology, CMHS should exercise a leadership role to bring together other federal agencies, state agencies, community organizations, and consumer and advocacy groups. To improve mental health services and clinical training for working with older adults, CMHS should provide catalytic incentives to promote broader-based collaborative funding for clinical training, drawing from multiple sources: federal, state, local, foundations, and universities. High-quality, research-based mental health training programs are seriously needed.

6. CMHS should recognize and reward those training programs that have made noteworthy achievements in clinical geropsychology, producing substantial numbers of graduates, making

[2] Although these recommendations were originally directed to NIMH, they now apply to CMHS, part of the Substance Abuse and Mental Health Services Administration (SAMHSA) which now has responsibility for the mental health clinical training program after the reorganization that occurred October 1, 1992, under Public Law 102-321, the ADAMHA Reorganization Act.

substantial improvements in their curriculum, and/or developing model programs.

7. CMHS should increase programs to develop more ethnic minority faculty and students with a commitment to clinical geropsychology.

8. CMHS should vigorously support collaboration in interface areas among clinical training, services, and clinical/services research on older adults by encouraging clinical research as parts of all appropriate clinical training grants. Likewise, services and clinical research grants that are appropriate should be required to include clinical training as a component of significant scope.

9. CMHS should improve programs for clinical geropsychology faculty development. Such new faculty development grants should permit short-term and long-term training; they should be given as institutional training grants as well as individual development grants.

10. CMHS should re-establish standing committees to review clinical aging training grant applications. These committees should be multidisciplinary and expert to review applications regarding training for work with older adults.

Recommendations to Congress

Shortages of well-trained psychology personnel are one of the major reasons why millions of older Americans do not receive adequate mental health services. This gap can be expected to increase dramatically in the 21st century when members of the "baby boom" reach old age.

The primary goal of clinical training in clinical geropsychology is to increase the quantity and improve the quality of services to older Americans. In addition to traditional mental health facilities, clinical geropsychologists provide services in hospitals, long-term care facilities, and the community.

Psychologists have expertise that can aid older adults in coping with psychological and health-related problems and enhance the ability of our current health-care system to provide effective, cost-efficient care. Clinical geropsychological services include assessment and intervention in a variety of therapeutic settings for a variety of issues including, but not limited to, serious emotional disorders, such as depression and anxiety and alcohol and substance abuse; emotional and behavior sequelae of neurological diseases, such as Alzheimer's disease and other dementing disorders; guardianship and competency issues; and aiding older adults in coping with aging, such as bereavement, chronic illness, health-care decisions, and retirement.

The 20–25% cuts in funding of NIMH clinical training programs in 1987, 1989, and 1992 have undermined and destabilized training efforts to provide clinical services for underserved priority populations. Programs for training in clinical geropsychology have been significantly affected.

1. Congress should appropriate more adequate funding for presently available institutional clinical training grants in order to attract new professionals to careers in public mental health, including aging and mental health. In particular, every effort should be made to restore the fiscal year 1993 CMHS/(NIMH) clinical training program at least to its 1986 level of $20 million.

2. Congress should provide funding support for new initiatives in clinical geropsychology training to meet the mental health services objectives of the 1990s and beyond, as recommended in recent conferences.

3. Congress should direct CMHS to systematically improve geropsychological services and clinical training for the older adult with mental disorders, just as it now does for severely mentally ill adults and children.

4. Congress should mandate that CMHS support a new Clinical Training in Geropsychology Grant that would feature payback obligations for trainees in preservice training; inservice training and continuing education; and university/medical school responsibility for high-quality, research-based mental health training programs.

5. Congress should support and expand present training programs in clinical geropsychology conducted by the Department of Veterans Affairs.

6. Congress should mandate that the Health Resources and Services Administration include clinical geropsychology training among the clinical training programs it supports for various health professions.

7. Congress should direct CMHS and/or other appropriate federal agencies to improve programs

for faculty development in clinical geropsychology, and provide funding to support such initiatives.

8. Congress should ensure the implementation of a Medicare provision authorizing psychologists to receive direct payment under Medicare. Although Congress enacted changes to the Medicare statute to allow psychologists to be directly reimbursed as independent mental health service providers to the older adult, Medicare-eligible population, this intent has largely been thwarted by the interpretation of the statute. Thus, older adults are deprived of needed mental health services and are threatened with further deprivation.

CHAPTER

5

Ethnic Minorities with Mental Disorders

Hector F. Myers
University of California, Los Angeles

The United States, as it approaches the turn of the century, is experiencing major social, economic, and demographic pressures that pose unique challenges for mental health care providers and for those who prepare clinical psychologists to be effective participants in this industry. The current economic recession and conservative social policies have severely limited the resources for both clinical services and training. At the same time, dramatic shifts in the ethnic composition of most urban communities and in the population served by public mental health facilities have increased the demand for more cross-culturally competent clinicians. The combination of reduced resources and increased demands for new clinical competencies provide the impetus for rethinking how clinical psychologists are trained (i.e., curriculum innovation) and how clinical programs are structured to optimize the fit between the needs of provider settings and the knowledge and competencies of clinical psychology trainees (i.e., innovative training models). In this chapter, which summarizes issues raised in an earlier volume (Myers, Wohlford, Guzman, & Echmendia, 1991), we argue for diversifying the curriculum in clinical psychology to ensure multicultural competence in all clinical psychologists. We also argue for forging more effective linkages between academic and public service settings to ensure that psychologists are trained to conduct appropriate research and provide effective mental health services.

In this chapter, first the population pressures that justify the need for changes in the personnel and curriculum in clinical psychology are described. Then, the implications of these population changes for mental health service delivery and for clinical training are discussed. Finally, some of the conceptual and pragmatic obstacles to making necessary changes in the curriculum are discussed, some of the models that have been developed to increase multicultural representation in clinical training programs are described, and innovative strategies for forging new collaborative relationships for clinical and research training to meet the demands for more multiculturally competent clinical psychologists are proposed.

We believe that the current social context is ideal for achieving the illusive objectives of recruiting and training more ethnic minority clinical psychologists and incorporating more culturally relevant content into the clinical curricula. As Pedersen and Marsella (1982) argued, the issue of multicultural training for treatment and research can no longer be considered simply a political issue; it is also an ethical one. In order for clinical psychologists to function as responsible professionals in the provision of clinical services and in the conduct of clinical research on an increasingly multicultural population, they must meet criteria of basic competence with the unique

The preparation of this manuscript was supported in part by NIMH Clinical Training Grant No. MH19269. Dr. Myers is professor of psychology and director of the Minority Mental Health Training Program in Psychology, UCLA and director of the Biobehavioral Research Center, Department of Psychiatry, Charles R. Drew University of Medicine & Science.

clinical problems they will face with these populations.

Population Pressures for Personnel and Curriculum Change

In two articles, Jones (1990b) and Myers, Echemendia, and Trimble (1991) provide strong arguments for the need for training more ethnic minority psychologists and for training all psychologists to be effective therapeutic agents. They note that in the past decade, the United States has experienced a dramatic increase in the proportion of the population that is non-White. This shift is driven mainly by the influx of people from Southeast Asia, the Middle East, and Latin America. According to the initial reports from the 1990 census, people of ethnic minority backgrounds now constitute 28.7% of the population of the United States. This includes 12.1% African-Americans, 2.9% Asians, 9.0% Hispanics, 0.8% Native Americans and Alaska Natives, and 3.9% other ethnic groups ("Analysis Puts," 1991). This greater ethnic diversification is especially evident in the Northeast, Southeast, the West Coast, Hawaii, and the District of Columbia. Non-Whites already constitute significant pluralities in these regions and are projected to become the majority by the turn of the century.

However, these figures do not capture the full impact and implications of these demographic shifts because they do not reflect the diversity among the various ethnic groups in terms of language, culture, national origin, immigration status, reason for immigration, level of acculturation to the United States, or pattern of geographic dispersal. For example, a state like Alabama with a large population of African-Americans (25%) is not as ethnically diverse as New York, which has proportionately fewer African-Americans (16%), but more Asians (3.9%), Native Americans (0.35%), and Hispanics (12%). To capture this more important difference, Phillip Meyer ("Analysis Puts," 1991) developed a diversity index[1] from the U.S. Census Bureau data to estimate the population mix in each of the 50 states. These analyses identified 16 states and the District of Columbia as more ethnically diverse than the country as a whole (i.e., diversity ratings > 40). It is also worth noting that even among these more ethnically diverse states, the proportion of persons of color range from a low of 19.1% (Arizona, with a diversity rating of 45) to a high of 70.4% (Washington, D.C., with diversity of 51; "Analysis Puts," 1991). These data suggest that the problem we face as a field is not simply to appreciate the differences between minorities and Whites but also to appreciate the range of differences among the various ethnic groups characterized as ethnic minorities. These groups are likely to be as different among themselves as they are from Whites. Furthermore, we must begin to recognize that being a member of one ethnic group does not ensure familiarity, sensitivity, or competence with members of other ethnic groups.

Implications for the Provision of Mental Health Services

Mental health epidemiologic data (Karno et al., 1987; Robins et al., 1984) and data on the pattern of mental health service utilization (Cheung, 1991) underscore even further the complexity of the challenge posed by the increasing ethnic diversity of the U.S. population. These data highlight differences between the groups in their need for appropriate mental health services as well as their varying patterns of use of the available mental health services. Cheung (1991) in her review of mental health utilization rates noted that although the need for mental health services is high in all ethnic minority groups, there are significant differences among the groups in how these services are used. Hispanics and Asians appear to be underutilizing mental health services, whereas African-Americans and Native Americans appear to be overutilizing services, especially inpatient services. These patterns of differences in service utilization have been attributed to such varied factors as culturally reinforced stigmatization of psychiatric problems (Kitano, 1982; Lum, 1982), factors that appear to influence the timing of seeking help (Jackson, 1981; Sue, 1977), and factors that influence the choice of mental health care providers (Neighbors, Jackson, Bowman, & Gurin, 1983).

There is also growing clinical and epidemiologic evidence that indicates ethnic and socioeconomic differences in factors that enhance vulnerability

[1] The *diversity index* is defined as the probability that two randomly selected people in the same geographic area are likely to be ethnically different from each other. This index acknowledges that all ethnic groups are different from each other and not just different from Whites. The diversity rating for the United States as a whole is 40, and states are defined as high or low in diversity in reference to this score.

to psychopathology (Kessler & Neighbors, 1986; Myers, 1982; Neff, 1985), in symptom presentation (Neighbors, Jackson, Campbell, & Williams, 1989; Trimble, 1991; Williams, 1986; Zane & Sue, 1991), in factors contributing to substance use and to comorbidity for substance use (Kleinman & Lukoff, 1978; Singleton, 1989; Trimble, 1991), in response to pharmacologic agents (Lin, Poland, & Lesser, 1986; Strickland et al., in press), and in factors that can affect psychotherapy processes and outcomes (Atkinson, 1985; LaFramboise, Trimble, & Mohatt, 1990; Lopez, 1983; Malgady, Rogler, & Constantino, 1987; Sue & Zane, 1987).

Implications for Clinical Training in Psychology

The increasing ethnic diversity of the U.S. population, the growing socioeconomic marginalization of ethnic minority communities, and the growing evidence of ethnic differences in vulnerability to psychopathology and in factors that affect treatment processes and outcomes pose a significant challenge to the clinical competence of most clinical psychologists. Mental health professionals of all races will be called on to address the mental health needs of clients who are more likely than ever to be different from them. Therefore, cross-cultural familiarity and experience will become an important criteria of clinical competence. The recent decision by the APA Committee on Accreditation to make diversity in clinical training a requirement for the accreditation of clinical training programs is an important step in ensuring that future psychologists will have greater ethnic exposure. In addition, because it is not feasible to expect that most clinical professionals will develop sufficient knowledge and skill with more than one or two cultural groups, it is clear that more ethnic minority and bilingual and bicultural clinicians and researchers will need to be trained.

Unfortunately, however, both the science and practice of clinical psychology have been slow to respond to the mental health issues and needs of our growing multicultural and multiethnic society. After decades of debate over the need to increase diversity in both the personnel and curriculum in clinical psychology, we see some important but modest changes. According to Jones (1990a), the number and visibility of ethnic minority psychologists have increased substantially since 1977, and detailed descriptions of some of the predoctoral and postdoctoral clinical training programs that have increased the diversity of their trainees and their training curricula are now available (see Myers, Wohlford, Guzman, & Echemendia, 1991). Also, the number and quality of research by minority scholars and on ethnic issues in psychology have increased, and this indicates that the psychological study of ethnicity and ethnic populations continues to gain credibility as a legitimate field of scientific inquiry.

However, as noted by Jones (1990a), excitement over these gains must be tempered by the realization that the percentage of minorities in graduate school (15%), the proportion of new minority doctoral-level graduates in psychology (8%), the percentage of minority members of APA (< 5%), and the percentage of minority faculty in psychology (< 5%) have remained relatively stable since the early 1980s. Also, there is growing evidence that the number of African-American and American Indian students equipped to enter graduate training in psychology has either hit a plateau or has dropped. If this trend continues, we may see either net reductions in the number of the ethnic minority doctoral-level psychologists produced during the 1990s or a shift in the ethnic distribution of each graduating class (i.e., increases in the number of Asian and Hispanic psychologists and decreases in the number of African-Americans and American Indians). Thus, for the foreseeable future, the average clinical psychologist will still be White and will continue to be trained primarily by White faculty. Although the APA accreditation guidelines should ensure greater ethnic diversity in clinical training, most clinical psychologists will still be trained to use assessment and diagnostic tools and treatment approaches that have demonstrated utility mainly with White patients. The average new doctoral-level psychologists will still formulate research questions guided by monocultural conceptual models and will still design and conduct studies on predominantly White samples. When non-Whites are included in the study sample, measures with no evidence of validity with multiethnic samples will still be used, ethnically relevant variables will continue to be ignored, and unsophisticated conceptual and analytic strategies to probe for race and socioeconomic status effects will continue to be the norm. Students working with ethnically diverse populations will develop greater conceptual, clinical, and research sophistication when the faculty and the training curricula achieve a higher level of sophistication in these areas than is presently the case. Thus, although some important gains have been made, clinical psychology in the 1990s remains very much a White science and profession.

Myers, Echemendia et al. (1991) noted several implications for the training of future clinical psychologists that can be drawn from these observations. First, there continues to be a need for more effective and aggressive education of ethnic minority communities about the appropriate and timely use of mental health services. However, these educational efforts must be linked to the development and dissemination of effective prevention strategies (Lorion, 1983) and to changes in the available treatment approaches to make them more culturally appropriate. Second, it is equally important that we continue to develop an adequate pool of trained ethnic minority clinical psychologists, especially those who are bilingual and bicultural. However, with minorities still accounting for less than 10% of new doctorates in psychology, White psychologists will continue to be the major providers of mental health services and to be the primary investigators of clinical problems that impact all segments of the population well into the 21st century. Therefore, it is imperative that we ensure that all psychologists are competent to provide clinical services to clients from a variety of ethnic and socioeconomic backgrounds. Furthermore, all psychologists must be equipped to contribute to the development and application of new knowledge that is informed by ethnicity, gender, and socioeconomic considerations. By this we mean that psychologists must develop a more sophisticated understanding of how ethnicity, culture, and socioeconomic influences contribute to psychological vulnerability and resilience, to the experience and expression of psychological distress, to the utilization of mental health services as part of their repertoire of help-seeking behaviors, and to processes and outcomes of treatment and prevention efforts.

Obstacles to Curriculum and Structural Innovations

Conceptual and Pragmatic Obstacles

There are several major conceptual and pragmatic obstacles to change in pursuing the ideals articulated above. The most significant obstacle to innovation exists in psychologists' way of thinking about clinical psychology. At the core of thought in clinical psychology is the belief that the principles and concepts that guide the field are universal, and therefore, any clinician who has mastered these concepts and skills is capable of working effectively with clients who differ on any of several demographic dimensions (e.g., race, gender, etc.). In addition, although there is recognition of ethnic group differences and the possibility that these differences may contribute to differential treatment outcomes, several unstated assumptions continue to limit the development of truly generalizable clinical principles, concepts, models, and tools. First, psychologists continue to assume that differences in treatment efficacy are largely attributable to the inability of the client to "do the work of therapy" rather than to problems with the fit and appropriateness of conceptual models and therapeutic approaches. Second, psychologists have advocated the development of special intervention strategies to meet the needs of ethnic or low SES clients, which is a pragmatic and effective first step. However, an unanticipated consequence of such special efforts is to reinforce the belief that the current models of clinical training need not be altered to incorporate these alternative clinical perspectives and approaches. Third, the assumption is made by many that ethnically focused training is only relevant to ethnic minority psychologists or to those with a specific interest in these populations and that this "specialized" training need not be part of the core clinical curriculum.

These beliefs and arguments are articulated even by well-intentioned colleagues who are generally supportive of efforts to encourage innovation. However, supporters who only favor superficial changes actually interfere with change because their supportive rhetoric often limits the extent and depth of discussion and the range of alternative strategies that might be considered. Such supportive rhetoric encourages quick fixes that defuse conflict but rarely lead to the type of substantive changes in perspectives and approaches that are necessary in order to train clinical psychologists who are truly cross-culturally competent.

Another important obstacle to change is a pragmatic one. The vast majority of clinical faculty who run training programs were trained in traditional university-based programs and received their clinical practicum experience in traditional clinical settings (e.g., university hospitals, veterans' hospitals, etc.). Consequently, most have little if any expertise or interest in ethnic issues in psychology and, thus, cannot teach what they do not know. This is not an insignificant problem. In fact, the lack of cross-cultural expertise in the faculty is not only a source of significant resistance to change but also poses a potentially serious problem when ethnically relevant material is incorporated into the clinical curriculum. For example, faculty may assign readings that perpetuate simplistic, unsubstantiated stereotypical notions about ethnic groups rather than teach students how to think about issues of individual or group differences that may impact assessment and diagnotic decisions, treatment processes and outcomes, and research. The latter requires substantially greater expertise than simply assigning readings in an uncritical fashion. It also requires courage to acknowledge one's limitations while encouraging students to gain this knowledge and engage in a critical struggle with these issues.

Structural Impediments to Change

There are also a number of structural impediments to forging new linkages between academia and the public mental health sector to improve clinical training. Clinical training is viewed, especially at the masters and predoctoral level, as the primary responsibility of academic programs. The appropriate curriculum, the sequencing of course and practicum requirements, the requirements for the degree, as well as the qualifications of faculty who guide training are all determined by the criteria, policies, and procedures of the academic institutions that confer the degree. On the other hand, mental health service settings, be they public or private, are important but secondary partners in the task of training clinical psychologists. These institutions address issues of training as secondary to their primary mission of providing direct services. These agencies are also governed by institutional guidelines and policies that are quite different from those of academia.

These differences in mission and institutional cultures make it very easy for these training partners to relate to each other from a distance and to perceive each other with suspicion. Academics think of their job as creating the basic knowledge in the field and view practitioners as applying this knowledge. On the other hand, clinical practitioners often view academics as creating knowledge that sometimes lacks relevance and utility to the problems and needs of psychiatric patients. These differences are especially noteworthy between academia and public mental health settings.

Current Approaches to Academic–Service Linkages

In the recent book on *Ethnic Minority Perspectives on Clinical Training and Services in Psychology* (Myers, Wohlford et al., 1991), a number of model minority mental health training programs in psychology were described. It is apparent that these programs reflect different philosophies and different approaches to achieving diversity in their student body and curricula. These programs reflect the unique character of each institution and the demographics of their location. For example, some programs target specific ethnic groups (e.g., Hispanics and Native Americans), whereas others have a more multiethnic focus. Some programs developed minority mental health specialty tracks within the broader clinical program, others have maintained their mainstream core curriculum and supplement it with specialized courses, and others have developed a combined approach that includes integrating ethnically relevant content into core courses and clinical practica, as well as offering special focus courses. Regardless of the model used, almost all of the programs were initiated by ethnic minority faculty and focused their initial efforts on minority student recruitment. Curriculum modification, which is more difficult to accomplish, was generally addressed later.

Regardless of the different models used, there is general consensus among program developers that increasing the pool of qualified ethnic faculty and curriculum reform are essential to the success of all multicultural training efforts. Ethnic faculty are a necessary but not sufficient condition for developing these innovative efforts because they provide the impetus and often carry the burden of leadership for social change. However, the active support and involvement of key nonminority faculty and administrators and the development of a critical mass of strong ethnic minority graduate students are also essential requirements. Unfortunately, the recent report by Stapp, Tucker, and VandenBos (1985) on the ethnic breakdown of psychologists indicates that only 5.0% of PhD psychologists who reported educational activities as their primary area of employment were non-White. These figures underscore the fact that there continues to be a critical shortage of this resource, and therefore, clinical training programs must place greater priority on preparing minority students for academic careers and not just for service careers.

There is also a growing consensus that the second major obstacle is still the limited availability of valid information on ethnic minority populations. Meaningful curriculum changes require that current information on the mental health of ethnic minority populations be critically evaluated to ensure its validity and applicability across ethnic groups. This information must be compiled and made readily accessible, additional lacunae in the knowledge base must be identified, and support and resources must be allocated to the creation and dissemination of new knowledge.

Finally, because the majority of mental health services and research on ethnic minority populations occur in the public sector, more effective public service–academic linkages need to be forged. Such linkages would ensure that clinical psychologists develop the competencies that are needed in the settings in which these populations are served. Such linkages would also ensure that the knowledge developed on the respective ethnic minority groups will be based on more representative community and public clinic samples rather than on minority college students.

The programs represented in the Myers, Wohlford, et al. (1991) volume differed in the success with which they developed effective linkages with the public sector. Several programs began this effort by establishing working advisory groups with representatives from the public service agencies where their students received practicum training. These groups provide valuable information to the faculty about weak knowledge areas of students and about changes in clinical problems and populations that are seen in the respective public agencies. In many cases, the directors of training at the public agencies are appointed as clinical professors at the university. Very often, however, these appointments are only symbolic and do not entail any meaningful role for the agency representatives in discussions about curriculum or related issues. In fact, many of these appointments are unremunerated.

Equally important is the fact that few programs have faculty who have any formal clinical or administrative ties at the public service agencies. Therefore, although faculty members may interact with service agency representatives about their students' training needs, university faculty have little real say in how such needs are to be met.

Therefore, achieving meaningful institutional linkages will require consideration of new and innovative institutional arrangements beyond those that have been forged to date. At the outset, both academics and public service personnel will need to recognize that modern clinical training requires establishing a real partnership of equals. Academic programs will be hard pressed to hire significant numbers of ethnic faculty with the expertise necessary to make the curriculum changes required for true multicultural training. Also, even if minority faculty were available in requisite numbers, current criteria for retention and promotion at major universities preclude the degree of involvement in clinical practice at public agencies necessary for them to maintain both their scholarly productivity and their effectiveness in the public setting. Therefore, other alternative approaches will have to be considered. One idea would be to formalize the affiliation of agency personnel as faculty in academic training programs. These faculty members could participate more directly in coteaching some of the core clinical courses or could teach some of the supplemental courses targeted at ethnic issues in assessment and treatment. Ethnic psychologists on the regular faculty could then concentrate on integrating ethnic content into core courses as well as conducting the research needed to upgrade the quality of the scientific knowledge on which to base curriculum changes.

Another way to utilize these linkages to achieve the stated objectives is to take advantage of the practical clinical expertise of public sector clinicians to upgrade the multicultural expertise of university faculty. Psychologists in the public sector could be hired as faculty in short-term, intensive continuing education programs that would provide university faculty with the information and skills needed to make effective changes in their core clinical programs.

On the other side of the coin, public service agencies suffer from a lack of skilled resources to conduct research that might be pertinent to their clinical services and to the fiscal viability of their agencies. Faculty also face considerable difficulties obtaining ethnically diverse clinical samples on which to test hypotheses. Therefore, developing formal collaborative research arrangements would also be beneficial to both parties. Faculty could provide the technical expertise necessary to design, obtain funding for, and conduct clinical research on questions of mutual interest. Faculty could also provide the necessary technical expertise to build the infrastructure at the public agency that is necessary for conducting high-quality research. In turn, the public agency would provide the facilities and serve as an effective conduit for more representative samples of patients for the faculty's research. Graduate students would then be able to obtain both their clinical practica and research training as part of this collaborative enterprise.

This is an ideal arrangement for training the next generation of psychologists to meet the unique demands for competent professional service, research, and teaching in a multiethnic, multicultural society. To do any less would ensure the continued production of very bright but culturally myopic clinical psychologists. It would also ensure that the field would continue to be ill-prepared to meet the mental health needs of modern American society. Since the early 1940s, American psychology has responded to the mental health challenges that have emerged from various national and worldwide crises. The new populations and worldwide economic changes pose a new challenge to the field. These challenges can be effectively met by changing the ethnic composition of the field, by incorporating more culturally appropriate content into clinical training curricula, and by fostering a more effective partnership for training between academic institutions and service agencies in the public sector. The modern clinical psychologist, regardless of race, must have a higher level of multicultural familiarity and competence. This standard of professional competency can best be achieved in psychology training programs that reflect a genuine respect and appreciation for cultural diversity. This respect should be reflected in the programs' philosophy and "culture," in the composition of the student body and faculty, in the content of the curriculum, and in the relationships established between the academic programs and the clinical practicum settings in which these students develop and polish their clinical skills.

References

Analysis puts a number on population mix. (1991, April 11). *USA Today,* p. 10A.

Atkinson, D. R. (1985). Research on cross-cultural counseling and psychotherapy: A review and update of reviews. In P. Pedersen (Ed.), *Handbook of cross-cultural counseling and therapy* (pp. 191–198). Westport, CT: Greenwood Press.

Cheung, F. K. (1991). The use of mental health services by ethnic minorities. In H. Myers, P. Wohlford, L. P. Guzman, & R. Echemendia (Eds.), *Ethnic minority perspectives on clinical training and services in psychology* (pp. 21–29). Washington, DC: American Psychological Association.

Jackson, J. J. (1981). Urban Black Americans. In A. Harwood (Ed.), *Ethnicity and Medical Care* (pp. 37–65). Cambridge, MA: Harvard University Press.

Jones, J. M. (1990a). A call to advance psychology's role in minority issues. *The APA Monitor, 21*(6), 23.

Jones, J. M. (1990b). Who is training our ethnic minority psychologists and are they doing it right? In G. Stricker, E. Davis-Russell, E. Bourg, E. Duran, W. R. Hammond, J. McHolland, K. Polite, & B. E. Vaughn (Eds.), *Toward ethnic diversification in psychology education and training* (pp. 17–34). Washington, DC: American Psychological Association.

Karno, M., Hough, R. L., Burnam, A., Escobar, J. I., Timbers, D., Santans, F., & Boyd, J. H. (1987). Lifetime prevalence of specific psychiatric disorders among Mexican Americans and non-Hispanic Whites in Los Angeles. *Archives of General Psychiatry, 44,* 695–701.

Kessler, R. C., & Neighbors, H. W. (1986). A new perspective on the relationships among race, social class and psychological distress. *Journal of Health & Social Behavior, 27,* 107–115.

Kitano, H. H. (1982). Mental health in the Japanese–American community. In E. E. Jones & S. J. Korchin (Eds.), *Minority mental health* (pp. 149–164). New York: Praeger.

Kleinman, P. H., & Lukoff, I. F. (1978). Ethnic differences in factors related to drug use. *Journal of Health & Social Behavior, 19,* 190–199.

LaFramboise, T., Trimble, J. E., & Mohatt, G. (1990). Counseling intervention and American Indian tradition: An integrative approach. *The Counseling Psychologist, 18,* 628–654.

Lin, K-M., Poland, R. E., & Lesser, I. M. (1986). Ethnicity and psychopharmacology. *Culture, Medicine & Psychiatry, 10,* 151–165.

Lopez, S. R. (1983). The study of psychotherapy bias: Some conceptual issues and concluding remarks. In J. Murray & P. R. Abramson (Eds.), *Bias in psychotherapy* (pp. 353–366). New York: Praeger.

Lorion, R. P. (1983). Evaluating preventive interventions: Guidelines for the serious social change agent. In R. D. Felner, L. A. Jason, J. N. Moritsugu, & S. S. Farber (Eds.), *Preventive psychology: Theory, research and practice* (pp. 251–272). Elmsford, NY: Pergamon Press.

Lum, R. G. (1982). Mental health attitudes and opinions of Chinese. In E. E. Jones & S. J. Korchin (Eds.), *Minority mental health* (pp. 165–190). New York: Praeger.

Malgady, R. G., Rogler, L. H., & Constantino, G. (1987). Ethnocultural and linguistic bias in mental health evaluation of Hispanics. *American Psychologist, 42,* 228–234.

Myers, H. F. (1982). Stress, ethnicity and social class: A model for research on Black populations. In E. E. Jones & S. J. Korchin (Eds.), *Minority mental health* (pp. 118–148). New York: Praeger.

Myers, H. F., Echemendia, R. J., & Trimble, J. E. (1991). The need for training ethnic minority psychologists. In H. F. Myers, P. Wohlford, L. P. Guzman, & R. Echemendia (Eds.), *Ethnic minority perspectives on clinical training and services in psychology* (pp. 3–11). Washington, DC: American Psychological Association.

Myers, H. F., Wohlford, P., Guzman, L. P., & Echemendia, R. (Eds.). (1991). *Ethnic minority perspectives on clinical training and services in psychology.* Washington, DC: American Psychological Association.

Neff, J. (1985). Race and vulnerability to stress: An examination of differential vulnerability. *Journal of Personality and Social Psychology, 49,* 481–491.

Neighbors, H. W., Jackson, J. S., Bowman, P., & Gurin, C. (1983). Stress, coping and Black mental health: Preliminary findings from a national study. *Prevention in Human Services, 2,* 5–28.

Neighbors, H. W., Jackson, J. S., Campbell, L., & Williams, D. (1989). The influence of racial factors on psychiatric diagnosis: A review and suggestions for research. *Community Mental Health Journal, 25,* 301–311.

Pederson, P. B., & Marsella, A. J. (1982). The ethical crisis for cross-cultural counseling and therapy. *Professional Psychology, 13*(4), 18–25.

Robins, L. N., Helzer, J. E., Weissman, M. M., Orvaschel, H., Gruenberg, E., Burke, J. D., & Regier, D. A. (1984). Lifetime prevalence of specific psychiatric disorders in three sites. *Archives of General Psychology, 41,* 949–958.

Singleton, E. G. (1989). Substance use and black youth: Implications of cultural and ethnic differences in adolescent alcohol, cigarette, and illicit drug use. In R. L. Jones (Ed.), *Black Adolescents* (pp. 385–402). Berkeley, CA: Cobb & Henry.

Stapp, R., Tucker, A. M., & VandenBos, G. R. (1985). Census of psychological personnel: 1983. *American Psychologist, 40*(12), 1317–1351.

Strickland, T. L., Ranganath, M., Lin, K. M., Poland, R. E., Mendoza, R., & Smith, M. W. (1991). Psychopharmacologic considerations in the treatment of Black American populations. *Psychopharmacology Bulletin, 27*(4), 441–448.

Sue, S. (1977). Community mental health services to minority groups: Some optimism, some pessimism. *American Psychologist, 32,* 616–624.

Sue, S., & Zane, N. (1987). The role of culture and cultural techniques in psychotherapy: A critique and reformulation. *American Psychologist, 42*(1), 37–45.

Trimble, J. E. (1991). Ethnic specification, validation prospects, and the future of drug use research. *The International Journal of Addictions, 25*(2A), 149–170.

Williams, D. H. (1986). The epidemiology of mental illness in Afro-Americans. *Hospital & Community Psychiatry, 37,* 42–49.

Zane, N., & Sue, S. (1991). Culturally responsive mental health services for Asian Americans: Treatment and training issues. In Myers, H. F., P. Wohlford, L. P. Guzman, & R. Echemendia (Eds.), *Ethnic minority perspectives on clinical training and services in psychology* (pp. 49–58). Washington, DC: American Psychological Association.

CHAPTER

6

Clients With Substance Abuse and Comorbid Diagnoses

Holly A. Hills
Florida Mental Health Institute, University of South Florida

Robert A. Zucker
Michigan State University

Steven L. Seitz
Center for Substance Abuse Prevention

Current estimates of substance use disorders as well as other types of mental disorder (Regier et al., 1984, 1990) claim that alcohol and other drug abuse and dependence account for 51% of conditions in the United States (American Psychiatric Association, 1980) and that these substance use disorders are as well a significant part of the clinical picture—by way of their comorbid occurrence—even when they are not the primary clinical concern (Regier et al., 1990). Although current evidence suggests that these problems have peaked (e.g., National Institute on Drug Abuse [NIDA], 1988, 1989), perhaps as a result of substantial federal efforts at prevention and intervention, the magnitude of the population that could benefit from intervention for these difficulties is still exceptionally large. Approximately 6% of the U.S. population (Helzer, Burnham & McEvoy, 1991) currently abuses or is dependent on alcohol, and 2.3% is involved in other drug use (Gerstein & Harwood, 1990). Other reports estimate that two thirds of those in treatment for alcohol and other drug abuse problems have other psychiatric diagnoses (National Institute on Alcohol Abuse and Alcoholism [NIAAA], 1990) and that the network of problems extends substantially beyond the formal treatment system. Thus, premature death and disability, disruption of families, criminal activity, and lost or diminished productivity, have all been tied to alcohol and drug abuse (Mayer, 1983; Millman, 1989; NIAAA, 1990).

This cluster of major social problems clearly warrants sustained and significant attention from the treatment community as well as from those who train the caregivers. Unfortunately, despite the magnitude of these difficulties, the administration and treatment systems associated with mental health and substance abuse service delivery have long been divided, and the educational and training communities have been largely inattentive to this domain. A number of authors have commented on the failure of mental health personnel to recognize the magnitude of substance abuse in the populations they treat. It is estimated that as many as 40% of all outpatients seeking psychotherapy have substance abuse problems that require intervention (Cummings, 1979). Among people with prolonged and severe mental illness, the numbers are even more dramatic, with approximately half of the individuals presenting (47% schizophrenia, 56% bipolar disorder) achieving diagnostic criteria for comorbid substance abuse or dependence (Regier et al., 1990). Despite this level of impact, the number of skilled professionals involved in this care is very small and does not meet the needs of this population (Millman, 1989). In addition, the number of psychologists working in the substance abuse field is also exceptionally small compared to the number of paraprofessionals (Schlesinger, 1984). Increasingly, however, professionals across disciplines are recognizing the need for specialized training for the diagnosis and treatment of substance abuse disorders (Fawcett, 1992).

In this chapter, we examine the factors that have kept psychologists on the sidelines with respect to treating these disorders. Historical systemic, training, and treatment issues will be discussed. Current trends in providing training in the areas of substance abuse and dependence and comorbidity will be evaluated, followed by a brief review of generalizable skills, methods, and measures. Finally, opportunities for psychologists in this field and recommendations for treatment and training guidelines will be briefly explored.

Historical Divisions

Differences in funding sources have historically kept the substance abuse and mental illness systems apart and have frequently compromised the coordination of care between these systems. The rigidity in these funding systems has also kept dollars from crossing boundaries between substance abuse and mental illness treatment. Thus, facilities have been built independently of each other, with separate personnel divisions and management, which has created geographic barriers. These different service delivery systems have historically maintained sharp boundaries, to the advantage of bureaucracies and not individuals (Thacker & Tremaine, 1989).

Beyond funding and geography, differences in orientation and conceptualization have maintained the division. What were formally narrow perspectives regarding etiology and treatment have broadened somewhat in recent years. Evidence suggests, however, that mental health workers and substance abuse professionals commonly retain their traditional approaches and are resistant to sharing and integrating treatment options (Thacker & Tremaine, 1989).

In psychiatric and, to some extent, psychological circles, a tendency remains to see substance abuse disorders as either secondary to other psychiatric illnesses or as a distinct and specialized symptomatic manifestation that requires the services of paraprofessionals or specialists rather than mainstream professionals (Fawcett, 1992). These interpretations, and continued ambivalence as to whether substance abuse is merely symptomatic of other underlying psychopathology, have also continued to promote divisions in treatment. Issues as to whether a disorder is primary versus secondary may have major etiologic importance; however, this distinction may have much less significance at the level of the individual requiring immediate help. At that juncture, both sets of problems must be addressed. Unlike work relating to other types of major psychopathology, the substance abuse field has a long history of partisanship. Treatment philosophies long promoted have, until recently, frequently emphasized the need for personal experience with the disorder before treatment credibility was established. Thus, psychologists without personal life experience were sometimes viewed as being unqualified (Lawson & Lawson, 1990). In addition, the issue of whether abstinence should be the ultimate goal of any substance abuse treatment program has also generated heated controversy and may have contributed to psychologists feeling they had to keep at arms' length if they had no compelling reason to adopt either position (cf. Marlatt, 1983; Schlesinger, 1984). Current reticence to enter the field might also be due in part to the lack of prestige associated with the counselors who typically do the one-on-one direct care in substance abuse treatment facilities, many of whom are recovering from their own addictions (Millman, 1989) and many of whom also lack professional training.

At the same time, there is another issue likely to be covertly driving this avoidance. Graduate school and even postdoctoral training is still notably weak in its teaching about dealing with externalizing disorders. Insofar as this clientele presents a different set of diagnostic and intervention issues for therapists, which their prior training has not prepared them for, they are likely to shy away from such problems thereafter.

The issue of whether psychologists are qualified by their training is currently being evaluated and tested. Certification programs (for addiction counseling) in many states have requirements not readily translatable to the experience gained in graduate psychology training. System differences have likely played a role in, or interact with the fact, that training in the treatment of substance abuse disorders has been highly variable, not only in psychology but across disciplines (Bacorn & Connors, 1989). Other disciplines (e.g., psychiatry) are evaluating how they have approached training in this area and have concluded that they have not adequately prepared students to diagnose or treat individuals with the substance abuse and dependence disorders alone, or with multiple disorders (Fawcett, 1992; Millman, 1989).

Lawson and Lawson (1990) suggest that the limited focus given to training psychologists in the area of addictions may be due to the interplay of political and economic forces and the complexities of treating these disorders. Perhaps also related to the relative unpopularity of this specialization is the implicit awareness that treatment of severe drug problems can be a difficult business that is more concerned with being a watchdog and a monitor (as in maintaining that one's patient stays drug free) than a change agent. From one perspective, there is some reality to this concern given the heavy comorbid association between both drug and alcohol dependence and antisocial personality and the concomitant observation that to engage in a treatment relationship with individuals with such problems is likely to lead the therapist into dealing with problems of criminal behavior as well as those of substance abuse (Gerstein & Harwood, 1990; Regier et al., 1990). Nonetheless, people presenting with substance abuse disorders are stigmatized because of the perception that they are all difficult to treat and "unattractive" (Millman, 1989). The notion that people with substance abuse disorders are on a progressive downward spiral that is not amenable to intervention is pervasive. Rather, research evidence supports the view that there is typically a variety of problems operating here, including psychological dependence and impairment in social, interpersonal, and occupational functioning. Sometimes those problems are accompanied by increasing tolerance and withdrawal episodes, in other cases substantial medical complications arise as chronicity progresses. Not all substance abusers share all of these difficulties. In addition, each of these areas is potentially addressable and remediable, but such work requires a broader perspective on the diagnoses involved and a broader armamentarium of professional skills than many professionals have immediately available.

Increasing Awareness of the Dually Diagnosed

The awareness that the division between mental health and substance abuse may exist in bureaucracies but not at the level of the individual has arrived. Numerous studies have described the high prevalence rates of substance abuse co-occurring among the chronically mentally ill (Drake & Wallach, 1989; Safer, 1987). In commenting on national epidemiologic data pertaining to these comorbidities, Regier et al. (1990) note that the Epidemiological Catchment Area (ECA) "data provide clear and persuasive evidence that mental disorders must be addressed as a central part of substance abuse prevention efforts in this country" (p. 2517). The authors point out that "the early recognition and treatment of mental disorders is a promising primary prevention strategy" (p. 2517). As Thacker and Tremaine (1989) note, many individuals with substance abuse disorders are not being accurately diagnosed, which likely predicts that they will not be effectively treated.

Clinicians and researchers in the area of dual diagnosis have lamented the fact that training programs have failed to adequately address this area (Pepper & Ryglewicz, 1984) and are pushing an agenda to increase these efforts. Bacorn and Connors' (1988) survey of program content revealed that dual diagnosis was spontaneously listed by site directors as a topic relevant to interns' alcohol treatment training, as was psychopathology among alcoholics. Thacker and Tremaine (1989) point out that mental health personnel have not been able or perhaps willing to take effective strategies and translate them to the comorbid population. Awareness of the vastness of this population and the economic factors pushing for the merger of these systems have created a circumstance whereby the evaluation of substance abuse disorders must be an integral part of graduate psychology training.

Current Status of Predoctoral Training

Coursework and Practica

A 1984 study by Schlesinger concluded that a concentrated focus on substance abuse issues was nearly absent. In his survey of clinical and counseling psychology academic and internship programs, exposure to "substance misuse" was a required part of the experience in 24.7% of programs. Elective experiences in these areas were available in approximately half of the programs surveyed (51.8%). Overall, 23% offered no exposure in their curricula. Methods by which students or interns obtained this exposure was highly variable. It was found that the training was typically received as part of other courses or internship rotations (60%), whereas a small minority had a single course or rotation on this topic (23%), and even fewer (17%) had a sequence of coursework and practica experiences. Furthermore, his investigation revealed that only 3.2% of academic programs and 8.5% of internship programs required this training before granting a degree or before "successful completion." Most programs had no plans to seek substance misuse treatment training grants (87%) and had no plans to add a faculty or staff member with a specialty in substance misuse to their institutions (90%) (Schlesinger, 1984).

Lubin, Brady, Woodward, and Thomas (1986) investigated the state of training in alcoholism and other substance abuse in doctoral programs in clinical and counseling psychology. The authors replicated a study by Selin and Svanum (1981). In their investigation, they concluded that the number of graduate-level courses in substance abuse had actually decreased over the years between 1979 and 1984. The number of settings offering more than two courses had also declined. Most programs offered substance abuse information as a component of other courses, however, and these courses were typically required. The faculty-estimated percentages of students having an interest in the substance abuse area remained low (11%). The authors conclude that students in these programs are receiving only minimal training in the areas of alcoholism and substance abuse.

Zalewski and Piotrowski (1992) surveyed clinical psychology PhD and PsyD programs in the United States to evaluate their training in the area of substance abuse assessment. They found that substance abuse courses were offered at 51% of programs responding, with 5% offering courses specifically in substance abuse assessment. Directors of these programs indicated that coverage in these areas occurred in the context of general courses. Doctoral programs granting PhDs and those granting PsyDs appeared to approach this task similarly. Lawson and Lawson (1990) propose that graduate coursework should include coverage on

> the history of substance abuse, theories of etiology, psychopharmacology, treatment methods, group and family therapy with the chemically dependent client, issues of special populations (including adolescents, women, ethnic and cultural minorities, military personnel, the elderly, and other high-risk groups), legal issues, related problems (e.g., physical and sexual abuse, AIDS, and fetal alcohol syndrome), and prevention. (p. 38)

Sayette and Mayne (1990) investigated the trends in the current training of clinical psychologists, including the research being performed and the opportunities for clinical training in their survey of all graduate programs in clinical psychology. Their findings revealed that research into the area of substance abuse was the third most prevalent topic being investigated after behavioral medicine and family systems and was tied with studies of depression. Forty-one percent of all programs studied indicated that they had funded research and faculty time involved in this pursuit. Correspondingly, however, substance abuse, as a specialty clinical training option, ranked as the sixteenth most common. Polcin (1992) comments that the bias toward individual psychotherapy in graduate psychology training programs is another factor that inhibits psychology's movement into the substance abuse treatment system.

Internship Opportunities

Bacorn and Connors (1989) investigated components of training provided through American Psychological Association (APA)-approved internships in the area of alcohol treatment. Programs that offered either a major (n = 136) or minor (n = 131) rotation in chemical dependency were examined. A portion (34%) of the group surveyed responded that they did not have this training to offer, despite their Association of Psychology Postdoctoral and Internship Centers (APPIC) description. The remainder were asked to evaluate whether interns were being exposed to certain content areas during the course of their alcohol training rotation. Six content areas were found to be the predominant methods (covered more than 80% of the time) given exposure on this rotation. They included group psychotherapy, relapse prevention, Alcoholics Anonymous, cognitive therapy, aftercare, and marital and family therapy. Two other areas, social skills training and stress management, were related as highly relevant; however, interns received less exposure to these areas. The finding that Selin and Svanum put forth in 1981 continues to ring true: Only a very small percentage of individuals receive direct clinical experience in substance abuse treatment centers (Selin & Svanum, 1981). Little has been written about the postdoctoral internship opportunities in this area.

Generalizable Skills and Methods

The findings of these training evaluations suggest that students are exposed to diagnostic information, some etiological theory, and minimal discussion of treatment interventions with the substance abusing population, with little evidence that the problems of people presenting with dual disorders are covered. This apparently remains true despite a decade of description and documentation of the overlap between traditional mental illness and substance abuse disorder diagnoses.

Some may consider this level of training appropriate, whereas others may evaluate it negatively because of its apparent lack of intensity and specificity. Still others may feel that it is more substantial training than that possessed by those individuals without degrees who are intervening based on their personal experience. Irrespective of these positions lies the fact that practicing psychologists possess many skills and techniques that are readily generalizable to the treatment of substance abuse disorders (Ziegler-Driscoll et al., 1980). Significant emphasis is placed on the assessment of major psychopathology, interviewing skills, and diagnostics in graduate-level training. Students are typically exposed to many interventions that are widely used in the treatment of people with prolonged and severe mental illnesses.

Miller and Hester's (1986) extensive review of the substance abuse treatment literature summarized the methods that have received controlled outcome research support. These include aversion therapies, behavioral self-control training, the community reinforcement approach, marital and family therapy, social skills training, and stress management. Though these interventions are being presented from an addictions perspective, these methods make up some of the fundamental training received by students to treat a broad spectrum of disorders.

However, it is surprising to find that the list of methods that have received support in controlled research, are elements that are "very rarely used in American treatment programs" (Miller & Hester, 1986, p. 122). The chasm between what is known and what is being done is striking. In contrast, the methods considered "standard practice" in alcoholism programs include Alcoholics Anonymous, alcoholism education, confrontation, Disulfiram, group therapy, and individual counseling. Miller and Hester (1986) comment that treatment modes in the United States have appeared to be "impervious to emerging research evidence" (p. 162) and that none of the methods in the latter category have been soundly supported by research.

Many models and methods for the assessment and treatment of substance abuse disorders are being generated; one example is the formalization of the relapse prevention model (Marlatt & Gordon, 1985). Although a review of this literature is beyond the scope of this chapter, many assessment and treatment methods are widely recognized. Traditional interview screening tools (CAGE: Have you tried to cut down?; have you been annoyed at another person suggesting you drink/drug too much?; have you felt guilty about your drinking/drug use?; have you had an eye opener?) are used, as are some of the more elaborate screening questionnaires (e.g., Alcohol Use Inventory [AUI], Michigan Alcohol Screening Test [MAST], and Addiction Severity Index [ASI]). Though these measures and methods have been used with the population of individuals with primary substance abuse disorders, few studies have documented the comparative effectiveness or validity of such methods with people of varying comorbidity. The lack of validated methods being used in the treatment of substance abuse or dependence, as pointed out by Miller and Hester (1986) and the frequent lack of awareness of comorbidity in the treatment of people with dual disorders, leaves educators to shoot in the dark as to what models and methods should be taught. Still, according to Mayer (1983), it is likely that "psychologically oriented treatment can have a substantial and long-term effect on reducing the patient's alcohol consumption, including total abstinence" (p. 119); treatments serve the purpose of encouraging individuals to reduce their intake and cause them to have fewer relapses and readmissions. Nevertheless, much still remains to be done to develop and validate a broad armamentarium of treatments that will be effective for the wide variety of people with dual disorders (Zucker, in press).

Training Issues

Substance abuse coursework has been included in curricula for marriage and family therapists (Heath & Atkinson, 1988). However, psychology has not yet taken the lead in training professionals to deal with problems related to substance abuse (Lawson & Lawson, 1990). We are not alone; physicians are estimated to receive only 2 hours of instruction on addiction in 4 years of medical school (Lawson & Lawson, 1990). There is likely to be some resistance to the inclusion of expanded training in the area of substance abuse disorders into what many training directors feel is an already overburdened curriculum. The mythology that this group of disorders are not distinct enough to merit training for specific competency, or that they warrant a highly specialized treatment focus (Schlesinger, 1984), will have to be overcome if effective training is to take place.

Training funds to support a focus on substance abuse intervention have not been appropriated at a level that would imply that this training is considered a priority. Until that is done, it remains unlikely that the professional programs will change their focus (Schlesinger, 1984). Workshops and conferences are likely to serve a consciousness-raising function but may fall short in being able to create "a new clinical specialization" (Thacker & Tremaine, 1989).

Development of curricula will have to be done carefully and with the respect to a broad spectrum of orientations. Presenting issues from a narrow perspective is likely to generate strong debate about the origins of abusing behavior; issues of etiology and most effective treatment focus still are frequently matters of polemics, rather than matters to be settled by an awareness of the existing scientific evidence (Heath & Atkinson, 1988). Comprehensive postgraduate training may reach practicing professionals through addictions certification courses developed by APA in conjunction with National Training Systems of Silver Spring, Maryland (Kent & Baker, 1992). Jack Wiggins states that APA "rode the horse of general licensure in psychology" (Curley, 1992, p. 1) but now feels compelled to address issues of specialization, especially in the area of addictions. The need for intensive training in this area, in the minds of insurance companies and third-party payers, and its relationship to emerging certification guidelines, keeps this a very controversial area of debate (Kent & Baker, 1992).

Certification for chemical dependency counseling varies widely and often requires no more than personal experience (Lawson & Lawson, 1990). Few psychologists have applied for the Certified Addiction Counselors Certification (CAC) (Kent & Baker, 1992). In addition to APA's efforts, some states have taken the lead. In California, guidelines have been put forth from the Psychology Examining Committee regarding required course content in the area of substance abuse for individuals entering programs after September 1, 1985. The California Association of Alcohol and Drug Abuse Educators is working with professional organizations to formulate possible certification guidelines (Lawson & Lawson, 1990).

Roles for Psychologists

Intervention, Assessment, and Prevention

The issue of psychologists functioning in the prevention field has received much recent attention. Psychologists clearly have a role in intervening in adolescent risk taking as it relates to substance abuse. They may be able to discourage involvement in health-compromising behaviors, prevent involvement that occurs from having seriously negative outcomes, and delay the onset of risk taking until judgment is better formed and risks can be more appropriately evaluated (Mayer, 1983). Psychologists are in an excellent position to provide early intervention for patients with substance abuse or dependence problems, because it is the social and behavioral manifestations rather than the laboratory tests that are the best and most easily identified diagnostic indicators of these disorders.

The conceptualization of the nature of substance abuse has evolved from a moral to a disease model, with behavioral models now increasingly prominent (Schlesinger, 1984). Psychologists typically have considerable training in the analysis of behaviors. They are, therefore, likely candidates to develop and implement treatments around modifying or extinguishing maladaptive behaviors. This may occur at many different points of intervention and involve a full spectrum of theoretically based techniques.

Workplace settings, such as employee assistance programs, are employing psychologists to treat alcoholism and other drug abuse disorders. Thousands of programs are in existence to provide early intervention and referral to workers with abuse and dependence disorders (Mayer, 1983).

Possible roles for psychologists in the area of family therapy were outlined by Heath and Atkinson (1988). They include providing a viewpoint on how substance abusing families function; identifying substance abuse patterns in families already in treatment; intervening with these families; providing interpersonal and contextual perspectives to treatment; offering alternatives for family members not connected to traditional substance abuse support programs; and finally, working with families to evaluate their problem-engendering interactions (Heath & Atkinson, 1988). These are, again, skills based in mental health treatment and are directly translatable to the comorbid population.

Psychologists can broaden their identification with this population through their participation in community health promotion or Alcohol and Other Drug Abuse (AODA) prevention efforts (Morgan, Wallack, & Buchanan, 1988). This might involve speaking to groups, providing training, or participating in community prevention planning efforts.

Global Training Guidelines

Graduate training programs require information regarding general global training guidelines that should be achieved. Several authors have commented on worksite training goals (Brown & Backer, 1988) that may be translated to graduate school curricula. Areas of coverage include

- providing instruction in evaluating a person's substance abuse history, understanding the spread of new street drugs, and understanding that even a small amount of drugs can be dangerous for people with comorbid disorders;

- exposing students to staff from both mental health and substance abuse treatment backgrounds;

- including curricula that deal with the topic of dual disorders such as drug and alcohol effects on psychotropic medications and symptom presentation, the role of the family, assessment strategies, and information about multiple addictions, and disease or self-help models of treatment;

- understanding the role of self-help or support groups;

- discussing information about different treatment models, including detoxification, therapeutic communities, recovery homes, methadone maintenance, 12-step programs, and inpatient and outpatient settings;

- evaluating negative attitudes regarding these issues and clients (e.g., are clients seen as unmanageable, manipulative, etc.);

- discussing information regarding special client populations, including women, the homeless, and the HIV-positive;

- using relapse prevention approaches in treatment; and

- discussing therapeutic approaches to working with family systems.

More specifically, psychologists need to screen for the presence of substance abuse disorders in all client contacts. Based on what is known to date, they should anticipate that a significant percentage of individuals will be using or abusing substances (Regier et al., 1990). In settings serving the seriously mentally ill, this number is estimated at close to 50%. The signs, symptoms, and behavioral indicators of the presence of ongoing substance abuse should be reviewed. Psychologists should continuously evaluate the increased suicidality in this population and refer clients for inpatient treatment of their substance abuse problems if their behaviors present a clear and imminent danger to themselves or others (i.e., suicidal behaviors). Clients should be educated as to the effects that alcohol or drugs may have on the presentation of their symptoms of mood, psychotic, or anxiety spectrum disorders. Fuller descriptions of treatment guidelines are available in Minkoff (1989) and Pepper and Ryglewicz (1984).

Future Directions

Bringing disciplines together to work on policy planning and funding initiatives in mental health and substance abuse can likely create greater "permeability" in the systems (Thacker & Tremaine, 1989). Professional organizations have been emerging across disciplines to bring together individuals who focus on evaluating and intervening with the substance abusing population. These include the Society of Psychologists in Addictive Behaviors, the Academy of Medical Educators and Researchers in Substance Abuse, and the American Society of Addiction Medicine.

Interest and investment in integrating substance abuse perspectives into the professional organizations already in existence must continue. Until recently, no separate APA division dealt with substance abuse issues, although some divisions (e.g., Division 28) focus on it in part (Lawson & Lawson, 1990). In 1993, APA established a new division in this area, (Division 50 on the Psychology of Addictive Behaviors), which currently holds "candidate status." There is concern, however, that the American Psychological Society (APS) has not demonstrated its interest in this area. The 1990 APS call for programs did not mention addiction as one of a possible 46 suggested presentation topics (Lawson & Lawson, 1990). Of 65 subject areas listed in the 1993 APS call for proposals, none specifically addressed addictions or substance abuse.

Moving substance abuse into the core of training in psychopathology is imperative. It has been suggested that inadequacies in graduate training in psychology likely predict the field's dissatisfaction with the psychological services (Lubin et al., 1986). However, very few programs surveyed in the past decade were making significant plans to include substance abuse treatment practica or coursework in their curriculum (Schlesinger, 1984; Selin & Svanum, 1981). To make a successful transition into the arena of substance abuse or dual disorders treatment, students need to be trained from various theoretical viewpoints with expanded clinical orientations and repertoires (Osher & Kofoed, 1989). Students will require exposure to traditional substance abuse treatment settings so as to be able to learn the dialect, rituals, and language of these facilities (Heath & Atkinson, 1988). Treater resistance to providing service to individuals with other diagnoses (be it mental illness or substance abuse) may also contribute to less-than-adequate client outcomes (Thacker & Tremaine, 1989) and must be overcome.

Millman (1989) calls for the development of training institutes affiliated with medical centers and universities that could prepare a "cadre of well-credentialed clinicians, counselors, researchers, and administrators who might command more respect, higher salaries, and more attractive career tracks" (p. 989). He is speaking to the field of psychiatry but his ideas are generalizable to psychology. He also calls for the expansion of public programs and greater insurance carrier responsibility. Fundamentally, service providers would have to come together to see the similarities between their services through the maze of differing jargons and models of etiology (Thacker & Tremaine, 1989).

Psychologists practice in diverse settings, serving virtually all social groups, classes, and ethnicities in private practices, public and private schools and colleges, community hospitals, and social service agencies. They, therefore, almost certainly access large numbers of individuals who are both abusing substances as well as suffering from some mental disorder. It is time that the reality of existence of these comorbid processes be recognized and effectively treated.

It appears that the public perception that psychology has something to offer the field of substance abuse treatment will be determined by increasing the training focus (Lubin et al., 1986). Employment opportunities for people with a background in the treatment of alcohol and drug abuse are thought to be expanding, and psychologists should be among those competing for these positions if they are appropriately trained (Heath & Atkinson, 1988).

And in Michigan, responding to concerns about the inadequacy of the CAC as a certification procedure, the States' Center for Substance Abuse Services (CSAS) is in the process of implementing a new entry level examination, to be required of all persons working with a substance abuse clientele. The new exam is based on a broadly conceived compendium text, authored by a multidisciplinary committee of psychologists, physicians, and pharmacologists (Zucker et al., in press). Successful passage of the exam is to be required of all individuals working in this area, regardless of professional background and degree. At the same time, the knowledge base being tested requires understanding of a broadly conceived, multiple factor perspective in both causes and interventions. Implementation of this new policy will take place sometime in 1994.

Psychologists have a role in communicating their interests in substance abuse to the public, research agencies, and insurance companies (Lawson & Lawson, 1990). Differences in approach have resulted in a gross lack of understanding, research, theory development, and cooperation between the fields when, in fact, each has a great deal to offer the other. "There is a place for everyone" (Heath & Atkinson, 1988, p. 416).

References

American Psychiatric Association. (1980). *Diagnostic and statistical manual of mental disorders* (3rd ed.). Washington, DC: Author.

Staff. (1992, July 13). APA poised to increase presence in addictions arena. *Mental Health Weekly, 2*(28), 1–3.
Bacorn, C. N., & Connors, G. J. (1989). Alcohol treatment training in psychology internship programs. *Professional Psychology: Research and Practice, 20*(1), 51–53.
Brown, V. B., & Backer, T. E. (1988). The substance abusing mentally ill patient: Challenges for professional education and training. *Journal of Psychosocial Rehabilitation, 12,* 43–54.
Cummings, N. (1979). Turning bread into stones: Our modern antimiracle. *American Psychologist, 34,* 1119–1129.
Curley, R. (1992). APA poised to increase presence in addictions arena. *Mental Health Weekly, 2*(28), 1–2.
Drake, R. E., & Wallach, M. A. (1989). Substance abuse among the chronic mentally ill. *Hospital and Community Psychiatry, 40,* 1041–1046.
Fawcett, J. (1992). Alcoholism and substance abuse disorder treatment can no longer be separated from psychiatric practice—are we ready for it? *Psychiatric Annals, 22*(8), 401.
Gerstein, D. R., & Harwood, H. J. (Eds.). (1990). *Treating drug problems; Volume 1. (Report of the Committee for the Substance Abuse Coverage Study; Institute of Medicine).* Washington, DC: National Academy Press.
Heath, A. W., & Atkinson, B. J. (1988). Systemic treatment of substance abuse: A graduate course. *Journal of Marital and Family Therapy, 14*(4), 411–418.
Helzer, J. E., Burnham, A., & McEvoy, L. T. (1991). Alcohol abuse and dependence. In L. N. Robins & D. A. Regier (Eds.), *Psychiatric disorders in America: The Epidemiologic Catchement Area Study* (pp. 81–115). New York: Free Press.
Kent, D., & Baker, L. (1992). APA addiction certification courses set to begin. *Mental Health Weekly, 2*(28), 2–3.
Lawson, G. W., & Lawson, A. W. (1990). Quality substance abuse education: To be or not to be? *Psychology of Addictive Behaviors, 4*(1), 37–39.
Lubin, B., Brady, K., Woodward, L., & Thomas, E. A. (1986). Graduate professional psychology training in alcoholism and substance abuse: 1984. *Professional Psychology: Research and Practice, 17,* 151–154.
Marlatt, G. A. (1983). The controlled drinking controversy: A commentary. *American Psychologist., 38,* 1097–1110.
Marlatt, G. A., & Gordon, J. R. (Eds.). (1985). *Relapse prevention.* New York: Guilford Press.
Mayer, W. (1983). Alcohol abuse and alcoholism: The psychologist's role in prevention, research and treatment. *American Psychologist, 38,* 1116–1121.
Miller, W. R., & Hester, R. K. (1986). The effectiveness of alcoholism treatment: What research reveals. In W. R. Miller & N. Heather (Eds.), *Treating addictive behaviors* (pp. 121–174). New York: Plenum Press.
Millman, R. B. (1989). Taking issue: Who will treat alcohol and drug abuse patients? *Hospital and Community Psychiatry, 40*(10), 989.
Minkoff, K. (1989). An integrated treatment of model for dual diagnosis of psychosis and addiction. *Hospital and Community Psychiatry, 40*(10), 1031–1036.
Morgan, P., Wallack, L., & Buchanan, D. (1988). Waging drug wars: Prevention strategy or politics as usual? *Drugs and Society, 3*(1–2), 99–124.
National Institute on Alcohol Abuse and Alcoholism (1990). *Seventh Special Report to the U.S. Congress.* (DHHS Publication No. ADM 281-88-0002). Washington, DC: U.S. Government Printing Office.
National Institute on Drug Abuse (1988). *National household survey on drug abuse: Main findings 1985.* (DHHS Publication No. ADM 88-1586). Washington, DC: U.S. Department of Health and Human Services.
National Institute on Drug Abuse (1989). *National household survey on drug abuse: Population estimates 1988.* (DHHS Publication No. ADM 89-1636). Washinton, DC: U.S. Government Printing Office.
Osher, F. C., & Kofoed, L. L. (1989). Treatment of patients with psychiatric and psychoactive substance abuse disorders. *Hospital and Community Psychiatry, 40,* 1025–1031.
Pepper, B., & Ryglewicz, H. (1984, July). The young adult chronic patient and substance abuse. *Tie Lines, 1,* 1.
Polcin, D. L. (1992). Issues in the treatment of dual diagnosis clients who have chronic mental illness. *Professional Psychology: Research and Practice, 23,* 30–37.
Regier, D. A., Farmer, M. E., Rae, D. S., Locke, B. Z., Keith, S. J., Judd, L. L., & Goodwin, F. K. (1990). Comorbidity of mental disorders with alcohol and other drug abuse: Results from the epidemiologic catchment area (ECA) study. *Journal of the American Medical Association, 264*(19), 2511–2518.
Regier, D. A., Myers, J. K., Kramer, M., Robins, L. N., Blazer, D. G., Hough, R. L., Eaton, W. W., & Locke, B. Z. (1984). The NIMH Epidemiologic Catchement Area study: Historical context, major objectives, and study population. *Archives of General Psychiatry, 41,* 934–941.
Safer, D. J. (1987). Substance abuse by young adult chronic patients. *Hospital and Community Psychiatry, 38,* 511–514.
Sayette, M. A., & Mayne, T. J. (1990). Survey of current clinical and research trends in clinical psychology. *American Psychologist, 45*(11), 1263–1266.
Schlesinger, S. E. (1984). Substance misuse training in graduate psychology programs. *Journal of Studies of Alcohol, 45*(2), 131–137.
Selin, J. A., & Svanum, S. (1981). Alcoholism and substance abuse training: A survey of graduate programs in clinical psychology. *Professional Psychology: Research and Practice, 12*(6), 717–721.
Thacker, W., & Tremaine, L. (1989). Systems issues in serving the mentally ill substance abuser: Virginia's experience. *Hospital and Community Psychiatry, 40*(10), 1046–1049.
Zalewski, C., & Piotrowski, C. (1992). Recent trends in family, aging, and substance abuse assessment curriculum in Psy.D. and Ph.D. programs. *Journal of Training & Practice in Professional Psychology, 6*(1), 22–29.
Ziegler-Driscoll, G., Sax, P., Deal, D., & Ostreicher, P. (1980). Selection and training of staff to work with the psychiatrically ill substance abuser. In E. Gotthiel, A. McLellan, & E. Druley (Eds.), *Substance abuse and psychiatric illness* (pp. 140–146). New York: Pergamon Press.
Zucker, R. A. (in press). Pathways to alcohol problems and alcoholism: A developmental account of the evidence for multiple alcoholisms and for contextual contributions to risk. In R. A. Zucker, J. Howard, & G. M. Boyd (Eds.), *The development of alcohol problems: Exploring the biopsychosocial matrix of risk.* Rock-

ville, MD: National Institute on Alcohol Abuse and Alcoholism.

Zucker, R. A., Bouknight, L., Clay, M., Glaser, F. C., Reed, B., & Schoener, E. P. (in press). *Fundamentals of alcohol and other drug problems: A manual.* Lansing: Michigan Center for Substance Abuse Services, Michigan Department of Public Health.

PART

II

Public Mental Health Service Responsibilities for the Mentally Ill

CHAPTER

7

The Role of the State in Public–Academic Linkages For Clinical Training

James P. Stratoudakis
Fairfax–Falls Church Community Services Board

Henry Tomes
American Psychological Association

Paul Wohlford
Center for Mental Health Services

James W. Stockdill
Maryland Mental Hygiene Administration

Because of its duties regarding the health and safety of its citizens, the state is ultimately responsible for providing services to people with serious mental illness. However, over the past 10 years or so, a number of important changes at the federal and local levels have changed the nature of those responsibilities and have made it necessary for the states to reevaluate their approaches to planning and providing public mental health care.

In this chapter, we shall first describe the state and local governments' complex and changing responsibilities for services to seriously mentally ill adults, seriously emotionally disturbed children and adolescents, and other priority populations. Next we shall discuss the planning process involved in carrying out those responsibilities. Then we shall present, from the perspective of state mental health programs, which are major employers of psychologists, the problems in mental health professionals' training. Finally, we shall recommend constructive changes to both bridge the gap between the public service system and academic training programs and, simultaneously, improve both clinical training and public services for seriously mentally ill adults and other priority populations.

Public Service System Responsibilities for People With Serious Mental Illness

The roles and responsibilities of state and local governments for the service needs of the seriously mentally ill are complex and changing. Because

The opinions expressed in this article are those of the authors and do not necessarily reflect the opinion, official policy, or position of the American Psychological Association, the Center for Mental Health Services, or the Maryland Mental Hygiene Administration.

states vary greatly from one another in size and style of operation, many important aspects of a state's role are unique. In spite of these differences, certain overarching issues are common to all state and local public mental health systems. These issues arise directly from deinstitutionalization and the political involvement of family members and consumers, plus a third fact of life in the public sector—the need to contain costs.

Starting in 1963 and continuing until 1982, the federal government constructed and then directly supported the operation of a network of hundreds of community mental health centers (CMHCs) throughout the country that were charged with providing a range of public services for the mentally ill. Although these services were often excellent, the federal grants were made directly from federal regional offices to the local CMHCs, and states often felt by-passed. Thus, in 1982, under the new policies of the Reagan administration, the CMHCs, along with many other federal programs, were shifted from federal control to state control through a block grant program. From 1982 to 1986, the states received federal block grant funds for mental health and substance abuse service programs with little direction as to the use of the funds. This shift reduced the total funding and gave states a freer rein in how they spent the federal mental health dollar.

State Mental Health Planning Under PL 99-660 and Later Laws

The change to state-administered block grants was only partially successful, at best, in encouraging states to adopt modern, community-based service systems for the mentally ill. Perhaps because of the greater freedom they had been given under the 1982 state block grant law, individual states varied considerably in the degree to which they adopted a new approach to the delivery of mental health services. As a result, in 1986, Congress enacted the State Comprehensive Mental Health Plan Act, known as Public Law 99-660 (PL 99-660). This legislation requires states to implement a comprehensive community-based system of care for seriously mentally ill individuals as a condition for receiving alcohol, drug abuse, and mental health block grant funds (Kennedy, 1990). The original legislation required the achievement of a total case management system by 1992. To help achieve this goal, federal technical assistance and planning grants were provided to each state during 1986–1992. In fiscal year 1990, the general alcohol, drug abuse, and mental health block grants to the states totaled $1,193 million. For the first time, a separate block grant for mental health was provided by the 1992 mental health law, and it totaled $278 million in 1993.

Consistent with a community-based approach, state plans must place special emphasis on case management and systems approaches. They must also devote a special section to services for children and adolescents, and all plans must accord families, consumers, labor unions, and other important stakeholders opportunities for participation in the planning process. Psychologists, other care providers, and all interested citizens should also have input into the formulation of these mental health plans (see Appendix C for details).

In 1990, Congress strengthened the state planning law through the amendment PL 101-639, which required the state to submit a separate plan for child and adolescent services. Two years later, PL 102-321 subsumed the preceding laws on state mental health planning as part of the responsibility for all mental health services under the new national Center for Mental Health Services (CMHS).[1] The new law specifically makes the state mental health block grant partly contingent on meeting the state planning requirements. Unlike earlier state mental health plans, both PL 99-660 and PL 102-321 have included severe penalties for noncompliance—5–10% of a state's block grant funds can be withheld as the result of a violation.

The development and implementation of comprehensive mental health plans have occurred in states with dramatically different structural, demographic, and policy realities. As one might expect, the states' plans and their progress in implementing them reflect that diversity. Details of their progress related to PL 99-660 are described in Appendix C of this book. There are those who are less than optimistic about progress under the state mental health planning process. They question whether states that are not in compliance will actually be penalized and whether such states might be excused for reasons of political expedience. Certainly, it will be interesting to follow the enforcement of state mental health planning provisions under the Clinton administration.

[1] PL 102-321, the ADAMHA Reorganization Act, went into effect October 1, 1992. It transferred responsibility for mental health services and clinical training from NIMH to the new CMHS. CMHS is part of the new Substance Abuse and Mental Health Services Administration (SAMHSA) within the Department of Health and Human Services.

Many others, however, see state mental health planning as mandated by PL 99-660 and PL 102-321 as an opportunity for states to integrate the Community Support Program (CSP), the Child and Adolescent Service System Program (CASSP), and the Human Resources Development program (HRD) synergistically to improve the entire service system (Kennedy, 1990; Pallak, 1990; Romeo, Mauch, & Morrison, 1990). These programs were discussed in chapter 1, and are described in more detail in subsequent chapters. The joint planning efforts required by the laws may enable states to identify and begin to communicate the knowledge, skills, and abilities required of staff members necessary to provide high-quality community-based care (Anthony, Cohen, & Kennard, 1990). A goal of the 1992 mental health block grant law, PL 102-321, is that future state mental health plans will accurately describe patient needs based on common definitions, project services to meet patient needs, estimate the number and kind of staff needed to provide these services, and estimate the cost of providing such services. It is expected that states will examine how they can redesign service systems based on CSP and CASSP principles and will redirect resources to run the new system. Regardless of the greater or lesser impact of PL 99-660, it is very clear that over the past decade, states have received increasing support.

President Clinton's national health care reform is expected to include mental health services. Such reform would create sweeping changes, awakening greater need for services while giving states more power. This process would develop a potential market for academic institutions to train psychologists to work with people who suffer from serious mental illness.

Patterns and Problems in University Education and Training

The state plans developed under PL 99-660 have been helpful by providing the service system vision and a philosophy that can be used as the context for developing more comprehensive clinical training and human resource development policies and priorities. This is important because academic programs are likely to be more willing and able to cooperate with states if the state mental health agencies have comprehensive human resource development policies that identify training needs, issues, and priorities.

So far, however, departments of psychology have been slow to respond to the states' human resource and training needs (Johnson, 1990). They are generally not graduating practitioners who have had exposure to and experience with service delivery management, research, and direct service skills based on the validated research on services for the seriously mentally ill. Also, most departments and schools are not planning for future curriculum and faculty development to prepare their graduates to meet the needs of this growing market.

There is a particularly urgent need for public–academic collaboration in the area of training in mental health administration. Psychologists and other clinicians who find themselves in administrative positions face a complex maze of funding mechanisms, regulations, human resource issues, planning and management requirements, and legal liabilities. As a result, there is a great need for new ideas on how to incorporate training in mental health administration into both preservice and in-service education. In 1986, the American College of Mental Health Administration and NIMH co-sponsored a symposium on the state of the art in mental health administration and had many excellent recommendations (White, 1987). The NIMH State HRD program has had a priority on training in mental health administration; current and former state and local administrators should be brought into academia to help develop such training. In psychology training programs, examples have been set by Carl Clements at the University of Alabama and Russell Bent at Wright State University, who have incorporated administration into their programs as tracks that advanced clinical students may choose.

Despite such innovative programs, the education and training of psychologists for practice usually follows a fairly standard pattern. Trainees acquire a set of theoretical ideas, constructs, and paradigms under the instructional control of a faculty, then subsequently are placed in a series of practical situations, under some degree of supervision, to acquire and hone practical professional skills (see Tomes, 1990, for further discussion). To apply the preceding analysis to training for service to the seriously mentally ill, the professional psychologist who is likely to be most effective in working with the seriously mentally ill is one who has been taught by a faculty who is knowledgeable about seriously mentally ill people, has acquired skills in settings in which seriously mentally ill people are found, and is supervised by knowledgeable and competent professionals to care for the mentally ill. Ideally, the acquisition of a professional demeanor, including attitudinal development, will be greatly influenced by the interaction of the trainee with faculty, supervisors, and obviously clients. Trainees who acquire their professional skills in public settings with a significant presence of seriously mentally ill clients are likely to have positive attitudes and may choose to devote their careers to working with this underserved group (Tomes, 1990).

Implementing this education and training paradigm requires involving trainees with knowledgeable faculty and competent trainers in appropriate public settings that serve the seriously mentally ill. Although there is no shortage of settings with the seriously mentally ill, there is a shortage of knowledgeable faculty and competent trainers in professional psychology who apply their skills in public settings serving the seriously mentally ill. This shortage, we hypothesize, stems from a lack of graduate faculty involvement in public mental health settings such as state hospitals, community mental health programs, and rehabilitative settings that provide services to the seriously mentally ill. The absence of such faculty involvement means that trainees seldom receive practical training in these public settings, because practica and internships are not usually developed in such settings. Thus, the application of psychological theory and practice to the publicly supported seriously mentally ill person is often left to psychologists trained only to the masters level. Reasons for lack of faculty involvement are many and likely involve issues of accessibility, knowledge, stigma, and lack of incentives (Tomes, 1990).

Now there is a significant and renewed interest at federal, state, and community levels in providing improved services to the seriously mentally ill; there is also renewed interest in doing research on these problems. However, there is a significant lack of psychology training programs for serving seriously mentally ill people in public settings. We believe that, because psychology has a significant contribution to make in providing and improving services to the seriously mentally ill, it is important that more psychology faculty and students become involved in knowing about and serving the publicly supported mentally ill client (Tomes, 1990).

Conclusions and Recommendations to Improve Public–Academic Linkages for Clinical Training

Consistent with a systems approach to improve services for the seriously mentally ill, a systems approach should also be used to improve clinical training. Just as constructive innovation should occur at each level, stage, or setting to improve services to the seriously mentally ill, so too should public–academic collaboration occur at each level, state, or setting to improve the clinical training of the next generation of psychologists providing services for the seriously mentally ill. This includes, but is not limited to

- faculty development and curriculum development;
- clinical competencies, administrative skills, and clinical research skills;
- academic training at all levels—undergraduate (where interest in helping seriously mentally ill people may first arise), graduate school, masters and doctoral coursework, and research;
- practica, predoctoral internships, and postdoctoral fellowships; and
- retraining and continuing education.

Both state and university programs have viewed the other party as the one responsible for not cooperating. In fact, change is difficult for both parties. Both universities and state–public systems of care constitute large, well-entrenched bureaucracies with their unique sources of intransigence. If this were acknowledged openly and undefensively by both parties, perhaps each could help the other to improve both the quality of services and the quality of clinical training simultaneously.

States' responsibilities are to articulate public sector needs and convey them to higher education and, specifically, psychology, based on the strategic planning process and the analytical use of data. States' responsibilities extend further, in our view, to invite academic preservice training programs to become part of the entire service system process, along with consumers, families, state and local agencies, and so forth. In extending this invitation, states should recognize that the training programs have institutional constraints that require some autonomy, but in this regard, training programs are no different from other players in the system such as consumers, families, labor unions, and so forth. Furthermore, states must realize that the genuine participation of academic training programs is just as vital for the success of the service system as that of the others.

In the interagency monograph, *Interdisciplinary Collaboration Between State Mental Health and Higher Education* (Davis & Sanchez, 1987), and in chapter 13 of this volume, Davis discusses in greater detail how the collaboration process can occur and the issues to be addressed. Above all, states have the responsibility to articulate clearly their human resource development needs, based on community service system principles and concepts. States have a responsibility to ensure psychologists receive exposure and experience in administration, treatment, rehabilitation, research, and political and social issues. States must work with higher education to ensure that students receive the exposure and the experience that will lead to expertise as providers and managers.

How can such collaboration be achieved? The most effective strategy to bridge the gap between preservice training and practice in public settings will be to develop programs that provide exposure of faculty and students to seriously mentally ill people in public settings (e.g., community mental health centers, rehabilitative day programs, and state hospitals). States and the federal government, in collaboration with universities, should develop incentives (e.g., financial support) for faculty and students to become involved in working and training in these settings. Faculty would be offered opportunities to practice and conduct research in public settings with an emphasis on the needs of seriously mentally ill people.

Additionally, predoctoral psychology internships and practica sites should be developed to involve publicly supported psychology staff in a training partnership with university faculty to develop meaningful internships in public settings that prepare students for work with the seriously mentally ill. An obstacle to such development in the field of psychology is the uneven level of, and sometimes poor communication between, doctoral training programs and internship programs. It would be particularly helpful if a new clinical training grant program was started that would require both state mental health authorities and academic training programs to be co-sponsors, with incentives for states to gradually assume some level of financial responsibility. Such a broadly collaborative program between universities and public mental health should accomplish the following:

1. Create opportunities for cross-appointments between state mental health departments, service delivery sites, and academic psychology programs in order to increase relevant role models; sensitize faculty, service program staff, and administrators to the others' settings; and develop more effective, reality based curricula and internship settings.

2. Encourage more academic faculty and students to engage in research on the seriously mentally ill, such as in the NIMH initiative, Public–Academic Liaisons for Research; community service systems research is especially important.

3. Persuade professional psychology programs to provide all students with a solid didactic foundation in the etiology and evaluation of, and intervention with, people with serious mental illness; the option to gain more advanced coursework on the seriously mentally ill; and the opportunity to learn clinical research approaches to problems, treatment, and rehabilitation of people with serious mental illness.

4. Create systems internship programs in the public sector that focus on both clinical skills and administrative skills, building functional competencies in each. Establish good working relationships between university psychology training programs and public mental health facilities that are practicing the latest community service systems work with the seriously mentally ill: at the preinternship practica, training for initial exposure to work with people with serious mental illness; at the predoctoral internship, training for experience in general clinical competencies in comprehensive service delivery, as part of a multidisciplinary team, as well as becoming aware of issues from the families' and the consumers' views; and at the postdoctoral fellowship, training for genuine expertise in advanced, specialized clinical competencies and a choice of either further training in clinical research or general training in mental health administration.

5. Enlist university faculties who already have relevant knowledge, competencies, and skills. They can then help state and local mental health authorities fulfill staff requirements of the state mental health plan provision of the state block grant program under PL 102-321. The staff should have the latest skills in community-based case management and psychosocial rehabilitation techniques through in-service training of all staff through workshops and follow-up support and supervision and through retraining of select staff through intensive training for periods of 2 months or more.

Although the funding of this retraining and in-service training would remain primarily a state responsibility, incentives should be provided for this through the establishment of regional centers of excellence for multidisciplinary clinical training.

Are these recommended new initiatives practical? Can they be implemented? Part III of this volume presents examples of how this has already been accomplished with children in North Carolina (chapter 14), with children and adults in Ohio (chapters 15 and 16, respectively), with the Vermont HRD program (chapter 18), and with postdoctoral psychology training in Denver (chapter 19). In some ways, Coursey's description in chapter 17 of a new statewide multidisciplinary training consortium in Maryland best illustrates what can be done if academic leadership in psychology will act decisively. In 1990, Coursey and others established a new training consortium that included representatives of each of the four core mental health disciplines as well as community providers, state officials, family members, consumers, students, and others. This consortium has already stimulated new directions and priorities for collaboration in clinical training for psychology and other disciplines. New linkages have been initiated in several communities between community service providers and university training programs.

Until now, psychology as a discipline has lagged in contributing to the care of the seriously mentally ill. Due to recent changes in the public service system, it now has an opportunity to make significant contributions. To interest psychologists to work in the public sector with seriously mentally ill people and to prepare them for this role will require fresh and innovative training as well as the perception of making a needed professional contribution to society.

References

Anthony, W. A., Cohen, M. R., & Kennard, W. (1990). Understanding the current facts and principles of mental health planning. *American Psychologist, 45,* 1249–1252.

Davis, M., & Sanchez, A. M. (Eds.). (1987). *Interdisciplinary collaborations between state mental health and higher education.* Boulder, CO: Western Interstate Commission for Higher Education.

Johnson, D. L. (Ed.). (1990). *Service needs of the seriously mentally ill: Training implications for psychology.* Washington, DC: American Psychological Association.

Kennedy, E. M. (1990). Community-based care for the mentally ill: Simple justice. *American Psychologist, 45,* 1238–1240.

Pallak, M. (1990). Community-based care for the mentally ill: Client outcome orientation in research, program planning, and service delivery. *American Psychologist, 45,* 1237.

Romeo, T. D., Mauch, D., & Morrison, E. (1990). A catalyst for change: The art of strategic mental health planning in Rhode Island. *American Psychologist, 45,* 1253–1256.

Tomes, H. (1990). The role of the graduate faculty in bridging preservice training and practice for psychologists in the public sector. In D. L. Johnson (Ed.), *Service needs of the seriously mentally ill: Training implications for psychology* (pp. 11–13). Washington, DC: American Psychological Association.

White, S. (Ed.). (1987). Proceedings of the State of the Art Symposium on Mental Health Administration. *Administration in Mental Health, 14* (3,4), 149–248.

CHAPTER

8

The Community Support Program and Psychology: Trends and Opportunities

Andrea K. Blanch
New York State Office of Mental Health

Numerous articles have been written about the role of psychology in the public mental health system and in services for individuals who would in the past have been referred to as chronically mentally ill (Hargrove, 1990; Lefley, 1990; Wohlford, 1990). Proposals have been made for curriculum changes, new clinical training experiences, joint research, and other mechanisms for bringing psychology and the public mental health system closer together (e.g., Anthony, Cohen, & Farkas, 1990; Hart, 1990; Sheridan, 1990). This chapter will suggest that the time is right to pay serious attention to implementing these recommendations. Substantial involvement on the part of psychology at this point in time could help determine the direction of a major and rapidly emerging component of the mental health system.

In this chapter, the term *community support programs* (CSP) refers to the broad range of services and supports that people diagnosed with severe, long-term mental illnesses may need to live up to their full potential.

The CSP concept was first articulated by the National Institute of Mental Health's (NIMH's) Community Support Program in 1977. The mission of the federal CSP initiative was to work with states and localities to improve opportunities and services for adults with severe and persistent mental disorders. To accomplish this, CSP funded state service system improvement grants to provide technical assistance to communities and agencies and to foster family support and consumer self-help activities. CSP also funded a variety of research demonstration projects that involved close collaboration between state mental health agency staff, local mental health and rehabilitation providers, and university-based researchers (B. Arons, personal communication, November 1, 1992).

Although the federal CSP initiative at NIMH remained relatively small, the development of effective community support programs has become a major priority for state mental health authorities. There are several reasons to believe that this situation will remain constant for some time.

First, the current economic climate has created, in some cases for the first time, the political will needed to close or consolidate unnecessary inpatient facilities. Although there remain substantial political barriers to hospital closure, it is increasingly difficult for state legislators to ignore the expense of maintaining excess inpatient capacity. It appears that there will be few increases in spending for mental health services of any nature until the dilemmas around inpatient care are resolved.

However, advocates, politicians, and administrators have all learned from their experiences with deinstitutionalization that there are substantial political, fiscal, and programmatic difficulties involved in developing community-based systems of care and that serious problems can result from downsizing facilities without adequate community service development. As states close facilities, they are likely to be vigilant in efforts not to be accused of "dumping." As a result, many states will be focusing considerable attention on the development of community support programs.

Second, the crisis in the health-care system has led to increased scrutiny of costs and utilization of all forms of inpatient and outpatient care. As policymakers experiment with Medicaid reform and various forms of managed care, increasing attention will be paid to groups who use very high amounts of service or who overuse the most costly forms of care. In mental health, a small subset of clients diagnosed with serious and persistent mental illnesses have been shown to consume up to 80% of the systems' total resources (Surles & McGurrin, 1987). It appears that the current configuration of outpatient services and hospital-based emergency and acute care is not meeting the needs of these clients in a cost-effective manner. New community support services that promote outreach, individualized interventions, and a crisis response capacity will remain a high priority for public mental health systems (Surles, Blanch, Shern, & Donahue, 1992).

Finally, passage of the Americans with Disabilities Act (ADA) has stirred new interest in the civil rights of current and former mental patients. The ADA, like its predecessor, Section 504 of the Rehabilitation Act of 1973, emphasizes access to the normal opportunity structure offered by society—jobs, housing, education, and so forth. As a result, state mental health authorities can be expected to focus increasing attention on reasonable accommodations and on developing the support systems necessary for effective community integration.

The development of community support programs requires attention to issues that lie at the core of community psychology. To be effective, community support services must reflect a sophisticated understanding of the specific symptoms, disabilities, and clinical issues involved in major mental illness and must do so in the context of nontraditional service delivery settings. CSP thus represents a convergence of community psychology, rehabilitation, clinical psychology, and community development.

Trends in Ideology

The discipline of psychology has had a profound influence on the development of community mental health ideology and structures. Three current trends suggest that basic tenets of psychology are playing a similar formative role in the emergence of a new CSP paradigm. These trends are (a) a new set of assumptions about long-term mental illnesses, (b) a new vision of community integration for people with disabilities, and (c) a growing recognition that limited resources will require services and financing to be organized around client outcomes.

Recovery and Empowerment

There is evidence that a significant shift is occurring in our understanding of long-term mental illness. This shift is reflected in a growing concern about the language that we use. For example, the term *chronic mental illness* is increasingly rejected as inaccurate and stigmatizing (Estroff, 1987). Current and former service recipients express a wide range of preferred terms to reflect their experiences and their status, ranging from *consumer* to *psychiatric survivor.* In addition, the term *recovery* is increasingly being used to reflect the possibility of a positive outcome without necessarily implying a *cure* (Deegan, 1988). In New York State, the Office of Mental Health has adopted a policy of inserting the words "persons diagnosed with" before references to mental illness or specific diagnostic categories in order to acknowledge that individuals who have received a diagnosis do not think of themselves as an "illness."

This concern with language reflects a change in thinking about people diagnosed with major mental illnesses and about appropriate interventions and expectations for this population. Increasingly, stereotypes about what "mental patients" can accomplish are being challenged. For example, professionals who have found ways to cope with the symptoms and disabling consequences of a major mental illness have begun to talk and write about their experiences (Deegan, 1988; Frese, 1989, this volume; Knight, 1991; Turner, 1990). Their message is clear: Some people can and do return to a very high level of functioning after experiencing the symptoms of major mental illness and even after lengthy hospitalization histories. Although these individuals do not represent the experience or potential of all people diagnosed with major mental illnesses, they do present a challenge to our current system of services for this population and to the way in which we think about these individuals in general.

The mental health self-help movement has also become quite vocal about what constitutes helpful interventions. In particular, the positive effects of approaches such as self-help and ex-patient controlled programs have begun to be discussed (Stanek, 1990). The importance of involving clients in making decisions about all aspects of treatment, including medication, has recently been highlighted (Corrigan, Liberman, & Engel, 1990). Similarly, current and former service recipients frequently point out the iatrogenic effects of services that reflect an imbalance of power between provider and consumer, particularly the misuse of involuntary commitment and the involuntary administration of drugs (Blanch & Parrish, 1991).

Although research in this area is sparse, it appears that services and approaches that give clients choices and help them to re-establish control over their own lives and symptoms are most helpful, whereas approaches that attempt to control or unilaterally "fix" the client are ultimately counterproductive. Studies of specific self-help organizations support this contention (e.g., Rappaport et al., 1985).

Underlying this growing emphasis on recovery and empowerment is an increasing recognition of the role of psychological factors in determining client outcomes. Consumers and ex-patients cite the importance of such factors as self-esteem, self-concept, self-efficacy, sense of mastery and competence, and participation in a valued role (such as that of helper instead of helpee) in their own recovery. Similarly, the internalization of stigma has been described by former patients as a disabling process not unlike learned helplessness (New York State Office of Mental Health [OMH], 1990).

The work done by Rappaport and colleagues on empowerment (e.g., Rappaport, 1987) is of enormous importance here. These concepts appear to have been embraced by psychology in reference to many of society's disempowered and disenfranchised groups but have infrequently been applied to the group that has been labeled "chronically mentally ill." However, some former patients have recognized on their own the importance of these factors and have started to define their experiences in ways that increase their personal control over subsequent events. For example, a former patient who has designed a "Self-Directed Rehabilitation Workshop" describes the onset of symptoms of mental illness as "unhelpful ways in which the mind tries to cope with feelings of anxiety and whatever is producing the feelings" (Knight, 1991, p. 8). Coping strategies taught as part of the workshop emphasize meaningful activities because "meaning is a buffer against stress and anxiety" (Knight, 1991, p. 8).

Public policymakers are increasingly paying attention to their constituents—both consumers and family members—who emphasize issues of empowerment and control. Rehabilitation programs that help people go back to college, resume careers, live in their own homes, and run their own services and businesses are being explored. Similarly, clinical interventions that respect people's abilities and autonomy are being developed. In New York State, for example, new Medicaid regulations require that all licensed outpatient programs provide education about the effects and side effects of psychotropic medications and teach clients the skills they need to monitor and manage their own symptoms. Clinicians and former patients are exploring techniques to help clients recognize prodromal symptoms and to manage positive symptoms through such strategies as stress reduction, meditation, and concentration exercises (Knight, 1991).

Symptom management is an excellent example of an area in which psychology has much to contribute. Many patients are anxious to explore the antecedent conditions of symptom onset and to develop wholistic intervention strategies. The tech niques of self-observation and self-monitoring developed by psychology could be of great assistance.

It is important to recognize that these emerging approaches do not represent a simplistic rejection of physiological aspects of mental illness. They also do not imply that psychological factors are more important than access to essential services and supports such as housing and jobs, which are commonly cited as the highest priority for people with psychiatric disabilities (Anthony & Blanch, 1989). Rather, they acknowledge the complications that inevitably occur when structures of meaning are imposed on experience, regardless of the initial cause of the experience. This is an arena in which psychology clearly has much to offer (Lazarus, 1991).

Psychologists are trained to teach people the skills they need to manage their behavior, especially in areas that relate to cognition and emotion. These skills can be of enormous benefit to people diagnosed with serious mental illness, who are struggling to control "unhelpful mental operations" and re-establish a sense of mastery and self-esteem. However, it appears that many clinical training programs equate skills training with token economies, behavioral programming of daily living skills, or vocational rehabilitation. The emerging empowerment paradigm in CSP clearly challenges this equation.

Community Participation

One of the first lessons learned through deinstitutionalization was that living in a community setting did not necessarily guarantee membership in a community. Many former patients living outside of hospitals are as effectively segregated by their community-based programs as they ever were in institutional settings. Moreover, a growing number of young people are avoiding participation in community programs for the same reasons they avoid state hospital care. As a result, planners and policymakers will be increasingly concerned with deinstitutionalizing community programs and will be defining community living to mean full participation in community life, including membership in community organizations and local political structures as well as access to normal jobs, housing, health care, and social services.

Creating a vision of full participation in community life immediately reveals the complex relationship between a person's symptoms and behaviors and his or her environment. People diagnosed with severe and long-term mental illnesses are generally poor; they often have untreated medical problems, live in substandard housing, and very frequently have been victims of violence or abuse (e.g., Rose, Peabody, & Stratigeas, 1991). Recent studies indicate that approximately half of all seriously mentally ill people today have concurrent substance abuse problems, and in one study, more than one third of young mentally ill women identified as the "most disabled and difficult to serve" had children under the age of 18 (Blanch & Surles, in press).

These changing demographics and social conditions will continue to challenge psychologists who work in community support programs. Significant clinical and organizational expertise will be required to handle increasingly complex and multidimensional problems. For example, it will require substantial skills and resources to help a single, non-English-speaking woman diagnosed with schizophrenia to handle her symptoms and to raise a family in a culture she barely understands or to help an individual from a seriously compromised inner-city neighborhood to deal with recurrent manic episodes while simultaneously working on job skills, dealing with an unstable community, and avoiding the drug culture. However, these are precisely the kind of complex problems that will be increasingly prioritized by the public mental health system. Response to these situations will require a systemic approach that incorporates clinical expertise with the capacity to understand and engage the structures of everyday community life, an approach that psychologists are uniquely suited for.

Achieving effective community integration for people diagnosed with long-term mental illness will require interventions that address the relationship between environmental stressors, social supports, and the manifestation of symptoms. Networking interventions and the teaching of specific self-advocacy, communication, and coping skills will be crucial. In addition, interventions that focus on group problem-solving, mediation, and other interpersonal dynamics will become increasingly important as community support programs bring CSP clients into the mainstream of life. In short, many of the techniques and interventions of clinical psychology will be in demand. However, they will need to be made available to individuals who experience serious and persistent symptoms, who are often angry at previous treatment, and who frequently reject services offered in traditional treatment settings.

Finally, developing effective community support programs will require effective interventions in social systems. Community living is by nature complex, variable, and risky. Some communities are openly hostile or rejecting to former patients. Others may be dangerous places to live, especially for people with social skills and communication deficits, and weak social networks.

Even safe and accepting communities can be complicated to negotiate. Successful community participation requires detailed and up-to-date knowledge about the community (e.g., norms of behavior, who controls the resources, and how to get things done). It also requires access to the decisionmakers and some stock of accumulated resources for exchange (e.g., knowledge, skills, and capital).

These aspects of community life are natural points of intervention for psychologists who are skilled in environmental analysis and modification. However, they are rarely addressed in therapy or in day programs. Many of the consultation and education techniques developed by psychology in other settings could be effectively brought to bear in this context.

Outcomes and Limited Resources

Across the country, health and mental health systems are caught in a situation of scarce resources and a growing demand for services. The politics of rationing health care has already become a dominant theme for the 1990s.

Strategies for better management of public expenditures are being developed and tested in all areas of health and mental health. However, for people with severe and long-term disabilities, inappropriately limiting community support services may lead ultimately to increased inpatient costs. To avoid this consequence, public mental health systems will increasingly emphasize systems of care that target or enroll groups of high-risk individuals and that monitor outcomes at the system, program, and client level.

Concepts like "rosters" of eligible clients, monitoring and funding services on the basis of measurable outcomes, and working to minimize the amount of intervention delivered are in some ways foreign to traditional clinical practice. However, the psychological traditions of behavioral observation and measurement could be extremely useful both in designing new administrative systems and in developing a new set of assumptions about clinical practice. Moreover, a psychological understanding of the behavior of systems will be increasingly important to administrators as our accountability structures shift from monitoring the production of a given type of service to ensuring outcomes for a defined target population.

Issues for the Future

The current climate in public mental health offers an opportunity for organized psychology to take a major leadership role in shaping mental health policy and program directions. From the perspective of CSP, there are several critical areas in which psychology could make a major contribution.

First, psychology has an enormous repertoire of skills in the areas described in this chapter. Many of psychology's historical contributions to public mental health have direct relevance to emerging community support systems. The future role of psychology in CSP may depend in part on our capacity to recapture our history and to reestablish a clinical practice paradigm that emphasizes both social context and the development of human potential for people diagnosed with serious, long-term mental illness.

Second, it has become clear in the past few years that CSP clients want and will eventually demand greater participation in the planning and delivery of services that affect them. Psychology could provide a model for this process by involving current and former service recipients in all arenas of professional life. The American Psychological Association (APA) has recently made laudable efforts to include people diagnosed with serious mental illnesses as part of an overall professional agenda (e.g., Johnson, 1990). However, there have been few forums to discuss future directions with clients themselves and few efforts to include current or former service recipients on committees or planning groups. Moreover, it is unclear how many clinical training programs have incorporated input from people diagnosed with serious mental illnesses into their curricula. Psychology has a long history of supporting a participatory process; CSP provides an opportunity to put this theory into practice close to home.

Third, organized psychology can influence the development of legislation and funding that support these principles. Community Mental Health Center (CMHC) legislation never adequately encouraged CSP interventions, nor did the block grant mechanism that replaced it. Moreover, few states have developed dedicated funding streams for this purpose. As a result, most community mental health programming was developed on a medically oriented, office-based outpatient model. This was further reinforced in some states by the use of Medicaid and Medicare to fund community mental health programs.

Health and mental health care financing are changing at such a rapid pace that it is impossible to predict the policy environment even 6 months into the future. However, it seems clear that although the inclusion of psychological services in Medicaid, Medicare, and other health-care financing systems will continue to be a major issue for psychology, establishing a consistent funding stream to support a community and competence-based practice paradigm could be equally important in the long run.

Recently, the federal government has taken some steps in this direction. The Alcohol, Drug Abuse, and Mental Health Reorganization Act was passed by Congress and signed into law by former President Bush in July, 1992. This bill, which authorizes changes in the ADM block grant as well as a reorganization of the Alcohol, Drug Abuse, and Mental Health Administration (ADAMHA). By mentioning rehabilitation and support as well as treatment, this bill specifically authorizes services based on CSP premises.

Finally, psychology can continue to develop and evaluate clinical interventions designed on CSP principles. Increasingly sophisticated outcome research will be needed to shape public policy decisions and to lobby effectively for new legislation and funding. In particular, multivariate research designs that analyze the impact of complex social systems interventions will be needed. Research examining the relationship between contextual variables and clinical outcomes will be critical as will continued research exploring the process of empowerment. Research in these areas must be clearly targeted to individuals diagnosed with serious and persistent mental illnesses, because many legislators and policymakers still believe that "seriously ill" people belong in hospitals and need permanent custodial care.

Conclusion

It appears that the public mental health system will see continued growth in community support programs in the coming years. The participation of psychologists in this process could have a substantial impact on the nature and effectiveness of new programs and services. In particular, many of the established techniques of community and clinical psychology have direct relevance to CSP.

Previous failure to implement these interventions on a widespread basis may have resulted from a lack of appropriate reimbursement mechanisms or from misconceptions about the capacities of people diagnosed with serious mental illness. Both of these conditions appear to be changing. Consumers and advocates are demanding community support services based on principles of rehabilitation and full community participation. As a result, policymakers will increasingly be looking for clinicians and program managers who are knowledgeable and skilled in these areas and who are willing to work in out-of-office settings. It is up to all psychologists, and especially APA and clinical training programs, to respond to this emerging opportunity.

References

Anthony, W. A., & Blanch, A. K. (1989). Research on community support services: What have we learned. *Psychosocial Rehabilitation Journal, 12*(3), 55–81.

Anthony, W. A., Cohen, M. R., & Farkas, M. (1990). Curriculum for the core disciplines for professional pre-service training in working with the long-term mentally ill. In D. L. Johnson (Ed.), *Services needs of the seriously mentally ill: Training implications for psychology.* Washington, DC: American Psychological Association.

Blanch, A. K., & Parrish, J. (1991). *Report on roundtable on alternatives to involuntary treatment.* Rockville, Maryland: National Institute of Mental Health.

Blanch, A. K., & Surles, R. C. (in press). Case management as a rehabilitation intervention. In J. Bedell (Ed.), *Psychological assessment and treatment of persons with severe mental disorders.* Washington, DC: Taylor & Francis.

Corrigan, P. W., Liberman, R. P., & Engel, J. D. (1990). From noncompliance to collaboration in treatment of schizophrenia. *Hospital and Community Psychiatry, 41*(11), 1203–1211.

Deegan, P. E. (1988). Recovery: The lived experience of rehabilitation. *Psychosocial Rehabilitation Journal, 11*(4), 11–19.

Estroff, S. E. (1987). No more young adult chronic patients. *Hospital and Community Psychiatry, 38*(1), 5.

Frese, F. J. (1989). *A consumer/psychologist's view of psychology.* Paper presented at the annual meeting of the American Psychological Association, New Orleans.

Hargrove, D. S. (1990). Key issues in training in psychology for service to the seriously mentally ill. In H. P. Lefley (Ed.), *Clinical training in serious mental illness* (DHHS Publication No. [ADM] 90-1679). Washington, DC: U.S. Government Printing Office.

Hart, I. H. (1990). A state-supported internship model: Camarillo state hospital and developmental center. In D. L. Johnson (Ed.), *Services needs of the seriously mentally ill: Training implications for psychology* (pp. 91–92). Washington, DC: American Psychological Association.

Johnson, D. L. (Ed.). (1990). *Service needs of the seriously mentally ill: Training implications for psychology.* Washington, DC: American Psychological Association.

Knight, E. (1991). How to deal with symptoms and medications now will be taught to many outpatients. *OMH News, 3*(2), 8–9.

Lazarus, R. S. (1991). Cognition and motivation in emotion. *American Psychologist, 46*(4), 352–367.

Lefley, A. P. (1990). Training psychologists to refocus on the seriously mentally ill. In D. L. Johnson (Ed.), *Services needs of the seriously mentally ill: Training implications for psychology* (pp. 25–28). Washington, DC: American Psychological Association.

New York State Office of Mental Health. (1990). *Task force on stigma and discrimination: Final report.* New York: Author.

Rappaport, J. (1987). Terms of empowerment/exemplars of prevention: Toward a theory of community psychology. *American Journal of Community Psychology, 15*(2), 121–148.

Rappaport, J., Seidman, E., Toro, P. A., McFadden, L. S., Reischl, T. M., Roberts, L. J., Salem, D. A., Stein, C. H., & Zimmerman, M. A. (1985). Collaborative research with a mutual help organization. *Social Policy, 15,* 12–24.

Rose, S. M., Peabody, C. G., & Stratigeas, B. (1991). Undetected abuse among intensive case management clients. *Hospital and Community Psychiatry, 42*(5), 499–503.

Sheridan, E. P. (1990). Preparing psychologists to work with the seriously mentally ill: Internships and postdoctoral fellowships with a research focus. In D. L.

Johnson (Ed.), *Services needs of the seriously mentally ill: Training implications for psychology* (pp. 93–95). Washington, DC: American Psychological Association.

Stanek, L. J. (1990). Consumer/expatient perspectives. *Resources, 2*(2), 8.

Surles, R. C., Blanch, A. K., Shern, D. L., & Donahue, S. A. (1992). Case management as a strategy for systems change. *Health Affairs, 11*(1), 151–163.

Surles, R. C., & McGurrin, M. C. (1987). Increased use of psychiatric emergency services by young chronic mentally ill patients. *Hospital and Community Psychiatry, 38*(4), 401–405.

Turner, B. A. (1990). Observations of a consumer–practitioner. *Missouri Mental Health Consumer Network, 2*(1), 1–3.

Wohlford, P. (1990). The role of clinical training in psychology to meet the needs of the seriously mentally ill. In D. L. Johnson (Ed.), *Services needs of the seriously mentally ill: Training implications for psychology* (pp. 7–9). Washington, DC: American Psychological Association.

CHAPTER

9

Public–Academic Collaboration in Training Child Mental Health Professionals

Lenore B. Behar
North Carolina Division of Mental Health, Developmental Disabilities and Substance Abuse

During the 1980s, there were major changes in children's mental health services. During this past decade, the foundation was laid for major shifts in attitude, philosophy, and policy that has begun to effect change in the strategies of service delivery. The impetus for these changes, as described below, has come from the increased visibility of the needs of children for mental health services, leading to major policy changes across federal and state agencies that provide for children and new models of service delivery for meeting these needs.

These evolving changes have presented a major challenge to the service delivery system, particularly the public mental health system, to identify new methods of identifying children in need of services, new methods of serving them, and new ways of assessing the quality of these services. A major requirement for meeting this challenge is having available the mental health professionals to deliver services, to design systems, and to evaluate services and systems. The public mental health system has reached the point of a worker crisis that must be addressed before the system can improve further. The remedy requires more than expanding the pool by training more professionals. The evolving changes in the service system require professionals who are trained differently, who believe differently, and who function differently; that is a major challenge for the universities. A critical strategy for addressing these challenges is through collaborative relationships between the public service system and the universities (Davis, 1990; Friedman, 1993). As a foundation for beginning to plan together, the types of changes in service delivery are described below, as are some areas of opportunity for mental health professionals.

Service System Development

In the past decade, progress has been made in child mental health services, bringing a significantly increased focus to the plight of children with serious emotional problems and to the wide discrepancy between their need for services and the availability of services. During the 1980s, the philosophy was solidified that community-based services are the essential and missing parts of the continuum of care that need to be put into place; the focus on the importance of providing services in the least restrictive, most appropriate treatment setting was intensified. This conceptual framework for service delivery, which has been the foundation for child mental health services since the publication of the report of the Joint

Commission on Mental Health of Children in 1969, was notably enhanced during the 1980s. The publication of *Unclaimed Children* (Knitzer, 1982) documented that across the country, 2 million of the 3 million children with serious mental health problems were receiving inadequate or no mental health services. This publication stimulated Congress to appropriate funds in 1984 to the National Institute of Mental Health (NIMH) for the Child and Adolescent Service System Program (CASSP), which had the congressional mandate to foster the development of new, expanded service delivery systems within the states. By 1990, CASSP had made grants and had a significant impact in all 50 states, the Virgin Islands, and the District of Columbia.

The impact of CASSP's funding to the states was enhanced by their joint funding, along with the Division of Maternal and Child Health of the Health and Rehabilitation Services Administration, of a technical assistance center at Georgetown University, and joint funding, along with the National Institute of Disability and Rehabilitation Research of the Department of Education, of two research and training centers. The research and training centers are based in the Florida Mental Health Institute of the University of South Florida and the Regional Research Institute for Human Services at Portland (Oregon) State University. The planning materials developed by CASSP, especially descriptive materials on planning a system of care (Stroul & Friedman, 1986) and on promising program models (Stroul, 1988) has made a significant contribution to the strengthening of children's services. The training seminars, newsletters, and professional publications by these three centers have added considerably to the knowledge base and have coalesced the field conceptually. The annual research conferences on children's mental health by the Research and Training Center at the Florida Mental Health Institute have made a substantial impact on the field, providing a well-attended forum for the exchange of current knowledge.

In 1989, the CASSP initiative was enhanced by the Robert Wood Johnson Foundation's child mental health initiative, which further primed the state systems to develop children's mental health services (Beachler, 1990). The Robert Wood Johnson initiative provided funds to eight states for 4-year demonstration projects that focused on further development of the system of care as a means of improving services for seriously emotionally disturbed children. In addition to providing funds for new services, the Robert Wood Johnson projects also engaged in efforts to restructure the financing mechanisms states used to pay for mental health services.

Additionally, during the late 1980s, state mental health agencies increased planning efforts, which is required by PL 99-660, to put in place expanded service systems. The CASSP technical assistance center at Georgetown has helped the states with their planning for child mental health services and has thus been instrumental in enmeshing the CASSP philosophy even further into the ongoing responsibilities of the states.

Through these efforts, a system philosophy has emerged that is shared by most mental health professionals and that has become the foundation for change in the 1990s. This concept of high-quality, comprehensive community mental health service systems for children and families is now shared across the state mental health agencies and includes the following deviations from traditional child mental health services.

New Treatment Strategies

Traditional concepts of treatment emphasized the importance of the client or the client's family seeking help and "being motivated to change." Over the past decade, the needs of children in this country have become more visible through published needs assessments and epidemiological studies (Brandenburg, Friedman, & Silver, 1990; Costello, 1989) or, according to many, the needs for treatment services have increased due to the changes in social and family pressures on children (Earls, 1989; Edelman, 1989; Friedman, 1993). The public mental health sector has been pushed in many parts of the country to assume responsibility for children formerly discarded as "untreatable." Beginning in 1980 with the lawsuit against the State of North Carolina on behalf of seriously disturbed and assaultive children, states were called on to develop new mental health treatment strategies for a range of difficult-to-serve populations. North Carolina's response to the lawsuit was to develop intensive, community-based, comprehensive systems of care across the state, emphasizing individualized treatment and rehabilitation plans for each client with intensive case management to keep the plan for each client organized (Behar, 1985). During the middle part of the 1980s, the Ventura County Children's Demonstration Project (Jordan & Hernandez, 1990), the Alaska Youth Initiative (VanDenBerg, 1990, 1993), and Project

Wraparound (Burchard & Clarke, 1990) emerged as new models with similar characteristics. In 1989, the largest demonstration of a comprehensive system of mental health treatment was begun by the North Carolina Division of Mental Health, Developmental Disabilities and Substance Abuse Services for the dependents of military families at Fort Bragg (Bickman, Heflinger, Pion, & Behar, 1992).

These demonstration projects shared the goal of keeping children in their own homes and avoiding out-of-home placements to the extent possible. Intensive treatment services are provided in nontraditional settings such as the home, as described below. Insight-oriented psychotherapy is usually not the treatment modality of choice, but behavioral approaches, restructuring of the environment, or re-education principles are more frequently used.

The Role of the Family

In the latter part of the past decade, in addition to the increased emphasis on the development of community-based services, a new attitude has emerged among professionals, partly from pressuring by parents. The importance of parents and families has taken on new meaning. Traditionally, parents were considered part of their children's problems and were, thus, necessary recipients of treatment along with the child. The shift now sees parents as the major caretakers of their children and, thus, as important partners in evoking positive change in their children. Parents are also seen as advocates for increased, appropriate services. The development of parent support groups such as the Alliance for the Mentally Ill—Child and Adolescent Network and the Federation for Families has moved this agenda forward.

With this new focus on families, the recognition has grown that separating children from their families in the name of treatment needs very careful assessment. In light of research that strongly suggests that many seriously disturbed children could be treated at home with new treatment strategies (Kinney, Haapala, & Booth, 1991), careful assessment is important. The idea of professionals providing intensive treatment services to help keep children in their homes grew into the idea that intensive services could and should include in-home services and a creative use of other sites outside the traditional clinic setting. The design of services to "meet the family on its own ground" brought into focus the need for professionals to gain a better understanding of ethnic and cultural beliefs, styles, and practices in order to relate better and provide better treatment outside the "culture" of the clinic.

The concept of in-home services addresses two types of services: (a) home-based services, which refer to more traditional counseling or therapy services provided in the family's home or in some other setting outside the clinic and (b) family preservation services, which refer to intensive, in-home crisis stabilization services designed to avoid removal of the child from the home (Kinney, Haapala, & Booth, 1991). The Family Preservation model is defined as crisis services that are offered in the home on a 24-hour-a-day basis, if necessary, and are limited in length (4–6 weeks); each professional also has a small caseload (2–4 families). Although these treatment strategies have clearly different approaches, both seem to be viable options for families and both expand the range of treatment services available. Family Preservation, according to evaluation studies, can make a significant difference for some families by helping avoid placing the child in a residential program or psychiatric hospital.

Cross-Agency Services

It is well known that the problems of emotionally disturbed children cut across the administrative structures that have been created to meet their needs; frequently, multiple agencies are involved with the same child. Therefore, it makes sense that agencies work together to help these children and their families. Most notable are the joint efforts needed between mental health agencies and schools, social services, the juvenile justice system, and substance abuse treatment programs. Although partially integrated, cross-agency services exist in some parts of some states, complete, coordinated services are still on the drawing board in most areas (Jordan & Hernandez, 1990; Macbeth, 1993; VanDenBerg, 1993). In her role of identifying children whose needs are neglected, Jane Knitzer has provided an additional spring board for the development of new initiatives. Her study of mental health services in schools (Knitzer, Steinberg, & Fleish, 1990) emphasizes how very little is being done in this arena where logically the most significant efforts should be occurring.

As these ideas have been put (slowly) into practice, creative yet tentative planning has emerged to join resources to provide better services across agencies. New financing strategies are emerging both out of the logic of the situation and out of the necessity to maximize what resources already exist. Most notable in the use of new financing strategies are the programs in Ventura County, California (Jordan & Hernandez, 1990) and in the eight demonstration sites funded by the Robert Wood Johnson Foundation's Mental Health Services Program for Youth (Beachler, 1990).

Program Evaluation

The evolving changes in planning and programming for children and their families has emphasized the need for better evaluation of programs, particularly the evaluation of treatment outcome. The treatment strategies, which are considered nontraditional, are subject to criticism. To some, they appear to fly in the face of one's professional training and therefore approach heresy; to others, they represent the logical extension and massaging of important principles of mental health treatment to address the changing needs of the population for which we are responsible, noting that the traditional methods were designed with other populations in mind. As a counterpoint, the traditional methods of treatment, especially hospital-based and residential treatment, are criticized as not being validated or substantiated as clinically effective. Thus, the evaluation of components of the service system, as well as some far-reaching assessments of the impact of the system of care are needed. Recognizing this important next step in changing methods of service delivery, NIMH built an important requirement for program evaluation into the CASSP program and has also made grants available for service system research. The first grant announcements were issued in fiscal year 1990 (FY90) to support research on the efficacy of innovative service delivery approaches and systems of care for children and adolescents with serious emotional disturbances. To enhance the success of these research endeavors, NIMH placed an emphasis on collaboration between university-based researchers and public policymakers in keeping with their 1988 initiative of Public–Academic Liaison (PAL).

CASSP has, since FY90, provided rich opportunities for interaction between public and academic settings. For example, in North Carolina, a CASSP-supported project, "Assessing Coordinated Care for Children and Youth With SED (serious emotional disturbance)" will study the effectiveness of case management services for children in the mental health system; the service system demonstration is being funded with a grant from the Robert Wood Johnson Foundation's Mental Health Services Program for Youth Project. A major strength of the evaluation project is the collaboration among the state mental health agency, two local mental health programs, the University of North Carolina, Duke University, and the Robert Wood Johnson National Program Office.

Manpower Needs and Academic Training

The changes that are occurring in the delivery of mental health services require significant changes in the functioning of mental health professionals and, thus, significant changes in the academic preparation new professionals receive. Friedman (1993) has pointed out

> that despite the fact that university settings are often thought of as a source of creativity and innovation, the changes in the public service delivery system have originated out of the needs of that system, rather than originating within university settings. (p. 303)

Friedman further explains that not only have the university training programs, for the most part, not responded to the changing approaches in public sector service delivery, they seem to have gone entirely in the other direction and emphasized the preparation of professionals for the world of office-based or hospital-based private practice. Thus, the gap between the need for professionals and the capacity of university training programs to respond to public service system needs has grown wider, both through the lack of training of professionals for the changing public systems and through the decreasing value placed on serving those using the public systems (Davis, 1990; Friedman, 1993).

A Time for Change

The public mental health systems have begun to focus on collaborative efforts with universities as one vehicle to remedy the problems described above. The focus is emerging as a two-fold strategy: first, a collaboration between state mental health agencies and the state-funded universities/

land grant universities, whose mission it is to support public purposes, in this case to prepare professionals to address the needs of the state's population; and, second, an emphasis from the federal level on PALs as a basis for funding research and demonstration projects. The next, very important step is for public–academic linkages to take place in the area of clinical training. With the creation of a new federal agency, the Center for Mental Health Services (CMHS) within the Substance Abuse and Mental Health Services Administration (SAMHSA), the opportunity exists to refocus federally funded training stipends and training grants on the preparation of professionals for public sector work. Currently, an initiative within SAMHSA provides funding to the states for addressing worker needs. Internal coordination with CMHS seems imperative to bring about a joint focus between these human resource development (HRD) programs that fund states and the clinical training programs that fund universities.

Recommendations to Universities

Build understanding. As noted above, there is a clear need in training professionals to make them aware of the philosophy, the goals, and the practices of the public system's services for children and their families. Several methods appear to be available to bring about such understanding, such as having public service system staff or parents serve as faculty, assigning readings relevant to public sector services, attending seminars and workshops provided in the public sector, and becoming involved in practicum and internships in public agencies.

Develop respect. Within some academic settings, the choice of public sector services as a career choice is not highly valued. This message comes from the existing faculty, for the most part. To effect change, new faculty members with background in public sector services would have much to offer, as would the infusion of public agency staff or parents on a visiting faculty or guest lecturer basis. Providing opportunities for existing faculty to consult with public agencies is another viable strategy.

Expand skills. By using visiting faculty or by exposing existing faculty more to public sector services, both noted above, provide training in the design and delivery of new treatment strategies, in the design and management of services and service systems, and in the techniques of field-based research and evaluation of services and service systems. Although the current curriculum has many requirements that seem essential, clearly new information needs to be included; this will be no easy task.

Expand activities. Through collaborative efforts with public sector professionals and agencies, develop joint practicum experiences, joint seminars, postgraduate programs, and research and evaluation projects. Professionals in training need to learn about the mental health system, but they also need to learn about other child serving systems, including (a) the child welfare system and protective services, foster care, adoption, and the entitlement programs; (b) the education system and the special education components; (c) public health programs such as family planning, infant health programs, and educational programs on sexually transmitted diseases; and (d) court programs such as juvenile justice, adoption activities, custody issues, and testifying in court. They also need to learn how to evaluate the impact of these agencies, both conceptually and formally.

Recommendations to States

Clarify needs. In forging collaborative relationships (e.g., teaching or guest lecturing) with university training programs, it is important to make clear what the manpower needs within the state actually are. Field placements should be made available for graduate students. They should be made aware of job opportunities in the state and should be given priority over out-of-state applicants.

Develop practicum and internship opportunities. It is important to find stipends for these activities. Explore federal funding, such as Title IV-E of the Social Security Act or Medicaid to finance training for those who commit to public sector service.

Develop joint initiatives in in-service training. By collaborating with university faculty in the design and delivery of in-service training curricula for those employed in child mental health programs, the training needs of the field can be articulated. Many of the same issues to be addressed for in-service training are relevant to preservice graduate training, such as the new treatment strategies for service delivery and new philosophies and attitudes. Such exposure for faculty could be helpful in the redesign of graduate programs. Providing funding to faculty for the in-service training activities, through state funds, federal grant funds, or Title IV-E, would enhance the relationship.

Develop joint initiatives in program evaluation. Recognizing the importance of evaluating new program strategies should lead to building an evaluation component into these programs. Funding needs to be identified as a part of program allocations. Federal funding can be jointly sought with university faculty. They can bring a level of expertise to program evaluation that public agencies frequently do not have. They should also bring students for this valuable exposure.

Recommendations to SAMSHA and NIMH

Coordinate clinical training program with CASSP and with the states. The public policies addressing child mental health services are reflected at the federal level by the CASSP policies. Thus, the coordination of training activities with CMHS overseeing CASSP, or the next generation of CASSP, would allow the needs of public sector services within the states to be considered as guidelines for training grants that are developed. As in earlier years, the requirement should also be continued that training grant applications be coordinated with and endorsed by the public agencies that are responsible for services to children.

Expand funding for PALs for program evaluation. Evaluations of field-based programs are increasing in number, as evaluators have recognized the importance of such work. The availability of funds for such evaluations certainly has increased the interest. However, funding is still marginal although the need for an empirical basis for further program development is strong.

Expand funding for postdoctoral training in services research and evaluation. Training in services research and evaluation is important to the longer term plan of expanding this area as a respected and valued part of the field. Further, to expect that the design of new services be based on empirical evidence requires that sufficient numbers of professionals be trained to conduct relevant studies.

The foundation for the expansion of mental health services to children and their families has been built over the past decade. To turn the plans for such expansion into a reality, manpower issues must be addressed. The three parts of the preservice training system have functioned independently for many years and changes will not come quickly; nonetheless, they must be pursued. The opportunities are endless.

References

Beachler, M. (1990). The Mental Health Services Program for Youth. *Journal of Mental Health Administration, 17,* 115–121.

Behar, L. (1985). Changing patterns of state responsibility: A case study of North Carolina. *Journal of Clinical Child Psychology, 14,* 188–195.

Bickman, L. B., Heflinger, C. A., Pion, G., & Behar, L. B. (1992). Evaluation planning for an innovative children's mental health system. *Clinical Psychology Review, 12,* 853–865.

Brandenburg, N. A., Friedman, R. M., & Silver, S. E. (1990). Epidemiology of childhood psychiatric disorders: Prevalence findings from recent studies. *Journal of the American Academy of Child and Adolescent Psychiatry, 29,* 76–83.

Burchard, J. D., & Clarke, R. T. (1990). The role of individualized care in a service delivery system for children and adolescents with severely maladjusted behavior. *Journal of Mental Health Administration, 17,* 48–61.

Costello, E. J. (1989). Developments in child psychiatric epidemiology. *Journal of the American Academy of Child and Adolescent Psychiatry, 28,* 836–842.

Davis, K. E. (1990). Collaboration between public mental health systems and universities. *Community Support Network News, 7*(1), 8–9.

Earls, F. (1989). Epidemiological strategies in child mental health. In P. Greenbaum, R. Friedman, A. Duchnowski, K. Kutash, & S. Silver (Eds.), *Conference proceedings: Children's mental health services and policy: Building a research base* (pp. 17–21). Tampa, FL.: Florida Mental Health Institute, University of South Florida.

Edelman, M. W. (1989). Foreword. In R. M. Friedman, A. J. Duchnowski, & E. L. Henderson (Eds.), *Advocacy on behalf of children with serious emotional problems* (pp. XII–XII). Springfield, IL: Charles C Thomas.

Friedman, R. M. (1993). Preparation of students to work with children and families: Is it meeting the need? *Administration and Policy in Mental Health, 20*(4), 297–310.

Jordan, D. D., & Hernandez, M. (1990). The Ventura Planning Model: A proposal for mental health reform. *Journal of Mental Health Administration, 17,* 26–47.

Kinney, J., Haapala, D., & Booth, C. (1991). *Keeping families together.* New York: Walter DeGruyter.

Knitzer, J. (1982). *Unclaimed children: The failure of public responsibility to children and adolescents in need of mental health services.* Washington, DC: The Children's Defense Fund.

Knitzer, J., Steinberg, Z., & Fleish, B. (1990). *At the schoolhouse door.* New York: Bank Street College of Education.

Macbeth, G. (1993). Interagency collaboration can be elusive: Virginia's experience using two approaches toward the development of a statewide interagency system of care. *Administration and Policy in Mental Health, 20,*(4), 259–282.

Stroul, B. A. (1988). *Series on community-based services for children and adolescents who are severely emotionally disturbed. Vol. 1: Home-based services.* Washington, DC: CASSP Technical Assistance Center, Georgetown University Child Development Center.

Stroul, B. A., & Friedman, R. M. (1986). *A system of care for severely emotionally disturbed children and youth.* Washington, DC: CASSP Technical Assistance Center, Georgetown University Child Development Center.

VanDenBerg, J. (1990). The Alaska Youth Initiative: An experiment in individualized treatment and education. In A. Algarin, R. M. Friedman, A. J. Duchnowski, K. M. Kutash, S. E. Silver, & M. K. Johnson (Eds.), *2nd annual conference proceedings: Children's mental health services and policy: building a research base* (pp. 59–72). Tampa, FL: Florida Mental Health Institute, University of South Florida.

VanDenBerg, J. E. (1993). Integration of individualized services into the system of care for children and adolescents with emotional disabilities or neurobiological disorders. *Administration and Policy in Mental Health, 20*(4), 247–258.

CHAPTER

10

The Human Resource Development Program: Improving Community-Based Mental Health Services

Susan E. Salasin
Center for Mental Health Services

Thomas E. Backer
Human Interaction Research Institute

Frank D. McGuirk
Western Interstate Commission for Higher Education

The mission of the Human Resource Development (HRD) Program in the National Institute of Mental Health (NIMH), from its inception in 1978 through the 1992 reorganization with the Center for Mental Health Services (CMHS), has been to enhance the capacity of mental health agencies to improve delivery and effectiveness of mental health services by supporting human resource development activities at the state, regional, and federal levels. HRD activities include workforce planning, education and training, management and evaluation, recruitment, retention efforts and sanctions and regulations. All of these focus on increasing the effectiveness of the mental health workforce in the context of a community-based mental health services system. This chapter provides a review of the history, goals, and current activities of the CMHS HRD Program, discusses how public–academic linkages are used in HRD activities, and provides examples of linkages in two of the program's current grant projects.

As in the private sector, HRD activities are directed primarily to improving performance of workers already within the system or to recruiting more qualified workers of certain types. However, training and development activities in public mental health also require interface with academic programs providing preservice training for mental health workers, especially those in the core disciplines of psychiatry, psychology, social work, and nursing. Coordination of preservice and HRD activities through public–academic linkages can greatly improve both of these elements of the overall system by which the mental health workforce is developed.

Increasingly, HRD activities also are seen as central to overall organizational change in the mental health service system. Systems change today is driven by pressures on mental health systems throughout the United States to be more effective and accountable in a time of continuing financial constraints that limit alternatives for services improvement. The HRD Program's grant projects are intended to play an instrumental role in increasing state capability to implement and evaluate the impact of these system change initiatives.

Efforts to enhance HRD in public mental health can take advantage of many similar trends elsewhere in both the public and private sectors. Moreover, larger societal, technological, and economic changes of the past 10 years all play into the emergence of human resources as a key factor in successfully bringing about organizational change.

Dramatic changes in public mental health services that have taken place in recent years call for a more thoughtful response from policymakers and program developers concerning how services are delivered and by whom. Just over a decade ago, planning for mental health services was very different. Historically, services had been provided in the state hospital, and services planning was largely limited to funding for the state hospital and a few outpatient clinics.

As the public mental health system has moved from a hospital-based system to a community-based one with hospitals as a significant part of the system, workforce needs also have changed in both hospital and community programs. Staffing patterns, as well as staff roles and functions, have undergone changes to accommodate the move to priority services for people who are diagnosed as severely mentally ill and to a philosophy of rehabilitation, community-based treatment, and continuing care.

Public mental health services are labor intensive. Services are provided by people, for people. At least 80% of the dollars spent for public mental health services goes toward paying the people who provide and support services to clients. Planning human resources to provide mental health services should be as basic a process as planning for the fiscal resources. However, mental health planners and program developers often downplay workforce issues when developing plans and proposals for services. It is often assumed that adequate numbers of staff with the necessary skills and characteristics are available in the local labor market and can be easily recruited, hired, and deployed. Moreover, it is also frequently assumed that plans or program proposals will have little impact on present staff. These assumptions are often erroneous, and many otherwise excellent program proposals falter due to inadequate attention to human resource issues. Planners and program developers may face some of the workforce problems listed below when developing mental health services for adults who are diagnosed with serious mental illness and for children who are diagnosed as seriously emotionally disturbed and whose care and treatment are the public sector's responsibility.

- Knowledge and skills that are not available in the current workforce or in the labor pool may be required in order to develop more appropriate services for adults and children who are diagnosed with severe mental illness and for special groups within these populations.

- Academic programs may not be adequately or appropriately training their graduates to work with the types of clients served by, or in the program models used by, the public sector.

- The shift of services from institutions to the community may require retraining and redeployment of staff.

- Competition from the private sector often requires re-evaluation of salaries and other incentives to enable state and community programs to recruit and retain staff.

- Bilingual and bicultural staff required to meet the needs of the growing numbers of ethnic minority clients may not be available.

- Staff, particularly from certain professions, may be unwilling to work in inner-city or rural areas in which new or improved services are needed.

- Use of an emerging, nontraditional workforce that includes consumers, ex-patients, survivors, and family members as service providers, administrators, and trainers may require special training and other accommodations for these new types of staff, as well as an attitude change on the part of present staff. Moreover, many consumer, ex-patient, and survivor self-help centers, drop in centers, and support groups are not publicly funded but could benefit from publicly supported training.

- Use of non-mental health staff such as corrections and parole officers, welfare workers, emergency medical technicians, school personnel, foster care providers, consumer and ex-patient self-help groups, and others to serve people who are severely mentally ill may require special interagency training.

HRD Program Development

From its inception in 1948, NIMH has provided support directly to individuals and academic institutions for preservice training and education of mental health workers in the four core disciplines (i.e., psychiatry, psychology, social work, and nursing). However, concern was expressed at both the congressional and agency levels in the mid-1970s about continuing such a significant amount of federal support for what was seen more properly as a responsibility of higher education, especially when the then-existing program did not directly strengthen state capacity to meet workforce needs and ensure workforce effectiveness.

To address the latter concern, NIMH, late in 1975, established a Services Manpower Task Force, leading to the creation in 1977 of the State Manpower Development Program. The Task Force conceptualized manpower development as "the activation of structures and processes to systematically and comprehensively undertake activities in four critical manpower areas including: (1) manpower planning and policy development, (2) manpower administration/management, (3) manpower education and training, and (4) manpower regulation/quality control" (Smith, 1976, p. 2).

Recommendations of the Task Force were translated into an authorization by Congress of NIMH's HRD Program in Section 803 of the Public Health Service Act (42 U.S.C. 242a). Through this authorization, HRD activities encompass professionals, support personnel, and consumers and family members working in all mental health operations for which the state mental health agency has direct or indirect responsibility. These include hospitals, community service agencies, consumer-run programs, and those entities that receive contracts or grants from the state mental health authority.

Since 1978, the HRD grant program has provided grants on a competitive basis to both state and multistate, or regional, projects. Each project is intended to promote linkages between mental health and related service agencies; linkages with institutions that educate, train, or otherwise prepare mental health personnel for the delivery of mental health services; and linkages with organizations responsible for licensure and certification or for reimbursement policies and processes affecting the deployment and utilization of the mental health services workforce. The program also is concerned with HRD issues affecting special service populations such as consumers and family members, women, minorities, people with disabilities, and people in rural areas.

HRD support for single-state grants, now called system development grants, emphasizes planning and evaluation, workforce management, and education and training toward the development of a community-based system of care. Evaluation of the impact and effectiveness of these activities is a core component of each grant. Multistate grants currently emphasize training of mental health administrators at the state and sub-state (e.g., county) levels, in addition to a variety of forms of technical assistance to participating states. Multistate projects also emphasize knowledge utilization approaches for promoting wider use of mental health innovations delivered through the HRD system already in place at the state level and for developing the capability of public mental health systems to incorporate selected innovations into their standard operating procedures.

The HRD grant program has been awarding funds to state mental health authorities since 1978. In 1992, 21 state grant programs, including 8 newly initiated Systems Development grants, were in operation, and 7 multistate projects were funded. The total grant program has been funded in excess of $3 million per year from 1978 to 1992. In 1990, the HRD program reached a goal of full coverage of all of the states through membership in one or more of the multistate project consortia. As federal funding dwindled, support of multistate projects for ongoing technical assistance to states appeared to be the most cost-effective approach toward ensuring equal access to federal resources.

In 1978, the first annual HRD Assembly was convened by NIMH to bring together HRD grant program administrators, state HRD administrators, and various experts in HRD. The Assemblies intended to promote technology and innovation sharing, collegial support and program advocacy, and knowledge exchange about pressing current problems. The Assemblies have been national in scope, usually attended by 175–200 individuals and have been convened in every region of the country. The 14th Assembly was held in Arlington, Virginia in November, 1992.

NIMH has evaluated the HRD Program in a sequence of studies, beginning with Carling's (1984) review of the first 5 years of NIMH's Center for State Human Resource Development (1978–1983). This study built on Kimmel's (1978) background paper on state services' worker development in mental health, which was targeted expressly to state agency officials. Both reports examined the progress of the HRD initiative in terms of its actual and potential culture-building contributions and in terms of the specific and concrete measures taken to further the achievement of HRD goals. Both studies stressed the need for knowledge dissemination and utilization in order to maintain the momentum of the HRD program and to keep HRD activities on the cutting edge of innovation. The Carling (1984) study summarized specific HRD accomplishments common across the states up to that time. These were classified in four general areas: (a) building state capacity to address critical human resource development problems, (b) meeting changing service system needs, (c) improving state human resource management, and (d) building ongoing system linkages. Carling also expressed concern about the need to develop better means of linking HRD activities directly to the decision-making processes of state commissioners.

In 1990, the NIMH HRD program awarded a contract to the Human Interaction Research Institute to (a) conduct an analytic review of state HRD programs, gathering information on successes and challenges experienced by the states in implementing these programs; (b) develop a portrait of these state-level initiatives, including an assessment of the circumstances under which the federal investment is achieving the greatest return; and (c) develop a set of implementation guidance criteria for HRD system development efforts related to community-based care. A strategic planning manual for HRD project staff and grant applicants was prepared to provide guidance for developing or enhancing a state HRD project (Goodstein & Backer, 1991b). In addition, a "white paper" was commissioned to create a vision for future enhancement of these state-level initiatives, including specific recommendations for action (Goodstein & Backer, 1991c).

The 1990 study (Goodstein & Backer, 1991a) identified eight factors critical for the success of state HRD grant projects

- knowledgeability about the basic processes of HRD and their potential for impact on mental health services,
- a clear definition of HRD goals and how to measure their achievement,
- use of a systems approach to relating the HRD effort to the overall state mental health service system,
- use of a strategic planning approach to implementing HRD activities,
- supportive circumstances in the state such as leadership by the state commissioner and highly visible program activities to which HRD efforts can be tied,
- systematic efforts to overcome resistance to change related to HRD activities,
- provision of ongoing resources for HRD in addition to what is available from the HRD grant, and
- availability of public–academic liaisons that are truly supported by the relevant academic leadership and are not just pro forma.

The study also provided a number of recommendations for state HRD grant project directors and for NIMH about how to better develop and conduct these projects.

HRD Program Goals

In May, 1990, under new program leadership, the NIMH HRD Program began the process of setting an "Agenda for the 1990s" to consolidate program achievements, lay out new activities reflecting the changing mental health system, and incorporate both private sector and technological advances in HRD activities. In addition, the time appeared ripe to incorporate knowledge utilization concepts and processes into HRD Program operations more fully and to develop mechanisms for ensuring improved HRD linkages with mental health commissioner concerns and decisions.

To determine future program directions, an informal survey was conducted, sampling commissioners, state HRD contacts, consumer and family groups, mental health professional organizations, and key contacts of the HRD Program. At the same time, the Human Resources Association of the Northeast (one of the multistate HRD grantees) completed a structured telephone interview process with over 100 leading mental health experts, regarding major trends expected in the field over the next 10 years and their implications for the mental health workforce. Results from these two studies, along with numerous focus group and constituency group discussions, resulted in the following overall program directions:

- HRD is now seen as the engine for systems change and development, with the HRD function tied directly to state commissioners and their decision-making structures and is seen as instrumental in the development of the State Mental Health Plan for Community-Based Mental Health Services under PL 99-660, PL 101-639, and most recently, under the 1993 state block grant provisions of PL 102-321.

• State mental health plans should be the basis for new HRD grant applications, and grant applications should have workforce implementation goals derived from the state plan to guide activities in their proposed project.

• An HRD Program policy and planning infrastructure should be developed and implemented. It involves regular meetings, consultation, and information exchange with each of the key HRD players, namely, HRD state and multistate project directors; state HRD contacts; the HRD Division of the National Association of State Mental Health Program Directors (NASMHPD); the HRD Division of the NASMHPD Consumer Advisory Group; and the CMHS services programs including the Community Support Program (CSP), the Children and Adolescent Service Program (CASSP), and the homeless programs. The linchpins of this infrastructure will, of course, be the state mental health commissioners.

• Knowledge utilization will be the theme that unites all of these elements, strategies, and processes; mechanisms will be developed to support and reinforce this goal; and knowledge utilization will form the basis for overall program evaluation (for more on knowledge utilization, see Backer, 1992).

Activities already initiated under these new goals include (1) a full revision of the competitive process by which HRD grants are awarded; (2) initiation of quarterly meetings with multistate project directors, yearly meetings with the state grantees, bi-yearly meetings with the NASMHPD HRD Division, and quarterly meetings with commissioner groups; (3) development of a special program at the 1991 Assembly in which NIMH services-related program directors interacted with Assembly participants to develop program linkages; (4) support for developing a guide on leadership for new mental health commissioners at the state and sub-state levels; (5) sponsorship of a national conference on gender and cultural diversity issues in the mental health workplace for the year 2000; (6) award of knowledge utilization supplements to state HRD grant projects that have promising findings to increase the likelihood of implementation of these significant innovations in new sites; and (7) development of an electronic bulletin board capacity for state HRD contacts, grantees, and other interested parties.

The HRD Program and Public–Academic Linkages

The genesis of the HRD program's public–academic linkages initiatives as a part of each HRD grant came through recommendations contained in the original 1976 task force report that established the HRD program:

> Basic professional education programs tend to be developed by university based practitioners. Too often this is done with very little consideration or in-put from the service delivery system. Graduates may then be ill prepared for jobs or jobs may not exist at all. Perhaps the major problems come about when graduates are trained in different role models or with different value orientations from those expected in agencies. . . . There is a need to bring professional education up-to-date regarding the trends in the delivery system so that they can provide more leadership and have credibility with the agencies. . . . there is a need for closer ties between the academy and the agencies. . . . Continuing education will need special attention to make it particularly sensitive to the programs and problems of agencies. (Smith, 1976, p. 20)

This was translated into a requirement that each HRD grant applicant addresses, in some manner geared to the particular needs of its state(s), the issue of building linkages between the state agency and the university for the purposes of preservice training, in-service training, or curriculum revision for training at all levels. In the initial years, these linkages were typically between the state agency and one department of the university, with one professor, for one purpose that was time-limited. These relationships were inherently unstable, because they were quite dependent on the two individuals from the state and the university who forged the linkage. If one of them left the job or was transferred, the linkage most often collapsed.

Concern arose about how to institutionalize these linkages in a more organized manner (see also Davis, chapter 13 of this volume). This often led to the formation of public–academic linkages advisory committees from the outset of a HRD grant; these committees were composed of representatives from both groups, with representation that went beyond the academic department and the mental health agency involved. As this representation broadened, consumers and family members were often added, as well as representatives from other units of government and levels of education.

As these advisory committees became more representative, they often created the impetus for multiple linkages with various departments in the university, at various educational levels, for various purposes. Eventually, community and technical colleges were also included in this purview.

Examples of Linkages in HRD Grant Projects

Two examples of public–academic linkages activities conducted by HRD program grantees (both of these happen to be multistate HRD projects, but many such efforts have also been developed by the single-state grantees) follow, to provide a fuller orientation to current public–academic linkages activities in the HRD arena.

The Center for Improving Mental Health Systems

In September 1991, a 5-year HRD grant was awarded to the nonprofit Human Interaction Research Institute to conduct a 6-state (California, New Mexico, New York, Oregon, Texas, and Virginia) HRD project, the "Center for Improving Mental Health Systems." Based in Los Angeles, the Center's parent organization is a nonprofit center that has conducted research, policy studies, and interventions on innovation and change in health and human services for over 30 years.

The six states just mentioned form a consortium for this center, which also includes the University of California—Los Angeles (UCLA) Center for Clinical Research on Schizophrenia and Psychiatric Rehabilitation and the National Alliance for the Mentally Ill (NAMI). In addition to an advisory board with state, topical expert, consumer, professional, and family representation, the Center has a 12-member Public–Academic Liaison Advisory Group, which helps to coordinate its public–academic linkage activities, described below.

The Center's overall mission is to enhance knowledge, attitudes, and practices of the mental health workforce in these six states and specifically to promote wider adoption of innovations in psychiatric rehabilitation and family involvement in community-based care. The Center's HRD activities emphasize validated approaches for stimulating and guiding innovation and change that increase the likelihood of innovation adoption (see Backer, 1992, for more detail). Successful Center outcomes from the six states may also be translated into national impact, because the Center's topical areas are of great interest to all public mental health systems.

The Center (a) assesses HRD needs in each topical area; (b) develops innovative systems for delivering knowledge, training, and technical assistance related to these needs; (c) develops knowledge packages and identifies validated "best practices" in each topical area; and (d) conducts and facilitates HRD training programs oriented toward innovation, adoption, and system change for mental health workers in each state.

During its first year of operation, the Center has developed training curricula, offered a number of training workshops, co-sponsored conferences, provided technical assistance (TA) consultations, identified more than 100 innovations in its topical areas (directories with brief descriptions of these innovations are now being prepared), and developed collaborative relationships with a number of state and national organizations. In-process activities include a series of large-scale training conferences with individualized TA follow-up in Southern California, emphasizing psychiatric rehabilitation for community-based facilities; a video-based training package on innovation and change in public mental health, based on the Southern California work; and a video conference resulting in a video-based training package on psychiatric rehabilitation services in rural areas, conducted in partnership with the state of Oregon.

A "systems change" project to develop skill-based competencies for involving families in service delivery is underway, with participation from the NAMI Curriculum & Training Network and family leaders and researchers from all states in the six-state consortium. A similar project is underway to develop and package a set of psychiatric rehabilitation competencies, with participation from the International Association of Psychosocial Rehabilitation Services. Once developed, these two sets of job competencies will be packaged in training formats so that they can be used for numerous training, TA, and system change applications.

Other Center public–academic linkages activities include (a) providing input to preservice education programs through, for example, a partnership with the state of Virginia on the

Forum for Improving Mental Health Systems, which is concerned with curricular reform on psychiatric rehabilitation and the Task Force on Families and Mental Illnesses, a preservice training enhancement project funded by the California legislature and operated by the California Alliance for the Mentally Ill; (b) developing collaborative relationships with academic programs to offer Center training programs in each of the six states (e.g., UCLA academic personnel are on the Center's staff, and public–academic linkages advisors act as trainers for Center programs in all six states); (c) promoting effective relationships between academic institutions, public mental health agencies, and family and consumer groups on continuing education efforts in the Center's topical areas (e.g., in the Center's co-sponsored conferences on psychiatric rehabilitation, already held in five of the six states); and (d) coordinating two job competencies projects with related professional association and academic activities (e.g., committees of both the American Psychological Association and American Psychiatric Association, of which Center staff are members).

As Center products emerge, such as the job competencies manuals and the two video-based learning packages described above, additional opportunities for public–academic linkages activities may develop. For instance, implementation of these products would be possible in settings that involve both academic and service agency personnel or that combine preservice and in-service training.

The Western Regional Center for Human Resource System Development

In 1992, the Center for Mental Health Services awarded several multistate projects to carry out an expanded role in assisting states in their workforce planning and systems change efforts. One of these awards was for the development of a Western Regional Center for Human Resource System Development operated by the Mental Health Program of the Western Interstate Commission for Higher Education (WICHE), a nonprofit organization of 15 western states established in 1953 to accomplish common purposes in higher education. These states are Alaska, Arizona, California, Colorado, Hawaii, Idaho, Montana, Nevada, New Mexico, North Dakota, Oregon, South Dakota, Utah, Washington, and Wyoming. The primary purpose of the 5-year grant is to develop and maintain a Western Regional Center for Human Resource System Development in order to address gaps in knowledge and practice concerning workforce development and planning in the western states. The Center will facilitate access to information, knowledge, and innovative practice and products that are necessary for implementation of the workforce requirements of a community-based system of mental health care for adults with severe mental illness and children and youth with serious emotional disorders.

The goals and objectives of the project are designed to develop, disseminate, and promote utilization of knowledge and technology on workforce problems that cut across individual state boundaries. This Western Regional Center promotes collaborative efforts in workforce development by bringing together the participating states to work jointly in solving mutual problems.

There are six major goals for the project:

1. to strengthen workforce planning for community-based systems of care to serve severely mentally ill adults and seriously emotionally disturbed children and adolescents in support of states' efforts to meet the state mental health plan requirements of PL 99-660 and PL 101-639, and the state block grant provisions of PL 102-321;

2. to establish and maintain an interstate information clearinghouse that promotes workforce development knowledge utilization by state mental health agencies, service providers, and academic programs in the West;

3. to explore and develop effective engagement of mental health academic discipline programs in response to public mental health sector service delivery and workforce development needs;

4. to improve utilization of mental health systems research findings that have implications for workforce planning and human resource development;

5. to assist states' efforts to increase the numbers and proportions of ethnically diverse staff in the workforce in order to provide appropriate services to the increasingly ethnically diverse client population of western state mental health systems; and

6. to facilitate states' efforts in the areas of leadership, management, and administration in the public mental health system.

Knowledge utilization and transfer activities include needs assessment; prioritization of needs;

screening of research findings and development of knowledge packages; identification of exemplary practices; exchange of information through a variety of print, electronic, and face-to-face mechanisms; identification and dissemination of consultant information; provision of technical assistance; development and utilization of human resource databases; and public sector linkages with academia.

Anticipated outcomes and accomplishments for the 5-year project include more in-depth, long-term engagement with higher education faculty; integration of HRD with WICHE's work in the decision support and Mental Health Statistics Improvement Program areas; staffing databases leading to staffing models and staffing standards; increased involvement of families, consumers, and nontraditional service providers; delivery of new technologies to the area of human resource planning (e.g., comparative databases, automated staffing models, electronic bulletin boards); and engagement of administrative and nonclinical staff in the HRD mainstream.

Plans for the Future

Since the 1992 reorganization of Alcohol, Drug Abuse, and Mental Health Association (ADAMHA), a number of changes are being made in the HRD Program, which now resides at CMHS. The HRD Program's priorities are currently being re-examined, particularly with reference to the recently published report of the National Task Force on Human Resource Development (1993), which has been exploring new directions for the Program for the past year. For instance, more active interface with preservice training activities is planned; this will also increase public–academic linkage efforts. The 1993 resources funding was sharply reduced and will probably continue to be constrained in the near future.

With these changes, the base of knowledge, training paradigms, and living networks developed by the HRD Program over the past 15 years become ever more important, both for continuity and for continued viability of the Program despite limited resources and changing direction. The need to develop skills and values of the current public mental health workforce remains, and both the traditional and emerging models from the various activities of the HRD Program can contribute to meeting this need. Current projects in the HRD Program concerned with multicultural competence, training for county-level leadership, and managed mental health care are just a few of the initiatives that will continue to have application value. The 1993 national task force report makes a number of recommendations for how the HRD Program could be further enhanced and expanded in impact as resources permit. Emerging models such as the innovation and technical assistance focused approaches of HRD projects described above may also have potential for much wider use, especially because these methods are well-integrated with public–academic linkages activities and blend together preservice and in-service training paradigms.

The workforce of the public mental health system is in a time of great stress. Shifts toward increased services for severely mentally ill people in the community and the increase in ethnic and cultural diversity among the client population are powerfully impacting the types of staff needed to provide services. Insufficient public fiscal support for mental health services has strained the ability of most public systems to hire enough staff with appropriate skills and knowledge to provide effective mental health treatment, rehabilitation, and support services for these clients. The small staff-to-client ratios desirable for programs that serve severely mentally ill individuals are beyond the reach of most public mental health programs. Because a typical agency expends three quarters or more of its budget for staff, the size, composition, and training of the mental health workforce are important management and service issues. Promotion of improved collaboration between higher education and public mental health service systems is vital to any effort to enhance and strengthen the public mental health workforce.

Increased collaboration and mutual respect and understanding are elemental for *all* involved in the development of human resources for serving mentally ill people. Those hiring professionals into the public mental health system workforce must find new ways to attract the interest and involvement in university-based educators. Those involved in training psychologists and other mental health professionals must immerse themselves in the realities of the lives of people suffering from severe mental illness and begin to modify values and curriculum to ensure more understanding and responsive graduates. Recent efforts at the national Center for Mental Health Services to integrate clinical training and human resource development give hope for more effective care for populations with severe mental illness.

References

Backer, T. E. (1992). Consulting on innovation and change with public mental health organizations: The Caplan approach. In W. P. Erchul (Ed.), *Consultation in community, school and organizational practice: Gerald Caplan's contributions to professional psychology* (pp. 149–160). New York: Hemisphere.

Carling, P. J. (1984). *Human resources for mental health: History, current status, and future directions of the National Institute of Mental Health's Center for State Human Resource Development.* Burlington: University of Vermont.

Goodstein, J. G., & Backer, T. E. (1991a). *Final report: HRD system development grant study—Implementation guidance for community-based care.* Los Angeles: Human Interaction Research Institute.

Goodstein, J. G., & Backer, T. E. (1991b). *Strategic planning manual for mental health HRD system development project planning.* Los Angeles: Human Interaction Research Institute.

Goodstein, J. G., & Backer, T. E. (1991c). *White paper: Enhancing the NIMH HRD system development grant program.* Los Angeles: Human Interaction Research Institute.

Kimmel, W. A. (1978). *State services manpower development in mental health: Introductory perspectives.* Rockville, MD: National Institute of Mental Health.

National Task Force on Human Resource Development (1993). *Strategies for public mental health workforce development.* Rockville, MD: Center for Mental Health Services.

Smith, B. (1976). *Role of the National Institute of Mental Health in relation to state mental health services manpower. Task Force report.* Rockville, MD: National Institute of Mental Health.

CHAPTER

11

The Role of Community Mental Health Centers in Public–Academic Linkages

David S. Hargrove
University of Mississippi

Recent wars and regional conflicts have demonstrated all too clearly that issues of collaboration are determined by who is, and perhaps more importantly, who is not at the negotiating table (Porter, 1975). Including certain parties and excluding others in efforts to link public mental health systems with universities for training or research will obviously determine the nature and results of the relationships that do develop. Consequently, it is vitally important that all stakeholders in the field are seated at the table when roles, resources, and responsibilities are negotiated.

Davis (this volume) has defined collaboration and outlined some procedures for developing collaborative relationships. He defines *collaboration* as

> a planned strategy in which two or more systems form a cooperative relationship around one or more ... functions ... designed to improve the chances that each system will reach its ... mission and ... goals as [these apply to] the severely mentally disabled. Functions are defined here as tasks or activities that must be initiated or completed if a system is to reach or approximate its mission and goals. (Davis, chapter 13, this volume)

As linkages between public mental health agencies and universities are encouraged by the National Institute of Mental Health, stakeholders have developed certain postures that influence the shape of the potential relationships. Representatives of public providers, for example, may say, "If you want to have collaboration, give us the money and collaboration will result." Advocacy groups for consumers and their families, who have increased in power in the last decade, have advocated an almost exclusive use of public funds for the seriously mentally ill population, thereby possibly reducing assistance for people with less serious disturbances. The universities, in their concern for academic freedom, want support for research and training with few strings attached so that a broader range of options may be pursued. These examples point out the diverse interests of the parties who currently are involved in public–academic linkage.

Absence of CMHCs

There is an important stakeholder not present in the current negotiations of public–academic linkage: the local community mental health center (CMHC), or its national organization, the National Council of Community Mental Health Centers. It is hard to find CMHCs or organizations of CMHCs at meetings about linkage relationships between state mental health agencies and university training and research programs. Undoubtedly, conferences designed to enhance negotiations for public–academic linkages would profit from the inclusion of CMHCs. Organizations such as the National Council of Community Mental Health Centers and the individual state and regional affiliations, which participate in national policy development and represent local providers, could also play an important role in the success of collaborative efforts.

The reasons for the absence of community mental health organizations lie in the historical context and evolution of the nation's mental health system coupled with the developmental tasks that CMHCs faced in their early years. Political alliances and changes during the 1980s shifted the balance of authority in mental health systems development away from a federal–community relationship to a federal–state relationship. These new alliances had an enormous impact on the continued development of the system.

In the early 1960s, when community mental health centers were begun, the National Institute of Mental Health (NIMH) focused predominantly on local communities to initiate programs. State mental health authorities were not primarily involved in the development of the centers, but typically played a supportive role. As CMHCs matured into a growing system of care across the nation in the 1960s and 1970s, their experiences were forged by President Jimmy Carter into a National Mental Health Systems Act (1980). This act would have emphasized collaborative activities between several levels of government and helped local, state, and federal systems share responsibilities for administration.

As Cutler (1992) points out, the Reagan administration allowed this bill to die without appropriations and substantially reduced funding for community programs by converting federal funds into block grants that would be distributed to the states without much restriction. The results of this were devastating. NIMH staffs were removed and service supports were drastically reduced. Many CMHCs complained that their service capacity was reduced because of staffing reductions (Estes & Wood, 1984). The "new American federalism" focused the block grants on the states, enabling them to have enormous influence on the operation of community programs.

These funding cuts caused a shift in power between the states and community programs, which had followed more than a decade of community–federal relationships with little state intervention. Suddenly, in the early 1980s, states were thrust into the community mental health arena. Many states greeted this new responsibility with little enthusiasm, particularly because, in many cases, they had had relatively little prior involvement. In some cases, states were asked to assume responsibility for programs in which they had little investment. State mental health authorities were faced with managing total systems of care as opposed to self-contained state psychiatric hospitals.

This decline in prominence of CMHCs in the 1980s added to a lack of enthusiasm for public–academic collaboration on the national level. Locally, however, many CMHCs had already met their training needs through collaborative projects with training institutions in their own regions. Many CMHCs developed strong training and programmatic relationships with educational institutions for the four "core" professions of psychiatry, psychology, social work, and nursing. Some went so far as to develop formal residency and internship training programs for integration into academic curricula.

Local collaborative efforts were not limited to the four core professions. Collaborative efforts also were developed with a broader range of educational institutions. For example, community colleges and vocational-technical schools play important roles in training many direct service providers in treatment of mental health problems as well as in substance abuse and mental retardation. They also trained people for important support roles in public agencies. The use of paraprofessionals and indigenous workers in the 1960s and 1970s was supported by training programs in these local institutions.

Although community mental health centers have been conspicuously absent from the negotiation tables of public–academic linkage in recent years, they have a rich history of collaboration in program development, training, and research. The absence is significant both in terms of its politics and the substantive contributions that can be made. The shifting sands of intergovernmental relations, including the preeminence of state governments in managing mental health systems and the simultaneous reduction of the role of the federal government, threaten the balance of power among public mental health providers.

Shared Power

Porter's (1975) report of the development of a power-neutral, round negotiation table for the talks designed to end the Vietnam war suggest a configuration for the continued evolution of public–academic collaboration. The round table provides a rich metaphor for an inclusive group of local, state, and federal partners of providers, consumers, and advocates to design training, research, and programmatic involvement between hospitals and administrative units and university training programs. There are several advantages to such an inclusive perspective. First, each group is in more intimate contact with the issues that the others confront. This assists each group to maintain much more relevance. For example, if academic training faculties interact on a regular basis with the consumers of mental health care, their training and research perspectives will be influenced. If state-level administrators understand academically-based research as one means of solving some of the systems' problems, they are much more likely to have serious, ongoing relationships with colleges and universities.

A second advantage of the inclusive perspective is that more creative solutions to the problems faced by the mental health system, university training programs, consumers, and advocates are likely to be devised. The more people there are with diverse perspectives to bring to problems, the greater the likelihood of fresh approaches. For example, the use of consumers as employees in the mental health workforce forces academic training programs to reconsider criteria for admission and re-examine curricula. The need to be responsive to the issues that consumers bring to training programs requires faculty to provide assistance to students in creative ways.

A third advantage of an inclusive perspective is that the various components of the system, including colleges and universities, community programs, hospitals, consumers, and advocates, have the opportunity to coalesce. A university training program can provide the impetus for a state psychiatric hospital to relate to a community mental health center in new ways that enhance the transfer of clients from one facility to another.

Collaboration between university programs, community mental health centers, state mental health agencies and hospitals, consumers, and advocates provides a broader base for the discovery of solutions to many of the system's problems. The collaboration is only meaningful, however, if it includes all of the players. If all the parties are not at the table, collaboration will not take place, and the solutions will be limited and less effective.

References

Cutler, D. L. (1992). A historical overview of community mental health centers in the United States. In S. Cooper and T. Lentner (Eds.), *Innovations in community mental health* (pp. 1–22). Sarasota, FL: Professional Resource Press.

Estes, C., & Wood, J. (1984). A preliminary assessment of the impact of block grants on community mental health centers. *Hospital and Community Psychiatry, 35,* 1125–1129.

Porter, G. (1975) *A peace denied: United States, Vietnam, and the Paris agreement.* Bloomington: Indiana University Press.

CHAPTER

12

Consumer Impact on Mental Health Services, Clinical Training, and Public–Academic Linkages: Some Personal Reflections

Frederick J. Frese
Western Reserve Psychiatric Hospital

With the formation of the National Alliance for the Mentally Ill (NAMI) 10 years ago and the beginning of the National Alternatives Consumers' Meetings 5 years ago, mental health professionals are beginning to experience important developments in caring for the seriously mentally ill. Developments are occurring in a dimension that was virtually ignored previously.

In this chapter, I would like to share with you some personal perspectives on the importance of the consumer movement in changing the attitudes of both those who currently work with the mentally ill and those who are being trained to do so. I am a psychologist who has been working with seriously mentally ill people in Ohio state hospitals for some 2 decades now, and I have been serving as the director of psychology at the large state hospital in the Cleveland–Akron area for over 10 years. In these capacities I have had daily contact with seriously mentally ill people and have also had the responsibility of training practicum students from area graduate programs in clinical and counseling psychology. These students have come primarily from Case Western Reserve and Kent State Universities, where I hold faculty appointments, but also from the University of Akron and Cleveland State University. From my experience with these students and patients I have formed opinions as to the value of these new academic programs. I am also a former patient and have carried the diagnosis of schizophrenia, or some other form of psychosis, with me for the past 25 years (Buie, 1989; Holmes, 1991).

I worked with the mentally ill for a long time; most of that time, my co-workers appeared to understand very little about the problems of the seriously mentally ill. Several years ago, I attended a local meeting of the Alliance for the Mentally Ill. I was amazed at the people's understanding of what mental illness was really like. They were not preoccupied with theory or ideology; their thoughts and concerns seemed to spring from first-hand experience with the illness. I was very impressed. A few years later, I attended the annual meeting of primary consumers in Cincinnati and found that a lot of recovered people, like myself, had an in-depth understanding of serious mental illness. Since my initial involvement with these groups began 5 years ago, I have come to appreciate the value of consumer and family member input into the operation of facilities for the mentally ill; this input is also valuable in training professionals to serve this population.

During the past 30 years, 80%–90% of those who were, or would have been, in public mental hospitals have been released and are now living, or at least existing, in the community (Torrey, 1988). Certainly the tens or even hundreds of thousands of homeless mentally ill people who dwell in our cities have received considerable attention in the popular press. Thousands of others are now kept in jails and prisons and nursing homes, whereas many others are living with their families, too disabled to support themselves without assistance. However, one group of former patients receives little attention for having been so successful. These are the people, like myself, who have recovered well enough to sustain themselves and who have integrated themselves reasonably well into the social and vocational fabric of society.

After generations of hiding from the shame of insanity in the family, family members and recovered people themselves are increasingly speaking out and demanding changes in the way the mentally ill are treated and perceived.

After being diagnosed with schizophrenia at age 25 and spending the next 10 years being repeatedly involuntarily hospitalized in numerous kinds of psychiatric facilities, I am particularly encouraged to see the growth of NAMI and the evolution of the primary consumer movement. In attending the past five Alternatives conferences, serving on the boards of various consumer and mental health organizations, developing and delivering presentations from a consumer and professional's perspective, and most importantly, interacting on a regular basis with other recovered people and their family members, I strongly believe that the experiences and opinions of consumers and family members must be accommodated and incorporated into the overall approach to the care of the seriously mentally ill.

In early 1988, Paul Wohlford invited me to attend the National Institute of Mental Health-sponsored (NIMH) national conference on improving psychological services for the seriously mentally ill, hosted by Dale Johnson at the University of Houston. At that conference I presented a paper (Frese, 1988) in which I called for a partnership among professionals, family members, and most outrageously, consumers themselves, in forging a new approach to the delivery of psychological services for the seriously mentally ill. In that paper I wrote in the first person plural ("we") when referring to the seriously mentally ill. However, when I was presenting the paper, I found that I could not publicly identify myself as a seriously mentally ill person. I pronounced the "we's" in my paper as "they's." Nevertheless, psychologists are fairly perceptive people. I am certain that many of them understood my message. At the end of the talk one "could have heard a pin drop," as one of the participants later said. The topic of serious mental illness in your own family and particularly in yourself has been taboo and too emotional a topic to discuss openly. This, however, is changing. At subsequent conferences I have been more open about my background, and others, like me, are also becoming more open about their conditions.

Areas for Change

As a consumer and professional, I would like to suggest three broad areas where consumers feel changes need to be made in training professionals who serve mentally ill people.

Eliminating Stigma

First, there is the area of stigma. This takes many forms, but one of the most egregious is in the use of pejorative and derogatory terms. When I have students arrive at the hospital, their conversation is not infrequently laced with such phrases as, "I must have been crazy to have thought such a thing," "That guy has got to be nuts," "Look what those schizos in Washington are doing now," and so forth. Mentally ill people believe that using these terms in everyday conversation is cruel. However, students serving the mentally ill use these terms with abandon. I find that I always have to lecture students about using such terms around patients. I stress that no mental health professional should ever be using such cruel terms in everyday conversation. But then I wonder why I have to tell students such an obvious thing. Why don't professors stress these matters? Students being trained to work with us need to be reconditioned.

Along these same lines, psychology reports are often written in a manner that is demeaning to the mentally ill. As is true for terms used in conversation, the wording used in professional reports should be dignified and nondiscriminatory. Too often I see psychology reports that are mostly an exercise in name-calling. The reports can and often do contain valuable information, but serious work needs to be done on the manner in which these reports are written.

Encouraging Employment

Employment is another area in which stigma is rampant for mentally ill people. Many employers are reluctant to hire people who have spent time as an inpatient in a mental hospital, particularly a public mental hospital. Ironically, this prejudice against recovered mentally ill people is probably greater in the mental health system than in the general marketplace. Consumers strongly feel that we can contribute to the mental health field and that the mental health system should take the lead in hiring us. At universities, the mental health professions need to take the lead in accepting us for training as mental health professionals. In many quarters there is great resistance to this concept. I have frequently heard senior psychiatrists, psychologists, and mental health administrators employed in the public health system adamantly declare that they "will not have any psychos working in their organization" (or words to that effect). This resistance also exists in academia. Consumers feel these attitudes need to be changed and indeed that affirmative action-type programs need to be implemented in which recovered people are encouraged to prepare for work with others such as themselves.

Developing Curricula

A second area consumers feel can be improved is in the development of curricula that incorporate views of recovered people and their families. Many recovered people are relatively articulate and have things to say about their experiences that students should be exposed to. Recent books by William Styron (1990), author of *Sophie's Choice;* the feminist author, Kate Millett (1990); and particularly the young psychiatrist, Carol North (1987), are all excellent examples of volumes that portray the experience of serious mental illness from the perspective of the person who is experiencing it. David Zelt (1981), Esso Leete (1989), and numerous anonymous authors give excellent subjective descriptions of their experiences with psychosis in issues of *Schizophrenia Bulletin.* Family members, too, have produced some well-written descriptions of their experiences that students should be exposed to. These include articles by Mona Wasow (1989), Paul Aronowitz (1989), and others. Family members, through the National Alliance for the Mentally Ill organization, also publish a list of several dozen recommended publications that they feel reflect the views of family members. This list appears in each issue of the *NAMI Advocate.* All these materials should be made available to students.

Understanding All Factors of a Disorder

A fourth area graduate programs in psychology can improve, is in the study of factors that contribute to mental illness but that may not be considered traditional psychological material. One of these areas is the psychophysiological. Serious mental illness is a brain-based disorder. Recent research makes it quite clear that there are definite physiological correlates of serious mental illness (Gershon & Rieder, 1992). Students should be exposed to these physiological and biochemical factors. After all, the NIMH has declared the 1990s the "Decade of the Brain." Serious work that will be done with the mentally ill must acknowledge the importance of organic factors in these illnesses and must recognize that serious psychological disabilities are also physical disabilities. People who are seriously mentally ill should be seen as having a disability that impairs their functioning just as blindness or paralysis handicaps those with such disorders that have traditionally been viewed as physical. Appreciation of the importance of medication, the propensity for relapse, and an understanding of the psychological deficits that we have even after we have "recovered" all demand that professionals have a thorough understanding of what our physiological deficits are. Indeed, professionals should be teaching us about our psychological deficits and their physiological correlates. Too often, students believe that "the pills only calm the patients down so that the real problem can be addressed" or they have other superficial views of the nature of our disorders. Certainly there are behavioral, cognitive, and perceptual concomitants of these disorders, but to dismiss or downplay the importance of biochemical factors is not taking advantage of the advances in research that have been made in this area during the past few decades. Furthermore, there has been much discussion of the possibility of psychologists being granted prescription privileges for mentally ill people. Obviously, if psychologists are to begin taking on such a responsibility, much more training concerning the pharmacological and biochemical aspects of these disorders must be addressed.

In addition to not being adequately knowledgeable regarding organic and physiological aspects of these disorders, I also find that students and recent graduates tend to lack understanding of the legal and bureaucratic mechanisms that are so important in determining how the seriously mentally ill will live. Concepts such as guardianship, trial competency, mens rea, and diminished capacity are too often foreign to young and prospective psychologists. Students are often untrained as to the importance of the world of Medicaid, Medicare, and SSI (supplemental security income for the aged, the disabled, and the blind). An understanding of these bureaucratic entities is extremely important even when dealing indirectly with the funding streams from which mentally disabled people can receive economic assistance. Psychologists should have a better understanding of the importance of these funding mechanisms. Psychologists all seem to appreciate the efficacy of behavioral systems and "token economies," but generally fail to see that the "token economy" in which their patients must exist is a very complex and changing one that all members of the mental health community should be prepared to help patients negotiate.

Overall, it seems that those who are already supposedly educated have much to learn. Former patients must teach educators, students, and professionals about sensitivity in order that those with mental illnesses will be accorded respect and allowed to maintain the dignity that is of utmost importance for all individuals.

References

Aronowitz, P. (1989). A brother's dream. In *NAMI Publication No. 2—The experiences of patients and families: First person accounts* (pp. 77–78). Arlington, VA: National Alliance for the Mentally Ill.

Buie, J. (1989). Psychologist prevales despite schizophrenia. *APA Monitor, 20,* 23.

Frese, F. (1988). The role of psychologists in serving the seriously mentally ill: A call for partnership between the served and the servers. In D. L. Johnson (Ed.), *Service needs of the seriously mentally ill: Training implications for psychology* (pp. 33–36). Washington, DC: American Psychological Association.

Gershon, E. S., & Rieder, R. O. (1992, September). Major disorders of mind and brain. *Scientific American, 267*(3), 126–133.

Holmes, D. S. (1991). *Abnormal psychology.* New York: HarperCollins.

Leete, E. (1989). How I perceive and manage my mental illness. *Schizophrenia Bulletin, 15,* 197–200.

Millett, K. (1990). *The loony-bin trip.* New York: Simon & Schuster.

North, C. S. (1987). *Welcome silence: My triumph over schizophrenia.* New York: Simon & Schuster.

Styron, W. (1990). *Darkness visible: A memoir of madness.* New York: Random House.

Torrey, E. F. (1988). *Surviving schizophrenia: A family manual.* New York: Harper & Row.

Wasow, M. (1989). The need for asylum for the chronically mentally ill. In *NAMI Publication No. 2—The experiences of patients and families: First person accounts* (pp. 71–76). Arlington, VA: National Alliance for the Mentally Ill.

Zelt, D. (1981). First person account: The messiah quest. *Schizophrenia Bulletin, 7,* 527–531.

PART III

Models of Effective Public–Academic Collaboration

CHAPTER

13

State Mental Health Systems and Universities: A Conceptual Model for Collaborative Service

King E. Davis
Department of Mental Health, Mental Retardation, and Substance Abuse Services

In the past 5 years, collaboration between higher education and state mental health systems has attracted increased attention (Davis, 1990). This increased attention seems stimulated primarily by the efforts of state mental health systems to link their service systems to professional schools within universities. The impetus for this current shift toward collaboration comes from the need within state mental health systems to solve a number of interrelated human resource management and development problems: attracting, hiring, retaining, and distributing mental health professionals from various disciplines; acquiring a mixture of staff by race, ethnicity, and gender; and providing state-of-the-art continuing education to maintain and enhance the scientific knowledge and skills of staff.

The need and stimulus for collaboration by universities is less recognized, contributing to tenuous and imbalanced relationships, pursued and supported more directly by state mental health systems. Universities often fail to identify the research, educational, service, and financial benefits available through collaboration with the state mental health sector. The purpose of this chapter then, is to define and explore the concept of collaboration, as well as to compare and contrast its benefits and risks as a strategy for helping state mental health systems and universities resolve alternative human resource problems. In the concluding sections of the chapter, various models of collaboration are presented to demonstrate the value of collaborative versus competitive strategies.

State mental health systems are highly labor intensive, with up to 90% of finances invested in human resources. However, these systems continue to experience major human resource management and development crises from the point of initial recruitment through retention and continuing education.

Until recently, state mental health systems appear to have paid limited attention to their needs for comprehensive human resource management and development policies or strategies. Part of the reason for this inattention stems from the assumptions held within the state mental health bureaucracy that human resource management and development issues will be taken care of by market forces without intervention or guiding policy by the state mental health authority. A second assumption is that universities and colleges will routinely produce graduates with the requisite skills, knowledge, and interest in careers in the state mental health sector without explicit efforts by the state mental health authority. There is also an assumption that demand for employment among graduates of universities and colleges will be so constant that state mental health systems will be able to compete successfully with other sectors of the economy for their share of this labor pool. However, low salaries, inadequate attention to working conditions, and an overall laissez-faire approach tend to increase the turnover of staff within state mental health systems, contributing to instability and difficulty in recruitment.

State mental health authorities may have misinterpreted the influence of market theory and practice for their human resource problems. Certainly, where an excess of professional staff exists, state mental health systems may be successful with a laissez-faire approach. However, the reality of the current and previous decade is that well-educated professionals are in increasingly short supply and have considerably broader options than they had in the past. As the trend toward community-based services has increased simultaneously with a widening of those professional disciplines eligible for third-party reimbursements, the market position of public mental health services generally, and state systems specifically, has declined significantly. The allure of private practice and its prospects for higher salaries, greater prestige, and independence has cut drastically into the human resource pool previously available to the public sector. These same issues have reduced the availability of well-trained paraprofessional and professional staff within state hospitals.

Another constraining issue for state mental health systems has been the tendency to conceptualize human resource problems and issues from a narrow, internal training perspective only. Far less attention has been focused on long-term strategies for ensuring workforce mix, racial and gender equity, recruitment and retention, geographic distribution, workplace conditions, or the potential roles of families and consumers in the workplace. Additionally, state mental health systems have not paid enough attention to the content of the academic curricula in the professional schools within their states that produce the majority of their workforce. The majority of consumers of state mental health services are individuals with severe disabilities, requiring extensive and protracted rehabilitation. However, a significant proportion of the university curricula remains focused on training and education of professionals for work with acute psychiatric disorders of limited duration and disability. As a result, state mental health systems must expend considerable resources in retraining of professionals whose academic education was incongruent with the realities of service in the public sector.

Contrary to the laissez-faire role of the states, the federal government has taken a relatively active interest in human resource issues and problems for several decades. Part of their interest dates back to the Mental Health Act of 1944 and to subsequent mental health acts. Throughout much of the period between 1944 and 1987, the federal interest in mental health service employees was operationalized through a variety of training and employee development grants available to educational institutions and to state mental health systems. More recently, the federal emphasis on human resources has become circumscribed around the problems states are now experiencing in providing services to the severely mentally disabled in state facilities and community programs. The federal perspective suggests that the state mental health authority needs to engage in planned relationships with several other related systems (i.e., universities, private agencies, public agencies, and licensing and certification authorities) in order to enhance the quality of human resources available in the public sector (Public Law [PL] 99-660). Likewise, this perspective identifies and suggests more proactive roles and responsibilities for the state mental health authority that go far beyond that which has traditionally and historically been evident. Part of the federal perspective on these issues is reflected in PL 99-660, the State Mental Health Planning Act. In this public law, states are required to develop a variety of training programs that will increase the skills and marketability of staff within state hospitals who are being displaced by deinstitutionalization efforts.

State mental health systems and universities have maintained a variety of collaborative relationships for decades. However, these relationships have diminished significantly over the past 3 decades corresponding to the decline of the federally supported community mental health centers movement and policy (MacPheeters, 1983). Principally because of the labor intensive character of state mental health systems, there is a need to understand more clearly the concept of collaboration and its potential role in helping these systems to resolve their human resource management and development crises.

The Concept of Collaboration

To meet the human resource needs of state mental health systems and the educational priorities of universities, at least four optional strategies can be considered: merger, competition, conflict, and collaboration.

Merger

Merger implies a combination of two or more organizations into one enterprise. It is seen as a method of unification where the intent is to construct one organization by pulling together the resources and assets of one or more diverse organizations that could not compete or survive independently.

In a small number of states, university departments of psychiatry, psychology, social work, and counseling operate as a part of the state mental health system, obliterating the lines of distinction between the two (Talbott & Rabinowitz, 1986). This novel practice offers an empirical illustration of how the merger concept can be operationalized in a meaningful, productive manner. Merger as a strategy is designed to prevent fiscal or programmatic bankruptcy, collapse, loss of control, or disruption. It is an attempt to increase efficiency, lower costs, and increase overall levels of service. In the American landscape, mergers became quite common in the business community after World War II. Between 1945 and 1959, numerous mergers occurred in manufacturing and mining alone. Thousands of other companies sought mergers as a method of increasing their capacity for achieving specific goals and maintaining market position. Thus far, however, mergers between state mental health systems and universities have been infrequent. This is perhaps due to the fact that state mental health systems and many universities are dependent on public tax dollars; few have actually reached the point of fiscal collapse. Although merger has been a cogent strategy in business, its application in the public mental health domain seems limited. Application of mergers to state mental health systems and universities has the potential for obscuring the boundaries of both systems, stimulating conflict and potentially confounding their respective missions. The South Carolina mental health system comes close to this merged model of training and service. In their hybrid model, however, the state university and state mental health systems maintain key elements of their operational autonomy while merging together in a single, shared service component that maximizes cooperation.

Competition

At various times in their history, state mental hospitals operated residency training programs for various disciplines. In this regard, the state mental health system competed with universities for students, resources, and prestige. During the period in which such competitive training took place, there was a duplication of effort, increased costs for training, and perhaps a dilution of the training effort. Some state mental health commissioners (Bevilacqua, 1992; Tanaka, 1992) assert that this competitive model was more successful in meeting the human resource needs of state mental health systems. This assertion is based on the finding that some university training programs fail to include content in their curricula that is relevant to the state mental health system. When training programs were under the aegis of the state mental health system, some commissioners suggest the content was more directly relevant. Furthermore, some commissioners contend that university programs tend to resist changes in their curriculum yet expect state mental health systems to allocate increasingly larger amounts of money to support academic programs of questionable relevancy to the state systems' needs. Because of unfavorable outcomes, some state mental health authorities advocate for a return to competitive academic training programs offered by state mental health systems. A number of state mental health commissioners have become disillusioned with their efforts to develop or sustain meaningful collaboration with university departments and, increasingly, see these efforts as exploitative of the public mental health system. However, state mental health system-based training programs did not carry the prestige of university programs and eventually found it increasingly difficult to attract students. Additionally, the impact of the training emphasis on the service mission of the state mental health system has not been assessed. University deans, chairpersons, and faculty have also expressed concerns about relationships with state mental health systems (J. Silverman, personal communication, June 1990).

University faculty also voice concerns that collaboration with state mental health systems tends to be of short duration and far too vulnerable to budget reductions. Once academic programs are altered to more adequately address the needs of the state mental health sector, faculty fear that resources will be reduced or withdrawn, summarily leaving the university with only contractual obligations to new faculty and students. University departments are encouraged to avoid such risks because faculty tend to perceive such academic programs as unstable, thus decreasing the chances of recruiting outstanding faculty and students. In these instances, universities favor a more competitive posture in which they maintain autonomy from the state mental health sector.

Rather than developing and maintaining alternative educational systems, which have the potential of increasing costs and diluting services, an effort to simultaneously energize and yet provide the requisite long-term monetary support for university curricula seems more than justified.

Conflict

Competition between the university and the state mental health system also has the potential for developing conflicts over issues such as student recruitment, faculty recruitment, limited state financial resources, as well as competition for research grants from private and federal sources. In some respects, the human services system operates from the same competitive value orientation as business. In such competition the focus is on dollars, turf, status, power, and control. Deming (1992) warned that the failure of American business to recognize and reduce the destructive impact of this kind of competition in the profit and nonprofit sectors contributes to excessive costs, duplication, confusion, needless complexity, as well as lower quality of service. In this sense, competition between the university and the state mental health systems seems to represent an unacceptable strategy for resolution of human resource problems or for maintaining academic standards.

Collaboration

In this chapter, collaboration is seen as the most viable of the four current strategies for helping state mental health systems and universities meet their respective missions. *Collaboration* is defined here as a planned strategy in which two or more systems form a cooperative relationship around one or more common functions or areas. The collaborative relationship is designed to improve the chances that each system will reach its overall mission and human resource goals as well as improve the quality of life of the severely mentally disabled. *Functions* are defined here as tasks or activities that must be initiated or completed if a system is to reach or approximate its mission and goals.

Although there seems to be a logical basis for collaboration between universities and state mental health systems, several factors inhibit its development and maintenance. One such factor is the tradition of autonomy within both systems. Somewhere in the evolution of public policy, universities and state mental health systems have been allowed to conceptualize or perceive their respective missions, systems, and methods as dichotomous. As a result, such systems have a tendency to become insulated from each other, fail to see how their missions are coterminous, become overly protective of their boundaries, and fail to place a value on collaboration. In the short run, universities and state mental health systems tend to view the human services landscape as competitive rather than cooperative. However, in the long run, the broad systems of human services from mental health to education can become segmented, isolated, confusing to the public, duplicative, costly, and less than successful.

Functional Areas for Collaboration

Mental health systems and universities share approximately 15 overlapping areas in which collaboration occurs (Davis, 1987). These include the following:

1. administration
2. advocacy/protection
3. consultation
4. continuing education/staff development
5. curriculum design/evaluation
6. grant development/application
7. planning/policy development
8. program design
9. public education
10. recruitment/staff sharing

11. research and evaluation
12. resource sharing/financing
13. retention
14. service delivery/certification
15. teaching

A review of university departments and mental health systems in several states showed that collaboration tends to take place simultaneously in several of these functional areas (Davis, 1987). Although collaboration may be initially reflective of a single function or area, there is a tendency for the collaborative arrangement to broaden soon after its initiation. For example, in Virginia, the collaborative relationship between Western State Hospital and the University of Virginia is based principally around education and service. However, there are strong research elements within the relationship as well. At one point, the university actually provided administrative direction to the state hospital through the department of psychiatry. Perhaps more than in some settings, the collaborative relationship between the state mental health system and the University of Virginia extends into more academic departments than is noted in other universities. One of the major benefits for the state hospital involved in this arrangement is the extraordinarily broad range of professional staff that are recruited from the university's graduates.

In another illustration from Virginia, the initial collaborative relationship between Central State Hospital and the Medical College of Virginia focused on research and demonstration, but quickly expanded to include service, staff development, recruitment, and teaching. Within the past 2 years, the Medical College of Virginia has extended its service collaboration to two community mental health programs and has absorbed a small state psychiatric center for children and adolescents. The Medical College of Virginia has also collaborated with the state mental health system in advocating for changes in state insurance coverage for the mentally ill.

Other examples of general collaboration are apparent in Virginia Commonwealth University's School of Social Work. It collaborates with the state mental health system in curriculum development, systems planning, research, and teaching. Other university departments (Journalism, Business and Health Administration) have collaborated with the state mental health system in such areas as public education, supported employment, and continuing education in quality management.

Within Virginia's universities, collaborative arrangements have rarely been confined to a single functional area. In most instances, the range, mix, and complexity of collaboration increases as the relationship between the two systems grows stronger. As the base of the collaboration broadens, more university departments, students, and faculty become involved, increasing the perceived and actual merit to the university and the state mental health system. As the perception of merit increases (e.g., quality training, service, or accreditation), the number of students and faculty actively seeking to be a part of the collaboration tends to increase. For the state mental health system, assistance from the university in obtaining or maintaining accreditation, recruiting difficult-to-acquire staff, or providing highly relevant continuing education reinforces the value of their investment in collaboration.

Models of Collaboration

A review of the experiences and approaches used in several states (Talbott & Robinowitz, 1986) demonstrates that there is no universally accepted model for state and university collaboration that should be pursued. Rather, the models or approaches utilized within a state should be designed by the stakeholders to reflect their mission, needs, resources, policies, values, and expected outcomes.

Although there is no universal model, there are similarities in the patterns by which the collaborative relationships originate. Typically, the collaboration starts with the state mental health system (facility, staff member, community center, or central office) reaching out to a single university department for assistance with a specific problem. For example, the initial collaborative model may be simply an informal agreement between two individuals who recognize an area of mutuality and decide to pursue it. The initial stimulus here could be in research or a specific practice method or clinical entity. Because of the personal nature of this approach to collaboration, the relationship may only exist as long as the individuals who established it find value in its continuation. In this sense, the collaboration does not reach the level of systems and may have only minimal impact on the overall interactions between the two systems.

Collaboration may also be built around the solution to specific problems found in one or both systems. State mental health systems frequently approach university departments for assistance in solving staffing shortages or problems in recruiting. Most recently, in Virginia, these collaborations have focused on the recruitment of psychiatrists and nurses. In other instances, the collaborative models focus on continuing education or preservice training between a specific university department and the state mental health system. In one program, the preservice training was designed to introduce psychiatric rehabilitation content into the curriculum of a school within the university, while simultaneously increasing the interest of students in such career paths in the state mental health system. The state mental health authority provided student stipends, partial faculty support, and field sites, while the university provided the other portion of faculty support, courses, field supervision, and opportunities for family involvement in teaching.

Another model of collaboration includes multiple departments within a school of medicine rotating students through a state psychiatric hospital directed by the chairman of the university's Department of Psychiatry. At the University of Virginia, students from Medicine, Neurology, Psychiatry, Geriatrics, Nursing, Psychology, and other departments provided services and participated in research within the state hospital, while state hospital staff taught courses, participated in research, and provided supervision of students in training. The university and the hospital shared staff and resources and participated in joint training opportunities.

Figure 1 reflects the fluid nature and range of collaborative models that are proposed. Here, it is shown that three major components (university, functions, and state mental health) make up the collaborative dynamic. Additionally, each of the major elements has multiple subcomponents or parts that can be included in the collaborative effort. The elements and their parts are displayed as gears, suggesting that a wide variety of interlocking relationships are possible depending on the direction that is taken or stimulated. For example, the collaboration can range from a single department within a university interacting with a single division within a state hospital or overall state mental health system to multiple university departments interacting with an entire human services system. Either of these two extremes can revolve around single or multiple functions (see preceding examples).

The fluid nature of collaboration suggests that as the needs of the stakeholders change, there is a tendency for the collaborative model to change toward greater complexity and the inclusion of a greater number of individual stakeholders: students, faculty, administrators, researchers, consumers, and family members.

In Virginia, the Department of Mental Health Services has established collaborative relationships with 12 colleges and universities. In some instances, the collaborative model consists only of financial support for a faculty member or a student conducting research in an area important to the Department of Mental Health. Another model reflects the Department of Mental Health using grant funding to stimulate curriculum development to support services for minority children. A more expansive collaborative model involves research, teaching, practice, administration, continuing education, staff sharing, stipends, and multiple rotations between the state hospital and multiple departments within a single university.

Benefits of Collaboration

For collaboration to be sustained and enhanced, each of the stakeholders must realize benefits that move them closer to their expected goals. Generally, collaboration has the potential for strengthening each of the stakeholders in the relationship, but not necessarily at the same time or in the same way. The benefits from collaboration will also vary considerably in magnitude over time. For example, collaboration was shown to be the seminal factor in determining whether a state mental hospital in Virginia achieved accreditation. The same collaboration helped a university department to recruit a highly sought-after researcher who was interested in a research problem and population readily available through the state mental health system.

One of the major benefits of collaboration is the potential impact on services. Involvement of university faculty and students in state mental health systems can greatly improve the quality of services provided to consumers, either through the skills of faculty or through the continuing education provided to state hospital staff. At the same time, the clinical experiences provided to students and faculty can result in major modifications in the knowledge and skill base taught in the university. In other instances, difficult clinical cases can be reviewed by teams of state mental health staff

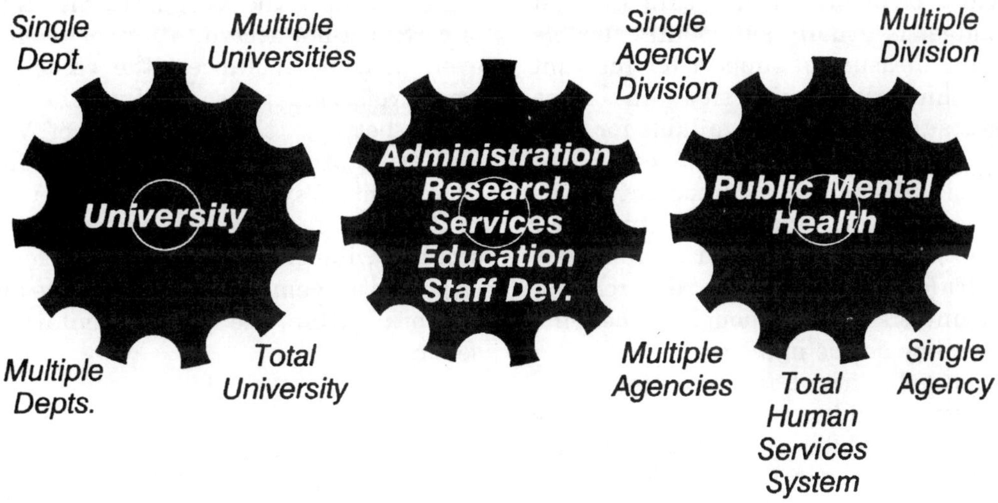

Figure 1. Models of Collaboration

and university faculty. In some instances, the university may have expensive technology that is otherwise not available to the state mental health system. The university may also be involved in specific clinical trials of medication that may be useful to consumers of state mental health services. Over the past 3 years, clinical trials of Clozapine have taken place in state hospitals with major involvement by university researchers from departments of psychiatry and pharmacology. This collaboration helped the state mental health system to formulate drug protocols for utilization of the medication within state facilities and community programs.

State programs have on-going problems in recruiting key professional staff. In several states, the major benefit of collaboration has been the improvement in the state system's ability to attract professional staff. In one state center for the mentally retarded, collaboration with an outstanding university research department assisted in filling a position that had been vacant for 2 years. In some instances, when the collaboration allows for joint positions within the university and the state mental health system, applicants express greater interest in such positions. The opportunity to spend a portion of time in practice, research, or other related areas has stimulated greater interest on the part of some potential staff.

The collaborative relationships have also allowed both systems to formulate more attractive or flexible financial packages for desirable applicants than either system could offer alone. Some state mental health systems may lack the salary flexibility and ranges available within the university. Collaboration that allows for transfers of dollars between the university and the state mental health system and the holding of joint positions can increase the prospects for successful recruitment and retention. In several states, this kind of collaboration occurs by contract and gives the university the responsibility for recruiting a faculty member to fill an important position within the state mental health system.

Universities can benefit from collaboration when the state mental health system provides financial resources to support faculty, students, or entire programs. Several examples are relevant here. The Virginia Department of Mental Health provides substantial support for the Division of Substance Abuse Medicine within the Medical College of Virginia. Substantial support is also provided by the department for the Institute of Law, Psychiatry, and Public Policy at the University of Virginia.

In Ohio, the state mental health authority provides support for a number of university programs through contracts that specify the expected outcomes for the state mental health system. South Carolina's Department of Mental Health provides substantial support, training opportunities, and space for the department of psychiatry. Because the state mental health authority is generally the largest provider of mental health care in most states, its budget is usually sufficiently flexible to provide some measure of support for relevant programs within the university. In some instances, this support may be available for pilot projects of new models, approaches, technology, medicines or skills potentially important to the state system and the university. In other instances, the state mental health system may provide support for long-term, basic research conducted by the university, even though the benefits for the system may not be immediate.

One of the most significant benefits of collaboration is its impact on student attitudes toward the severely mentally disabled and careers in state mental health. Within several years following the development and implementation of collaborative models in Virginia, there have been dramatic changes in the willingness of students to work with the severely mentally disabled. In several university medical schools, rotations in the state hospital became the most desired following the development of an extensive collaboration agreement between the hospital and the medical school. As a result of this relationship, the state hospital has been able to successfully recruit graduating residents.

Collaborative models also have the potential benefit of stimulating changes in each of the systems involved. Training programs tend to expand their curricula, investing more in directions of relevancy to the state mental health system, whereas the mental health system tends to alter its approaches to service delivery and research-based practice. State mental health systems tend to become more amendable to feedback from consumers; more open to questions about policies, services, and practices by students; and more willing to shift traditional approaches to be more congruent with newer practices.

Another benefit is the increased opportunity for research, owing particularly to the availability of cases in the public sector and the skills and structures for research in the university. As an additional benefit here, public mental health staff have increased opportunities to learn and participate in research and publication. Collaboration around research and training also has the potential for increasing the quality of services provided in the public mental health system. As collaboration increases, there have been noted gains in political, professional, and administrative support for the public–academic linkage. As a result of collaboration, each segment of the new relationship tends to increase in stature, recognition, and reward. In some instances, the recognition may take the form of certification, accreditation, or licensure. However, in some instances, the recognition comes from professional associations. The collaborative model between the University of Virginia and Western State Hospital received the Hospital and Community Psychiatry Award for Collaboration in 1986. The receipt of this award helped to underscore the importance of collaboration but, more importantly, demonstrated the value and rewards of work within the public mental health care sector.

Risks of Collaboration

Efforts to establish collaborative relationships are not without some substantial risks for both the universities and the public mental health systems involved. One of these risks is the potential for a loss of identity for one or both of the participants. Depending on the degree of relationship, the factors that distinguish each system may become blurred, giving rise to concerns by faculty or staff. Additionally, there is the major concern expressed within the university sector that affiliation with public mental health systems can result in a lowering of the quality of education for their students. The rationale that has been described by faculty stems from the belief that students may be used to supplant regular staff, thus leaving limited time for student learning and growth.

Mental health systems, on the other hand, often are fearful that their systems and consumers will be exploited by universities bent on research as a high priority. Public mental health systems express particular concern about research because of the highly politicized environment in which they operate. Research that involves substantial risks for the public mental health system is one factor that hampers collaboration between these systems. Universities often do not understand the differences in the political environments and expectations between their system and the public mental health system.

A further risk here is the resistance by faculty, public mental health staff, and university students to the idea of collaboration. There are numerous instances in which collaboration has been less than successful because of fears and concerns by these varied groups. Universities in particular express concern about a loss of status or prestige because of their affiliation with the public mental health system. A final factor that has been noted is fear on the part of the public mental health system that their substantial resources will be exploited by the university. The university, on the other hand, fears that the public mental health system will be unwilling to allocate resources over an extended period to sustain the collaboration.

Conclusion

The most significant factor that stimulates and sustains collaborative relationships is the degree of communication between the leaders of the university and public mental health systems. This communication requires a mutual understanding of the coterminous nature of their missions and the degree of mutual benefits to be derived from collaboration. Leadership from mental health commissioners, university presidents, deans, and chairpeople is a prerequisite for effective collaboration.

In many instances, the collaborative relationship is heightened and strengthened via written agreements that spell out the roles, expectations, contributions, and exchanges that are needed. The state of Ohio's mental health system is an acknowledged leader in building its relationships on a contractual basis. Virginia, on the other hand, has utilized a shared faculty position approach as the intermediary in establishing and sustaining collaboration. The Galt Visiting Scholar program in Virginia has proven very successful for stimulating the types of collaboration noted in this chapter.

In some instances, collaboration requires or is enhanced by executive or legislative mandates. One of the key ingredients for collaboration, as well, is the identification and sharing of resources. This resource sharing can be in the form of sharing faculty and staff positions, stipends, support for research, joint recruiting, or the sharing of funds for special projects. Collaboration has been demonstrated in a number of states to offer key advantages to public mental health systems and universities. The overall key appears to be the recognition by both systems that the eventual success of mental health care in the public sector requires the active participation, support, and investment of both systems.

Human service systems and educational institutions have been encouraged over the years to develop and pursue parallel tracks toward their missions. To some extent, state mental health systems and universities are distinguished further by their priorities. The most important priority in the state mental health system is service, whereas in the university system, the priority is on the generation and transfer of new knowledge. In some instances, this difference in priority may be seen as a deterrent to collaboration. In many university programs, teaching and education may be viewed as secondary to their research mission. In the state mental health system, research and education are generally of secondary importance to the service mission. In this kind of policy environment, it is readily understood how collaboration may not be recognized as a key strategy for either system. However, the challenges of solving human resources problems, meeting the public needs, and maximizing state resources common to both state universities and state mental health systems should provide a compelling mandate for exploring and testing collaboration as a viable system-enhancing and change strategy.

References

Bevilacqua, J. (1992, June). *Betty Smith Memorial Lecture.* Human Resources Conference, Arlington, VA.

Davis, K. E. (1987). *Final Galt Report—Virginia Department of Mental Health, Mental Retardation and Substance Abuse Services.* Richmond: Virginia Department of Mental Health.

Davis, K. E. (1990, December). Collaboration between public mental health systems and universities. *Community Support Network News, 1*(2), 2–3.

Deming, E. W. (1992, May). *Dr. Deming's plan for action for the optimization of services organizations.* Teleconference. Washington, D.C.

McPheeters, H. (1983, July). *Relationships between universities and agencies to better meet public needs.* Paper presented to the Commission of Mental Health and Human Services, Williamsburg, VA.

Talbott, J., & Robinowitz, C. (Eds). (1986). *Working together: State–university collaboration in mental health.* Washington, DC: American Psychiatric Association.

Tanaka, A. (1992, June). *Betty Smith Memorial Lecture.* Human Resources Conference, Arlington, VA.

CHAPTER

14

The North Carolina Children and Youth Demonstration Project: Increasing Professionals' Understanding of Service Systems

Lenore Behar
North Carolina Division of Mental Health, Developmental Disabilities, and Substance Abuse Services

Tom Bainbridge
North Carolina Division of Mental Health

Richard Munger
North Carolina Foundations for Alternative Health Programs, Inc.

In response to statewide concerns about the critical shortage of child oriented mental health professionals in the state of North Carolina, the Orange–Person–Chatham Mental Health Center (MHC) and the University of North Carolina at Chapel Hill (UNC) are collaboratively involved in the Children and Youth Demonstration Project. The Project evolved out of a joint effort by UNC and the North Carolina Division of Mental Health, Developmental Disabilities, and Substance Abuse Services (MH/DD/SAS) to obtain funds and operate the program. The chapter describes a public–academic partnership to enhance professionals' understanding of service continua in child mental health. The project's objectives are reviewed and details presented about (a) project administration, (b) project center-based services, and (c) project community-based services. Then, the training curriculum and financing of the project are discussed.

The Project's primary mission is to provide intensive training experiences within a community-based, client-centered continuum of care that is well integrated into a process of interagency coordination of service delivery. This training for-

This chapter is based on a paper that was presented as part of the symposium, "Innovative Training Models: Working With Children With Serious Emotional Disturbance," at the annual meeting of the American Psychological Association, San Francisco, August 18, 1991.

mat was developed as an alternative to previous options that were often limited to either a traditional center-based model of community mental health or to inpatient settings. The program is intended to assist trainees in the acquisition of those competencies necessary to support the effective operation of any community-based continuum of child mental health services. Figure 1 depicts the organizational structure of the Children and Youth Demonstration Project.

The MHC serves a three-county area with a population of 161,053. The catchment area is predomantly rural and agricultural except a portion of Orange County, where the University of North Carolina at Chapel Hill is located. North Carolina Memorial Hospital, the principal teaching hospital of the University of North Carolina School of Medicine, also is in Chapel Hill. The MHC has about 200 staff at the central clinic in Chapel Hill and in four satellite offices, including approximately 19 full-time equivalent staff working in child mental health services.

In addition to these 19 child mental health positions are 49 staff who provide an array of services in the "Willie M" Program. The statewide Willie M Program originated as a result of a class action suit filed against the state of North Carolina on behalf of children with emotional or develop-

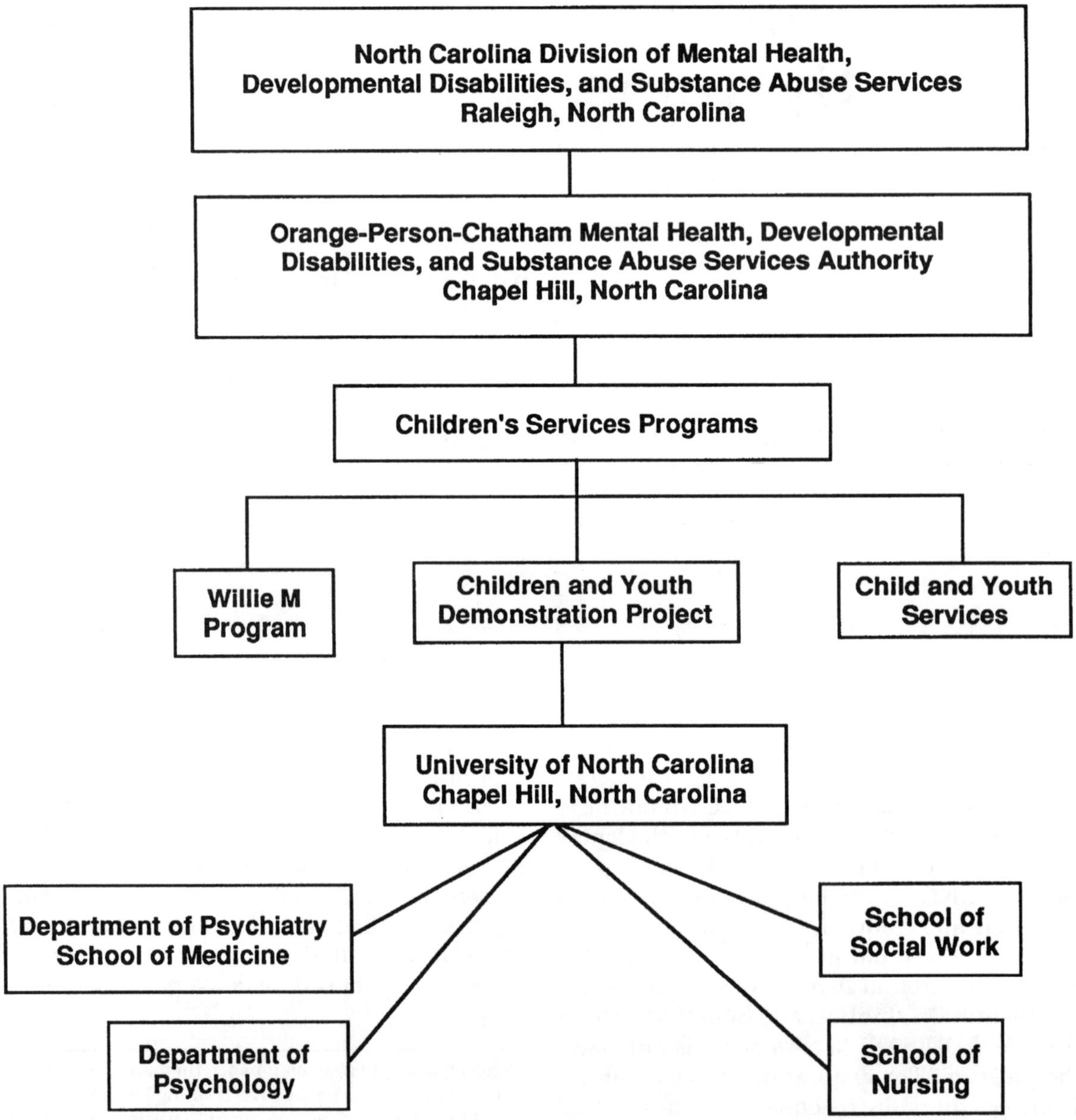

Figure 1. Organizational Structure of the Children and Youth Demonstration Project

mental handicaps who exhibited assaultive and violent behavior and who were not being appropriately served by educational and mental health agencies within the state. The state consented to provide services in the least restrictive setting appropriate for the child. At present, the MHC's Willie M Program has not been integrated into the Children and Youth Demonstration Project.

In order to pursue the Project's mission, objectives have been developed in three general areas: training, service enhancement, and community coordination of services.

Training objectives have focused on skill development in the following areas:

1. how to assess client need and identify corresponding resources;

2. how to utilize community resources and outreach interventions, as appropriate;

3. how to develop a realistic understanding of community systems, resources, organizational mandates, and so forth; and

4. how to participate in community-based interdisciplinary collaboration.

Community coordination objectives have focused on the following areas:

1. development of key staff positions that provide improved coordination of services and agency linkage, including case management and direct psychological services to Social Services and juvenile courts; and

2. both formal and informal mechanisms to support interagency coordination of services.

Service development objectives focus on expansion of the MHC's Child and Youth Services system of care in the following key areas:

1. shifted focus of treatment resources, where indicated, away from center-based interventions and toward services in the community;

2. developed community-based crisis management resources and alternatives to hospitalization; and

3. increased capacity to coordinate and advocate for crucial community-based services for the seriously emotionally disturbed child.

Prior to the initiation of the Project, Child and Youth Services at the MHC were primarily center-based. Case management resources were extremely limited. Interagency coordination was restricted to the initiative of individual MHC staff and was limited by severe time constraints. Specific services that have been developed, their utility as training experiences, and the nature of related interagency processes will be discussed below. Both trainees and faculty liaisons have simultaneously benefitted from involvement in this developing system while providing some of the staff resources necessary for its development and operation.

Project Administration

The following is an overview of the administrative structures of the Project, as illustrated in Figure 2.

1. The Project Coordinating Committee meets quarterly; the focus is on problem identification, problem solving, and planning related to administrative issues.

2. The interagency service functions of the Project Coordinating Committee have been vested with county-specific Interagency Coordinating Groups, which meet monthly. These groups assess service needs of seriously emotionally disturbed youth and develop coordinated, interagency service plans.

3. The Education and Evaluation Committee meets monthly to focus specifically on training outcomes.

4. The Child and Youth Clinical staff meetings convene weekly to assess client needs and make specific service allocation dispositions. This meeting is attended by most relevant child and youth staff and Project participants.

5. The role of the project coordinator is to function as a clinical coordinator for the integrated project and child and youth service. He or she has the function of providing direct supervision to the Project and child and youth staff for the purpose of ensuring the highest quality of client care and compliance with program goals and objectives.

Staffing Pattern

Reflecting the interdisciplinary, interagency focus of the Project objectives, the Child and Youth Dem-

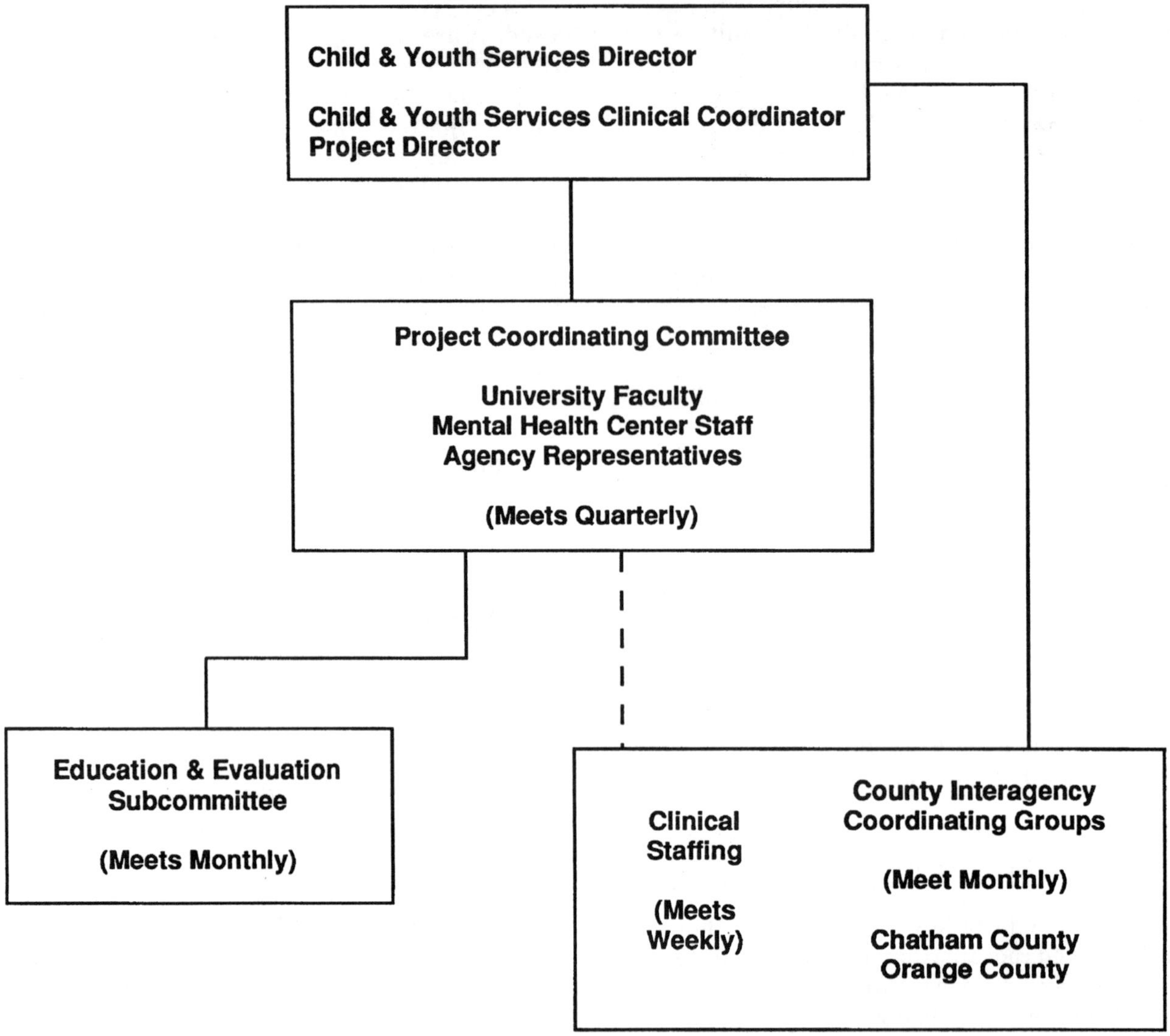

Figure 2. Administrative Structure of the Children and Youth Demonstration Project

onstration Project is staffed by faculty and trainees from four departments of the University of North Carolina at Chapel Hill, clinicians and administrators from the MHC, and staff providing liaison services to community agencies.

In 1990–1991, 15 faculty from UNC regularly contributed to Project training, service delivery, and administration. Nine faculty from the UNC School of Medicine, Department of Psychiatry routinely participated in Project functions. The Department of Psychology and the Schools of Nursing and Social Work were each represented by 2 faculty.

With few exceptions, Project faculty responsible for service delivery or for the supervision of trainees were housed at one of the MHC's five sites. Exceptions included some of the psychiatry faculty who remained at North Carolina Memorial Hospital while rendering or supervising emergency services.

Trainees

In 1990–1991, the academic departments placed a total of 12 graduate-level trainees in Project internships. The trainees included 4 child residents from the Department of Psychiatry, 3 postinternship doctoral candidates from the Department of Psychology, 2 masters-level students from the School of Nursing, and 3 masters-level students from the School of Social Work. In addition, a number of other graduate-level trainees participated in various Project training events throughout the year. These student interns, from North Carolina Memorial Hospital Department of Child Psychiatry, included general psychiatry residents, student nurses, and masters-level interns from the Department of Psychology and the School of Social Work. Additionally, general psychiatry residents participated in the provision of hospital-based emergency services supervised by Project faculty. This faculty time was funded by the Project.

MHC Staff

Several MHC employees are significantly involved in the Project. On-going Project implementation occurs under the general administrative supervision of the Child and Youth Clinical Coordinator. A senior member of the child and youth clinical staff serves as a liaison consultant between the Project and pre-existing MHC clinical services. The position is instrumental in the training of faculty and trainees in agency procedures. Additionally, a doctoral-level psychologist provides psychology services to the Department of Social Services and Juvenile Courts.

Community Agency Representatives

Four community organizations have participated in coordination and management functions of the Children and Youth Demonstration Project. These affiliated agencies include two public school systems, one county department of social services, and one juvenile court system covering two counties.

County Interagency Coordinating Groups

The interagency service planning functions of the Project have been vested in local interagency planning groups. Two such groups are now in operation. By establishing these groups locally, the level of community participation is broader, resulting in more effective client-centered discussion. As these groups become routinely operational, Project trainee participation will be beneficial. The overall process of community coordination of services is generally informed and guided by the objectives found in the National Institute of Mental Health's Child and Adolescent Service System Program (CASSP) model for "A System of Care for Severely Emotionally Disturbed Children and Youth."

Affiliated Agency Psychologists

Recognizing the need for psychological evaluation and treatment for the populations served by both Juvenile Court Services and Social Services, and in accordance with the interagency collaboration prescribed by the Project philosophy and objectives, two half-time equivalent clinical psychologists have been employed by the Project and housed part-time at these two agencies. In addition to providing assessment, consultation, and treatment to agency clients, the psychologists serve as structural linkages between their host agencies and the MHC, assisting staff and trainees in learning and negotiating unfamiliar systems, advocating across systems for clients, and participating in the Project's Coordinating Committee and clinical staff meetings.

Program Planning and Development

The full integration of the Project into the routine operation of the MHC is an on-going priority. The Project Coordinator role has been merged with the Child Clinical Coordinator position. The Child Clinical Coordinator has programwide responsibility for integrating the Project into service programming. Just as important, the individual has substantial responsibility for ensuring that all of the MHC's children's services conform, to the greatest extent possible, with the client-centered program objectives of the Project. The children's "continuum of care" that is emerging at the MHC and that operates as a foundation of the training experience will now develop and operate in an integrated manner, avoiding the conflicts and redundancies which are characteristic of dual systems.

Centered-Based Project Services

Project faculty, trainees, and staff have participated in the development and delivery of a range of clinical services. These services represent a significant expansion of those that existed at the Mental Health Center prior to the introduction of the Project. In many cases, the services were unavailable in the catchment area prior to Project implementation. In other instances, Project activities expanded previously existing services. In every instance, a measurable increase in the number of clients served has been realized. The full integration of Project resources and Child and Youth Services has established a momentum that enhances both the service and training functions. The present and future development of the emerging continuum of care will be guided by North Carolina's Child Mental Health Plan. In 1987, the North Carolina General Assembly adopted a 10-year plan for the expansion of services for emotionally disturbed children other than in the Willie M class. This 10-year commitment was based on the Child Mental Health Plan, which describes the continuum of care, the gaps in services, the cost of completing the continuum statewide, and the management supports needed to sustain it. The Child Mental Health Plan was created by a task force of professionals and citizens appointed by the legislature. Input was provided by all relevant agencies at state and local levels, and the Child Mental Health Plan was the subject of public hearings across the state.

Center-based project services are outlined in Figure 3 and are discussed below.

Crisis Team

A significant augmentation of the MHC child and youth crisis response capacity was realized with the implementation of the Children and Youth Demonstration Project. With Project funds, the MHC contracted with the University of North Carolina Memorial Hospital Department of Child Psychiatry for the supervision and provision of hospital-based emergency evaluation and intervention for catchment area children and youth. Prior to the Project, hospital-based emergency services for child and adolescent clients operated without supervision from Child Psychiatry faculty and without integration with child mental health at the MHC. With the implementation of the Project contract services, faculty child psychiatrists began to supervise crisis and emergency evaluations and interventions. Additionally, child specialists from other disciplines (psychology and social work) employed by Child Psychiatry became systematically available for crisis intervention. This step has been a significant transition from the historically institutional-based psychiatry training. Psychiatric trainees have reported becoming knowledgeable about alternatives to the hospitalization of youth in crisis and have begun to use a range of community resources with confidence, rather than relying solely on medical expertise to respond to emergencies.

Interface between North Carolina Memorial Hospital and the MHC has been a critical component of the crisis management services. The MHC Child and Youth Services staff provide community consultation to hospital staff as needed on an on-call basis. When called, the MHC staff assist in identifying and accessing community treatment resources. Project and hospital faculty have participated in the presentation of a series of seminars for hospital-based psychiatry residents on a range of related topics including "Differential Assessment and Intervention With Adolescents in Crisis" and "Identifying and Accessing Appropriate Child and Youth Treatment Resources." The purpose of these meetings was to inform residents of community services and enlist them in hospitalization diversion strategies.

A Department of Psychiatry faculty member has begun to provide a range of support services to the crisis team efforts toward hospital diversion. Operating out of the main MHC clinic, the psychiatrist is available to screen walk-in emergencies referred by the crisis team, provide quick response and follow-up evaluation to clients screened through the crisis team (who can be maintained in the community with immediate psychiatric intervention), and offer consultation to the crisis team staff and emergency room residents regarding the MHC services that are available for hospital diversion.

Psychopharmacology Clinic

A weekly psychopharmacology clinic provides assessment and treatment of children and adolescents with affective, behavioral, and attentional difficulties. The clinic operates for about 6 hours a week. Referrals to the clinic are made by parents, the MHC staff, Project staff, and community agencies. The psychopharmacology clinic offers a weekly multidisciplinary diagnostic team that provides evaluations by students and faculty members. This team offers comprehensive evaluations for children who present with complex diagnostic, management, and treatment problems. The MHC has realized the benefit of center-based medical evaluation and consultation; prior to the Project, psychiatric evaluation for children was available only through outside referral to hospital services or private providers.

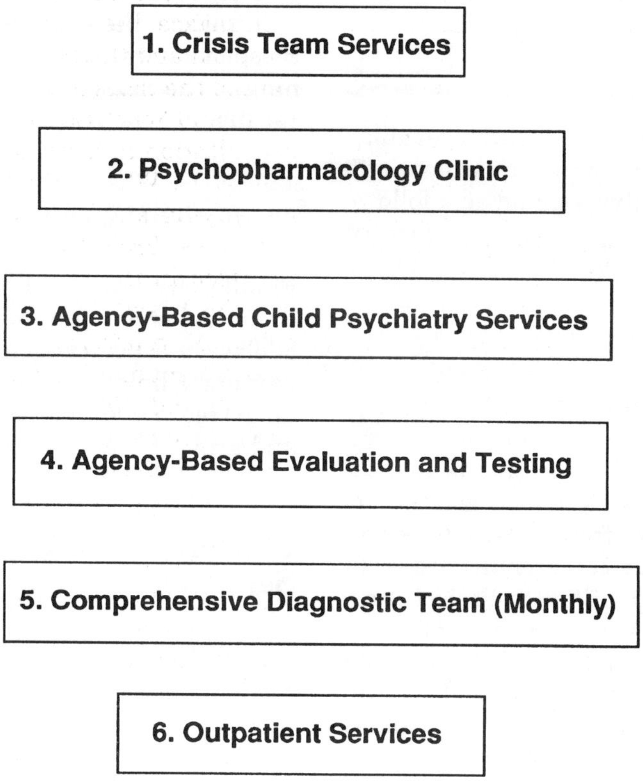

Figure 3. Center-Based Project Services

Trainees from the four disciplines are provided an opportunity to experience and practice multidisciplinary intervention in a community mental health setting in direct collaboration with representatives from related community agencies. The multiagency participation is successful in facilitating client compliance and community treatment collaboration.

Agency-Based Child Psychiatry Services

Prior to Project implementation, child psychiatry services were not available at any of the MHC sites and were available only through outside referral to hospitals and private providers. Child psychiatry residents and supervising faculty are assigned to three MHC sites, providing child psychiatry services to each of the MHC's three counties. One resident and one faculty supervisor is assigned to each site for approximately 4 hours per week. One of the rotations is the psychopharmocology clinic. As discussed above, additional psychiatry faculty time is available at the main MHC site for crisis management, intake evaluation, and treatment. The remaining three rotations differ from the psychopharmocology clinic in function. At these sites, psychiatry staff are available for consultation and evaluation of clients who are in treatment with nonmedical staff or who have been referred by community agency staff.

Psychiatry faculty report that the training experiences offered to the child residents in these four agency placements are unparalleled within the university's system. Training benefits cited include working with widely varying client populations among the MHC sites. Other valuable training experiences are said to derive from the opportunity to train in both urban and rural communities. Trainees in rotation in one county work with clients and staff of the therapeutic preschool (discussed in the Day Treatment section of this chapter).

Agency-Based Evaluation and Psychological Testing

Psychiatry faculty and trainees provide evaluation services through the psychopharmocology clinic, other site-based activities, and as a follow-up to crisis team screening. Psychology faculty and interns also provide psychological testing to clients.

Comprehensive Diagnostic Team

This monthly "difficult case" conference is an integral training and service event. Utilizing an interdisciplinary faculty team from North Carolina Memorial Hospital, these conferences are held monthly to discuss cases identified by Project clinicians and MHC clinicians as being in need of intensive assessment and treatment consultation. The conferences are attended by Project faculty, Project trainees, graduate-level trainees in hospital internships, MHC clinical staff involved in treatment of the client, and representatives from other agencies providing services to the client.

These conferences begin with a case presentation by a staff member who is involved with client treatment or service delivery. This initial presentation is followed by multiple concurrent interviews of the client and various groupings of family members. Interviews are conducted by pairs of faculty and trainees and are observed by the remaining participants through the use of a one-way mirror. On the completion of interviews and the departure of the client and family, conference participants reconvene for case discussion, consultation, and treatment recommendations.

The conferences have resulted in the development and implementation of effective interdisciplinary, interagency community-based treatment plans that have been seen as instrumental in preventing further hospitalization. Most clients who are staffed are experiencing crisis situations that in all probability would have resulted in inpatient or extracommunity placement in the absence of intensive, cooperative intervention. Several clients have been under consideration for hospitalization, and the team treatment assessments resulted in plans for community-based care and treatment, thus directly avoiding unnecessary hospitalization. The interagency consensus and collaborative intervention strategies that resulted from these conferences are seen as vital in appropriately serving and monitoring clients while maintaining them in the community. Occasionally, these monthly team meetings are devoted to planning or to a didactic presentation of relevant clinical theory and practice.

Outpatient Services

Finally, the outpatient program offers a full range of clinical and community services to children and adolescents, preschool to age 18, as well as to their parents. Clinical services include short- and long-term treatment on an individual, family, conjoint, and group basis.

Community-Based Project Services

Community-based project services are outlined in Figure 4 and are discussed below.

Case Management

Prior to the addition of designated child and youth case managers to the MHC staff, case management services were performed by outpatient therapists and were primarily limited to those clients in center-based treatment. Time and role constraints severely limited this service capacity. As a result of day-treatment funding through the Project, State Child Mental Health Plan funds previously applied to day treatment were reallocated for the provision of case management.

Child and youth case management services have been made available to seriously emotionally disturbed youth throughout the MHC catchment area. Case management activities have focused on maintaining clients in the most appropriate, least restrictive environment. This objective has been pursued through accessing services, facilitating interdisciplinary collaboration, linking agencies and institutions, advocating for services in the community, and maintaining appropriate family involvement.

Case managers have worked in close relationship with agency and Project staff as members of treatment teams, often providing the necessary continuity for teams composed of largely part-time

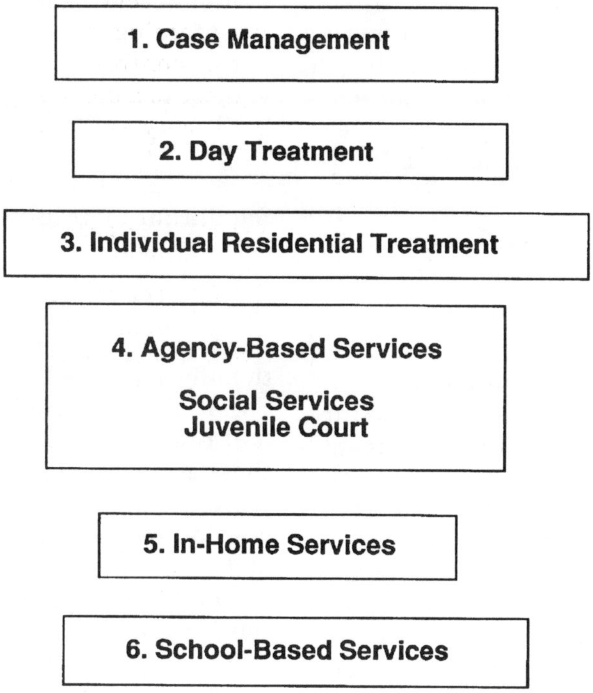

Figure 4. Community-Based Project Services

Project clinicians. When not directly involved in client treatment, case managers have also been available to staff, faculty, and trainees for consultation regarding community resources and systems. Additionally, case managers have been available to community agency staff for collaboration, consultation, and assistance in assessing appropriate treatment resources for catchment area clients. Finally, child and youth case managers have established productive linkages with regional treatment institutions including the child and adolescent inpatient units at the regional state psychiatric hospital.

Day Treatment

The Adolescent Day Treatment and Education Program (ADTEP) is jointly funded by the MHC and three participating school systems. The school systems provide funding for educational services and the MHC supports treatment efforts. Project funding ensures the MHC five placement slots in the ADTEP, thereby extending the range of services available to seriously emotionally disturbed children and providing Project trainees with a valuable community treatment resource.

Clients placed in ADTEP receive services including individual educational programming, individual and group therapies, social skills training, rehabilitation assessment and intervention, recreational and prevocational services, and group community socialization activities. Additionally, family consultation, support, and therapy are made available to receptive families. Through the mechanism of the integrated clinical staff meeting, ADTEP clients are now more readily served by additional treatment resources in the service continuum including the psychopharmacology clinic, case management, and outreach services.

A therapeutic preschool (TPS) program provides day treatment services to children in one county. This early intervention program is designed to remediate social and developmental deficits and involves parents in the treatment process. A psychology intern now provides a full day of services to the TPS and the local clinic, serving primarily preschool-aged children, most of whom have been victims of sexual, physical, or emotional abuse. In addition to evaluation, consultation, and treatment, the psychology intern is involved in interagency and court proceedings designed to focus attention on the needs of abuse victims. Additionally, a child psychiatry resident has provided weekly consultation and evaluation to the TPS clients.

Individual Residential Treatment

As a result of Project funding, the recruitment, training, and supervision of licensed therapeutic homes have been expanded in the MHC catchment area. In this program, children in need of out-of-home treatment are placed in private homes with trained families who implement carefully developed plans for residential care. A permanent part-time therapeutic home placement support position has been recently created and will help maintain children placed in this type of residential care. The children's services community residential care coordinator supervises the training and licensure procedures for the families (therapeutic parents) who are recruited. These efforts have resulted in the creation of a small pool of therapeutic home service providers that is expected to grow over time.

The implementation of individual residential treatment services has been an invaluable addition to the alternative services available through the MHC and Project clinicians. Under supervision, social work trainees have provided extensive placement support to therapeutic parents. Generally, Project trainees accessed this community-based residential alternative for their clients. They learn to differentiate between clients needing hospitalization and clients able to benefit from less restrictive, community-based therapeutic home placement. Individual residential treatment services enable clients to avoid both emergency hospitalizations and extracommunity placements while avoiding the attendant disruptions in community treatment, educational placement, and social support.

Interagency collaboration—especially with the Department of Social Services and Juvenile Court Services—has been a consistent characteristic of treatment planning, placement, and service delivery for seriously emotionally disturbed clients served through individualized residential treatment. Community agency staff have been responsive to the introduction of community-based individualized residential treatment, but consistently identify a need for expanded services.

Psychological Services to Affiliated Agencies

Significant interagency linkage to Project service delivery is accomplished through the provision of psychological services based at two affiliated agencies. In order to better respond to the diagnostic and treatment needs of the behaviorally and emotionally disturbed clients of the Department of Social Services and Juvenile Court Services, a half-time staff psychologist is provided to each of these agencies. Support provided by these psychologists includes direct services to agency clients and indirect services in the form of consultation and training provided to agency staff. Clients in need of more extensive treatment are referred to the MHC or regional treatment institutions.

Juvenile court. A psychologist provides services to the juvenile court, including comprehensive psychological evaluations, case management, competency evaluations, crisis assessments, and treatment to individuals, families, and groups. Client-related consultation is provided to court personnel and public school personnel. In-service training has been developed and provided for court personnel. Training topics have included "Social Skills Group Treatment" and "Assessment and Treatment of Juvenile Sex Offenders." In addition, a sex offenders treatment group has been developed that is ongoing and now serving clients identified through the court system.

Department of social services. Psychological services are provided to a county's Department of Social Services, including direct evaluation and treatment services to clients and client families. Indirect services include staff training, client related consultation, and program development consultation. Services are provided at numerous sites, including satellite offices, schools, and client homes.

Parent–child observation sessions are held for additional clients to inform them of treatment and placement recommendations. Treatment to Department of Social Services client families includes child, parent, and family therapies ranging from brief, situation-specific interventions to ongoing supportive therapy. The role of the psychologist in this setting has evolved over time and now places greater emphasis on consultation with staff around client needs and referral to appropriate service providers.

The Department of Social Services and juvenile court representatives continue to report that the psychological services and consultation provided have been extremely valuable in identifying and meeting the mental health treatment needs of children and youth served by their agencies. One of the psychologists has been involved in the integrated clinical staffing process discussed earlier that has resulted in the strengthening of the structural linkage between the Department of Social Services and the MHC.

The social work faculty and trainees also have established an ongoing parent support and skills group at one county health department. Trainees spend several months learning the routine of the clinic, developing an understanding of resources in the county, and establishing working relationships with clinic staff and clients. In addition to the group, trainees provide early assessment of developmental delays and referrals to other community agencies, and act as a link between the health department and the mental health system.

In-Home Services

In-home services are provided to the Project clients by the School of Social Work trainees. In-home family therapy is provided for families who, for a variety of reasons, were unable to access center-based family therapy. Psychology interns occasionally provide in-home services for clients' families assessed to be unable to participate in center-based family treatment. Psychology interns also have provided ongoing supportive contacts to clients placed at the regional state psychiatric hospital.

School-Based Services

Psychology and social work interns provide school-based services. As a direct outgrowth of services provided through the Project, a pilot program —the School Intervention Project—has been established though which group therapy is offered to students in the self-contained behaviorally and emotionally handicapped classes in one school system. Additionally, individual therapy slots are made available to selected students. Although not provided directly under its funding, the three psychologists delivering this service are associated with the Project. This pilot was arranged through a separate contract with the affiliated school system resulting from mutual awareness of a need that emerged from Project services. Additionally, through a Children's Trust Fund Grant, an early intervention program targeting children at risk for abuse and neglect has been established at one elementary school. The Project provides school-based individual and group therapy to students, as well as individualized, in-home outreach services to families of at-risk children. Consultation with school staff and interagency, community-based treatment planning also occur. Both programs are utilizing Medicaid reimbursement to fund programming. Both are integrated with, and have access to, the full range of support services available through the Project.

These are exciting examples of how the Project has contributed to the growth and development of child and youth services and of the increasing willingness of community agencies to engage in and support collaborative models for service delivery. Finally, the impact of the Project on fostering the development of more client-centered treatment approaches has been significant.

Training Curriculum

The development of a standardized, accountable system for tracking and evaluating training objectives has begun. This effort takes on the form of an individualized educational plan for each trainee that will include individual trainee goals, departmental or school goals, and a common core of objectives identified by the MHC. (See Appendixes A and B, this chapter, for some initial objectives and resources from the Project.) These objectives will operate as a core curriculum that will serve as a foundation for more specialized discipline or agency-specific curricula and evaluation of Project training outcomes. Additionally, as a result of the School of Social Work's participation in the Project, the North Carolina Division of Mental Health, Developmental Disabilities, and Substance Abuse Services (MH/DD/SAS) has begun working with the School to develop a child mental health case management curriculum. Although literature already exists on case management in general and on children's case management within child welfare services, it is believed that case management in the context of child mental health services must respond to very specialized needs. The ambitious collaborative project has produced a comprehensive curriculum for use in university settings and for the in-service training of mental health professionals.

Financing

In 1988, the North Carolina General Assembly appropriated $367,000 to UNC to implement the Project. The funding has been renewed each year at the same level. However, since the second year of the Project, the appropriation has been to the North Carolina Division of MH/DD/SAS and then contracted to the Orange-Person-Chatham MHC. The Division is actively pursuing other resources to subsidize the Project. Title IV-E foster care monies are one potential source of funds from the maintenance and supervision (that is, nontherapy and education) costs in the Project's residential therapeutic homes. Also, both Title XIX and Title IV-E provides for the reimbursement of costs for training mental health professionals who work directly with Medicaid and Title IV-E-eligible youth. The project is closely tracking these costs and will seek reimbursement.

Summary

In response to statewide concerns about the shortage of trained child mental health professionals in the state of North Carolina, the Orange–Person–Chatham Mental Health Center has established a demonstration site for training. The Child and Youth Demonstration Project's mission is to provide training experiences within a model that is consistent with state-of-the-art theory and practice of community mental health for children. Trainees from the psychology department (postinternship Ph.D. candidates), psychiatry department (residents in child psychiatry), and Schools of Nursing and Social Work (master's level), have been involved in the provision of selective clinical services under the intensive supervision of faculty-level staff (faculty liaisons) from each school or department. Services are provided to MHC clients in a variety of settings, including mental health center offices, schools, client homes, and community agencies. Trainees from the School of Nursing and the School of Social Work have concentrated on outreach services through the provision of in-home family therapy. Psychology trainees have participated in the provision of a full range of psychological services at MHC sites, as well as in the community and other agencies. These service and training experiences include individual, family and group psychotherapy, psychological testing, community education and consultation, case management, and interagency coordination. Psychiatry trainees have worked in a psychopharmacology clinic, assisted in center-based evaluations with a diagnostic and prescriptive orientation, and screened emergency clients through the crisis service.

The Project has provided resources to expand services at the MHC in the following areas:

- therapeutic foster care for clients in need of emergency respite and short-term therapeutic placement,
- emergency screening to more effectively serve children in crisis,
- a behavior clinic that serves psychopharmacological needs of children and adolescents, and
- an adolescent day treatment and education program.

Project faculty share responsibility for locating or developing training resources, modules, reading lists, seminar presentations, or mini-courses in targeted content areas. Each school or department and the MHC develops a list of discipline or agency-specific training objectives and desired outcomes regarding competencies in community-based mental health services. Through analysis of these objectives, a core curriculum is being developed that will serve as a foundation for more specialized discipline or agency-specific curricula.

APPENDIX A

Elements of the Training Curriculum

Core Principles

1. The task of providing a broad array of community-based services for children requires many skills in the community—negotiating systems change, working with advocacy groups, dealing with bureaucratic regulations, navigating complex funding streams, and so forth. The work of the mental health professional on behalf of seriously emotionally disturbed youth significantly involves the cultivation and use of these skills. Although counseling and other traditional skills remain essential, these other responsibilities must be looked on with equal importance.

2. There is a difference between a child being appropriate for a particular service versus being appropriate because an alternative service is not available.

3. The epidemiology of childhood psychiatric disorders is the preeminent determining factor in how intervention is pursued. The responsibility of public mental health services is to all severely emotionally disturbed youth. To use intervention technologies that can reach only a small portion of those in need is not a responsible use of public resources. The key responsibility is to use approaches that can realistically reach the greatest numbers of afflicted people.

4. A *system of care* is a fundamental concept because it encourages all agencies and informal helping sources to contribute to the treatment of the child, whereas a *continuum of care* implies that the preponderance of services are provided by the mental health system.

5. The question is not what kind of placement is appropriate but rather what is necessary to maintain a particular child in his or her own home and community.

6. The concept of empowering families is dynamic. On the one hand, it involves no longer blaming families or parents for a child's "psychopathology" and joining with parents as partners in the therapeutic process. But it is more. It means giving families the skills to seek ongoing supports that they need for their family. It means often helping families to obtain "things" that will reverberate throughout their lives to indirectly attenuate the disturbance of the their child.

Attitudes, Knowledge, Skills

Attitudes

1. Parents should not be blamed for their child's problems but rather are brought into the therapeutic process as partners.

2. Children should receive treatment in the least restrictive environment and one that approximates as closely as possible the most normal living environment.

3. Services should be accessible to families. For example, transportation to services should be readily available to clients, service costs should be based on ability to pay, outreach services should be available, and services should not be dependent on a client's motivation to be at an appointment at a designated time.

4. The most severely disturbed youth should be given the highest priority to receive services. Those youth should not be institutionalized so less disturbed youth can be treated with local resources. In most cases, youth who are sent away for residential treatment can be treated locally but require a much greater share of service delivery time.

Knowledge

5. The continuum of care is a central concept in the delivery of mental health services. A broad array of services must be available to children and offered in optimal ratios of capacities.

6. The system of care extends beyond the continuum (which focuses on mental health services) to include other agencies and informal resources that contribute to the resources needed for the emotionally disturbed child.

7. An ecological perspective is fundamental to a system of care. It broadens the context of assessment and intervention to include other relation-

ship systems beyond the family (e.g., school, workplace, etc). In this perspective, the individual's problem is not restricted to the family context but extends to other physical and social contexts within which he or she interacts.

8. Transition services—from child to adult services—for youth who turn 18 years old must be carefully constructed.

9. Creative funding of public mental health services is a necessity. The use of entitlements and other funding mechanisms can ensure monies for a broader array of services.

Skills

10. Cultural competence: Service providers must be familiar with methods and implications for cross cultural interactions.

11. Informal helping systems: Service providers must be familiar with methods of augmenting family supports by identifying and intervening with informal support systems.

12. Case management services are central to the operation of a system of care: All clinicians, not just specialized case managers, must have facility in case management skills. Case management skills and functions should be viewed as equal in importance to "psychotherapy."

13. Collaboration: Clinicians must prioritize interagency collaborations and develop skills to facilitate the interactions. Interagency collaborations are essential to the concept of a system of care.

APPENDIX B
Curriculum Resources

Training

Friedman, R. (1990). *University-based preparation of students to work with students and families.* Tampa, FL: Research and Training Center for Children's Mental Health.

Saxe, L., Cross, T., & Silverman, N. (1988). Children's mental health: The gap between what we know and what we do. *American Psychologist, 43,* 800–807.

Systems of Care

Greenley, J., & Robitschek, C. (1991). Evaluation of a comprehensive program for youth with severe emotional disturbance: An analysis of family experiences and satisfaction. *American Journal of Orthopsychiatry, 61,* 291–297.

Stroul, B., & Friedman, R. (1986). *A system of care for severely emotionally disturbed children and youth.* Washington, DC: CASSP Technical Assistance Center.

Cultural Competence

Sue, D. W., & Sue, D. (1990). *Counseling the culturally different: Theory and practice.* New York: Wiley.

Crisis Intervention

Gutstein, S., Rudd, M., Graham, J., & Rayha, L. (1988). Systematic crisis intervention as a response to adolescent crises: An outcome study. *Family Process, 27,* 201–211.

Psychiatric Hospitalization

Crespi, T. (1989). *Child and adolescent psychopathology and involuntary hospitalization: A handbook for mental health professionals.* Springfield, IL: Charles C Thomas.

Groze, V. (1990). An exploratory investigation into institutional mistreatment. *Children and Youth Services Review, 12,* 229–241.

Johnson, A. (1990). *Out of bedlam: The truth about deinstitutionalization.* New York: Basic Books.

Pfeiffer, S., & Strzelecki, S. (1990). Inpatient psychiatric treatment of children and adolescents: A review of outcome studies. *Journal of the American Academy of Child Psychiatry, 29,* 847–853.

Weithorn, L. (1988). Mental hospitalization of troublesome youth: An analysis of skyrocketing admission rates. *Stanford Law Review, 40,* 773–838.

Ecological/Systems Viewpoints

Combrinck-Graham, L. (1990). *Giant steps: Therapeutic innovations in child mental health.* New York: Basic Books.

Munger, R. (1991). *Child mental health practice from the ecological perspective.* Lanham, MD: University Press of America.

Informal Helping Networks

Belle, D. (Ed.). (1989). *Children's social networks and social supports.* New York: Wiley.

Pargament, K., Ensing, D., Falgout, K., Olsen, H., Reilly, B., Van Haitsma, K., & Warren, R. (1990). God help me: Religious coping efforts as predictors of the outcome to significant life events. *American Journal of Community Psychology, 18,* 793–824.

Pearson, R. (1990). *Counseling and social support: Perspectives and practice.* Newbury Park, CA: Sage.

Case Management

Moxley, D. (1989). *The practice of case management.* Newbury Park, CA: Sage.

Family Preservation and Home-Based Services

Cole, E., & Duva, J. (1990). *Family preservation: An orientation for administrators and practitioners.* Washington, DC: Child Welfare League of America.

Spinelli, L., & Barton, K. (1980). Home management services for families with emotionally disturbed children. *Child Welfare, 59,* 43–52.

Day Treatment and Education

Knitzer, J., Steinberg, Z., & Fleisch, B. (1990). *At the schoolhouse door: An examination of programs and policies for children with behavioral and emotional problems.* New York: Bank Street College of Education.

Zimet, S., & Farley, G. (1991). *Day treatment for children with emotional disorders.* New York: Plenum Press.

Therapeutic Homes

Meadowcroft, P., & Trout, B. (Eds.). (1990). *Troubled youth in treatment homes: A handbook of therapeutic foster care.* Washington, DC: Child Welfare League of America.

CHAPTER

15

Initiatives in Ohio With Seriously Emotionally Disturbed Children and Adolescents

W. Rodney Hammond and Betty Yung
Wright State University

The blending of state and federal support to develop a specialized training focus has resulted in a unique public–academic linkage program in Ohio. Using grant funding awarded by the Ohio Department of Mental Health as companion support for a grant from the National Institute of Mental Health, the School of Professional Psychology at Wright State University in Dayton, Ohio, has developed and begun to implement a program to prepare doctoral-level clinical psychology students for clinical services to children and adolescents with serious emotional disturbance. The NIMH award specifically has supported the preparation of ethnic minority students for service roles with this priority population, and the state awards have provided administrative support for detailed planning of the academic and experiential components of this specialized training emphasizing interdisciplinary elements as well as continued funding for teaching and supervision in the implementation phase.

This chapter will trace the evolution of this partnership program beginning with a description of the state's funding structure and the School's historical application of state resources. Factors influencing program design including the School's areas of strength and mission emphasis will be highlighted as background to a description of the planning and development of this new clinical training track.

Although the clinical psychology training program at Wright State University has always served as a unique resource to the public mental health system in Ohio, the full potential of the public–academic relationship was not realized prior to this initiative. In addition, the state-sponsored training efforts in which the School had participated were not directed toward the needs of a particular population. For several years, the Ohio Department of Mental Health has provided support for the following purposes:

- stipends for predoctoral students for practicum placements in public mental health settings,
- curriculum or seminar development,
- support for faculty to teach or supervise students in practicum placements,
- nontraditional placements,
- support for student attendance at mental health conferences,
- fifth-year residencies (clinical, research, or administrative),
- stipends for special population students, and
- in-service training.

Cross-cutting themes and priorities, as extrapolated from requests for proposals (RFPs) issued by the Department, have included interdisciplinary training; training to prepare students to work with special populations such as severely mentally disabled adults, forensic clients, individuals with deafness or severe hearing impairment, or dual diagnosis individuals (e.g., mentally retarded and mentally ill, or substance abuser and mentally ill); support for students or faculty who are minorities, mental health consumers, or individuals with deafness or severe hearing impairment; use of staff from the public mental health sector as faculty in university training; and use of an advisory committee representative from the geographic, cultural, and consumer populations to be served.

As shown in Table 1, prior to 1989, the Wright State University training program had previously used state grant support for somewhat traditional purposes (i.e., stipend support to place students in clinical practica at such locations as community mental health centers, inpatient treatment facilities, and forensic settings). Although these were valuable training experiences and in some cases resulted in a student's choosing the public mental health sector as a posttraining career path, clearly such programming did not address the state's full training agenda.

Overview of the University's Professional Training Program

The potential for an enhanced relationship between the academic training program and the state and local mental health service system can be best understood in light of the School's background and special areas of emphasis. The School of Professional Psychology prepares students at the doctoral level for clinical practitioner roles in psychology. Students in the program follow a managed curriculum requiring 3 years (12 quarters, approximately 140 quarter hours) of academic studies accompanied by systematic field practice experiences and a 1-year internship leading to a PsyD degree. The training focus centers on the areas covered below.

1. *Academic coursework,* which provides an initial foundation in empirical and scientific methodologies and basic behavioral and biological sciences.

Table 1. Wright State University School of Professional Psychology State-Supported Training Initiatives

Prior to 1989	After 1989	Types of state-funded program support available
X	X	Stipends for predoctoral students for practica in public mental health settings
	X	Curriculum or seminar development
	X	Support for faculty to teach or supervise students in practicum placements
	X	Nontraditional placements
	X	Support for student attendance at mental health conferences
	X	Fifth-year residencies (clinical, research, or administrative)
	X	Stipends for special population students
	X	In-service training
		Cross-cutting themes and priorities
	X	Interdisciplinary training
		Training to prepare students to work with special populations
X	X[a]	Severely mentally disabled adults
X	X[a]	Forensic
	X[a]	Individuals with deafness or severe hearing impairment
		Dual diagnosis individuals (e.g., mental retardation and mental illness substance abuse and mental illness)
		Support for students or faculty who fit into one of these categories:
	X	Minorities
		Mental health consumers
	X[a]	Individuals with deafness or severe hearing impairment
	X	Use of staff from the public mental health sector as faculty in university training
	X	Use of an advisory committee representative of the geographic, cultural, and consumer population to be served

[a] Provided through programs not discussed in this chapter.

2. *Research application and sophisticated consumption and use of research findings,* in which students develop skills in statistics, research design and methodology, and program evaluation through a research sequence.

3. *Practical training* in assessment, consultation, service delivery, general and specific proficiencies, and intervention skills in which students work closely with clinical practitioners in supervised experience. Clinical training has traditionally occurred in settings such as community agencies including community mental health centers, family and domestic courts, residential inpatient treatment centers, and medical centers; or the Psychological Services Center (PSC) managed by the School. In their PSC placements, students work under the direct supervision of School faculty. PSC operations are conducted both on campus in a medical center facility and in a recently opened facility in downtown Dayton. The new facility, called the Duke E. Ellis Human Development Institute, extends mental health services to a regional client population, with an emphasis on time-limited, focused assessment and intervention, as well as competency enhancement. Examples of PSC programs in which students may receive clinical training include a counseling center for university students, a psychometric laboratory (a program for gifted children and their families), a faculty-owned and -operated practice group, and special programs directed by School faculty.

Recently, the School has begun to offer special proficiency track studies that prepare students for specialization in particular areas such as pediatric and adolescent psychology, forensic psychology, health psychology, feminist psychology, organizational consulting, and general practice.

Since the School's beginning, its training approach has emphasized preparation for practice roles, in particular in services to underserved populations. In addition, the School was established with a specifically mandated legislative mission of increasing the supply of minority clinical psychologists. The School's written mission statement expresses this intent, and a central value has been placed on developing programs and policies to encourage and support the training of ethnic minority students. Areas receiving special attention have included a vigorous and multifaceted recruitment program, including specially developed multicultural recruitment materials; an equitable, value-based admissions process; a culturally sensitive training environment, including coursework and practica focusing on minority mental health issues and exposure to minority practitioner role models; a strong student support system, including academic and personal development; and innovative ways to support the financial needs of minority trainees such as using overhead from the faculty-owned and -operated private practice. Such programs and practices have resulted in a high degree of success in the training of ethnic minority students; they address a nationally recognized need for greater use of diverse strategies to promote more equitable participation in clinical psychology training and practice (Hammond & Yung, 1993). In particular, the School has graduated a large percentage of African-American students, as shown in Table 2.

These accomplishments in the training of ethnic minority students were instrumental in helping the School to compete successfully in 1989 for an award from NIMH that has provided essential fellowship support to ethnic minority students to prepare them to deliver mental health services to children and adolescents with serious emotional disturbance.

Planning Project Objectives

Because the administrative support for program development provided through the National Institute of Mental Health (NIMH) grant was very limited, in 1990 the School applied for and received a planning grant from the Ohio Department of Mental Health. This grant provided companion support for capacity building for this special proficiency training. In particular, it allowed for a broadening of the disciplinary base. The planning grant had two programmatic emphases: (a) development of new coursework that would incorporate academic content from related disciplines, and (b) planning for clinical experiences that would team the psychology trainees with multidisciplinary groups of mental health, education, and human services professionals in staffing patterns comparable to those found in settings serving children and adolescents with multiple needs and problems. The specific objectives of the Ohio Department of Mental Health-funded planning project included the following:

1. To develop coursework blending education and mental health curricular content in the area of behavior management of children and adolescents with severe behavioral handicaps and emotional disturbance.

Table 2. Ethnic Minority Participation in Clinical Psychology Training Wright State University School of Professional Psychology

Student groups	*N*	Ethnic minorities	*n*	%
Program graduates, 1982–1991	245		44	17.90
		African-American	38	15.50
		Native American	1	.04
		Hispanic	2	.08
		Asian American	3	1.20
Current trainees	108		27	25.00
		African-American	19	17.60
		Native American	2	1.80
		Hispanic	3	2.80
		Asian American	3	2.80

2. To develop coursework in multiservice systems for youth with serious emotional disturbance.

3. To determine curricular fit of the new courses into the existing clinical psychology training program and the special proficiency track requirements.

4. To identify potential practicum placement sites where students will receive experience in interdisciplinary teamworking and to conduct joint planning with site representatives to prepare for the placements.

5. To explore the feasibility of developing special services in the applicant's clinical training facility that can be used in training experiences for clinical psychology students.

6. To identify general curricular support for the special proficiency training.

7. To field test new courses with small groups of clinical psychology students.

8. To consult with faculty who are operating exemplary service and training programs related to the target population.

As a result of the planning grant, two new interdisciplinary elective courses were developed and provided to special proficiency trainees on a field-test basis. State grant funds allowed the hiring of adjunct faculty (previously unaffiliated with the School) from other professional training and service provider programs to develop and teach the new coursework. One faculty member is affiliated with the University of Dayton as faculty in their school psychology and counselor education training program; she provides special expertise in the area of behavior management of children and youth with severe behavior disorders. The District II director of the Children's Project for the Ohio Department of Mental Health was also used as faculty to develop and teach the course in Service Systems for seriously emotionally disturbed Youth. Her participation in the course development and training design (through service on the advisory committee) gave direct input to the project from the perspective of the state and local public mental health systems. Her course involves many classroom presentations and field trips giving students broad exposure to community mental health centers, community-based youth service agencies, criminal justice and child welfare systems, and intersystem collaboration and made extensive use of professionals working in these settings for clinical instruction.

In addition to the development of coursework, the planning project permitted the collection of a large bank of information on appropriate placement sites throughout the state that would give students practice experiences with the target population and would provide opportunities for the development of teamwork skills with practitioners of other disciplines. The potential placements included a wide range of educational, health, and mental health services such as residential treatment, parent or caregiver counseling and training, and outpatient services. Disciplines with which students might be teamed through these placements would include health-care providers (nurses, hospital social workers, neurologists, pediatricians, psychiatrists, and substance abuse counselors) or school personnel (school nurses, counselors, psychologists, and regular and special education teachers). Based on a needs assessment conducted through the project advisory committee, actual placement sites were reduced during the late spring and early summer, and formal arrangements were negotiated with the cooperating agencies so that placements could begin in the fall of 1992. In addition to the identification of practicum locations, the collection of this databank served additional useful purposes. It permitted the identification of sites for observational or experiential activities for students that constitute less than a full practicum but would broaden the trainee's understanding of services to seriously emotionally disturbed youth. Furthermore, it identified professionals from schools, hospitals, parent training programs, and other human service programs as resources for classroom presentations or for teaching of portions of courses.

During the planning grant period, the special proficiency training plan was formalized as part of the School's existing clinical psychology training program, with a curriculum committee having developed the specific guidelines for the academic and practicum requirements, approved the new courses, and identified faculty to teach the courses. In addition, a review of syllabi in existing courses in the School's curriculum was initiated to determine where content related to the special proficiency could be integrated into the regular course of study. The content for the child psychopathology course, and other child-related courses, was revised through this process. The curricular revision process has been continuous throughout the program and has been beneficial in that it allows the incorporation of content based on recent research findings related to the priority population. Modest support from both the state planning grant and the NIMH award was helpful in this regard because it permitted professional development activities such as conference attendance and consultation on model programs and research related to seriously emotionally disturbed children and youth.

A broad-based advisory committee to provide oversight to the training initiative was established. The advisory committee is made up of representatives from the following groups:

1. School of Professional Psychology faculty staff: Providers of, and expertise in, academic and clinical training.

2. School of Professional Psychology students: Consumers of academic and clinical training.

3. State and local mental health system: Providers of planning, policies, and funding for services to the target population.

4. Public mental health agencies: Providers of services to the target population and consumers of the services of trainees and graduates.

5. Private mental health agencies: Providers of services to the target population and consumers of the services of trainees and graduates.

6. Consumers: Recipients of services to the target population (parents of seriously emotionally disturbed youth; current or former youth clients).

An innovation in the experiential component of the training resulted from state budget cuts that reduced the size of the grant award for the implementation phase of the project. Because the cut was significant, initially it appeared that the ability of the School to offer the desired training plan at its optimal level would be threatened. However, the local mental health service providers on the advisory committee, who had become enthusiastic and invested in serving as placement sites, responded by requesting partial support from their affiliated agencies. Four trainees were supported from the practicum plan that evolved as a result of the funding reduction. This practicum, which has now become a permanent part of the training initiative, features a rotational placement of trainees within multiple, newly affiliated child service settings, allowing for diversity of experience across the continuum of care. The child practicum consortium also allows for a secondary level of collaborative on-site supervision from professionals in medical, nursing, special education, and allied health fields so that interdisciplinary teamworking knowledge and skills can be obtained. Table 3 illustrates the site rotation plan.

Building from this foundation, the basic training approach has stabilized. State and local financial support has continued, enabling the program to be carried forward despite the end of federal funding. Minor year-to-year refinements continue to be made in both the didactic and experiential training components. As the program has matured, the need for targeted development of advanced training experiences has been recognized. Internship and postdoctoral placements to develop higher levels of proficiency in the specialty study are especially needed. At present these needs are addressed through locating external child-related placements within the state or around the country. It would be helpful if federal support were available to develop and offer such placements in house so that sequential building of knowledge and skills could be assured.

Attention is also needed at the exit end of the training continuum. The development of the special proficiency training at the preprofessional level should be accompanied by efforts to prepare

Table 3. Child Mental Health Services Practicum Consortium

	Placement and Clinical Rotation Model			
Month	Site 1	Site 2	Site 3	Site 4
September	Trainee 1	Trainee 2	Trainee 3	Trainee 4
October	↓	↓	↓	↓
November	↓	↓	↓	↓
December	Trainee 4	Trainee 1	Trainee 2	Trainee 3
January	↓	↓	↓	↓
February	↓	↓	↓	↓
March	Trainee 3	Trainee 4	Trainee 1	Trainee 2
April	↓	↓	↓	↓
May	↓	↓	↓	↓
June	Trainee 2	Trainee 3	Trainee 4	Trainee 1
July	↓	↓	↓	↓
August	↓	↓	↓	↓

Note. Site 1: Severe Behavior Disorder Program, day treatment, jointly staffed through Community Mental Health Center and county school district; Site 2: Intermediate district preschool-age and school-age programs for children with moderate to profound developmental and behavioral disabilities and their families (County Board of Mental Retardation and Developmental Disorders); Site 3: Residential treatment center (programs for children and adolescents, including 6–12 mo lengths of stay); Site 4: Hospital-based treatment unit (emergency and acute care primarily for adolescents).

a career path for program trainees. We have tried to meet this need by keeping the state mental health department informed of the progress of trainees and encouraging them to locate or develop appropriate positions for upcoming graduates in the Ohio public service system.

Conclusion

The experiences of developing and implementing the special proficiency training in services to children and adolescents with serious emotional disturbance emphasize the need for flexibility and creativity in approach, given the differing missions and complexities of service and academic training systems and the economic realities of public funding. Out of these experiences, we have reached conclusions about the ongoing challenges facing both the academic and the public mental health service system, as follows.

1. It is important for the academic community to become more knowledgeable about state service plans, intervention philosophies, unmet service needs and underserved populations, and cost constraints.

2. It is also essential that state mental health service providers become better acquainted with university training programs including the differences between programs (philosophies and methods), and funding constraints and issues.

3. States should consider providing technical assistance to potential applicants and co-funding or matched support for federally funded programs.

4. There is a general scarcity of federal support for clinical training versus research training, assistance to training programs in recruiting and retaining minority and disadvantaged students, and administration of special training initiatives.

5. There is a need to address the problems and issues at the graduation and employment end of the training continuum; these include providing incentives for public service employment, better defined career pathways, and ways for graduates to serve the target population outside of the traditional public mental health system.

It is hoped that these conclusions will help other states formulate strong new linkages with clinical psychology training programs so that children and adolescents with serious emotional disturbance can benefit from the services of well-prepared practitioners.

Reference

Hammond, R., & Yung, B. (1993). Minority student recruitment and retention practices among schools of professional psychology: A national survey and analysis. *Professional Psychology: Research and Practice, 24,* 3–12.

CHAPTER

16

The Cincinnati Consortium: Training for Services to Seriously Mentally Disabled Adults and Their Families

David T. Hellkamp
Xavier University

Over the past 2 decades, an emerging body of research and practice has provided technologies for how to intervene with people with serious mental disorders. Anthony, Cohen, and Kennard (1990) have listed many of the different psychiatric rehabilitation technologies, and Hellkamp (1993) has discussed rehabilitative psychotherapies that exist for treating the seriously mentally disabled patients and their families. As Anthony, et al., 1990, stated about the technologies:

> they are developed to the point at which instructors can teach it, service providers can perform it, administrators can monitor it, researchers can evaluate it, consultants can shape it, and consumers and family members can observe it before they participate in it. Service models, training curricula, and consultation strategies exist. (p. 1252).

Very few graduate psychology programs in the United States currently train their students in these intervention procedures as applied to the seriously mentally disabled population. In 1989, a member of our Academic Steering Committee conducted an informal survey of graduate psychology programs in the United States and found that only a small number of clinical psychology programs had any curriculum incorporating psychiatric rehabilitation concepts. Discussions with the National Institute of Mental Health (NIMH) and the Educational Affairs Office of the American Psychological Association reinforced these findings.

Although technologies such as the psychiatric rehabilitation models have frequently been developed by psychologists such as Anthony, Cohen, and Farkas (1988) and Farkas and Anthony (1989), the technologies have generally not been integrated into mainstream psychology in journals and textbooks. For example, Halter, Bond, and DeGraaf-Kaser (1990) conducted a computerized search of the *Journal of Abnormal Psychology*

David T. Hellkamp is a professor in the Department of Psychology, Xavier University, Cincinnati, Ohio 45207. My thanks to Don Cosgrove and Susan Wideman for their comments on earlier drafts of this chapter. Similar appreciation is expressed to the Academic Steering Committee members of the consortium at Xavier University, the University of Cincinnati, and the Ohio Department of Mental Health.

and the *Journal of Consulting Clinical Psychology* between January 1985 and May 1989. Among 928 articles, only 49 (5%) were at best peripherally related to severe mental disorders. Most of these concerned assessment instruments, research design, and psychotherapy. Of the 184 articles appearing in *Rehabilitation Psychology* since 1982, only 15 (8%) have dealt with psychiatric rehabilitation. A recent examination of mainstream psychology textbooks also highlights the void in coverage of rehabilitation concepts in dealing with seriously mentally disabled people. In a content analysis of 28 introductory psychology textbooks published between 1983 and 1987, Halter et al. (1990) found significantly more space devoted to both drug treatment and hospital treatment than to any of the community treatments developed over the past 30 years. There was slightly more space devoted to lobotomies than to all community treatments combined. There was no mention of psychiatric rehabilitation. A content analysis of 14 textbooks on abnormal psychology published between 1980 and 1989 was only slightly more encouraging (Halter et al. 1990). The concept of a community support system was mentioned in only 2 (14%) of the abnormal psychology texts and none of the 28 introductory texts.

Although a multitude of psychiatric rehabilitation programs are in operation, very few have conceptualized a theoretical underpinning for their practice, with fewer yet having offered much empirical validation for their procedures. Nevertheless, one such psychiatric rehabilitation model with promise is the Boston University program (Farkas & Anthony, 1989). The Boston University rehabilitation model includes strategies and techniques for diagnosing, planning, and intervening in the rehabilitation of seriously mentally disabled clients (Farkas, 1990). Although these technologies were developed by combining principles and techniques from both the field of rehabilitation and the field of psychotherapy, the model cannot be reduced to either field alone. The strategies and techniques are different from how psychotherapy procedures are applied under more traditional, office practice conditions and are different from traditional rehabilitation procedures for people experiencing physical disabilities.

Clearly, one challenge to mainstream psychology in the decade of the 1990s is to consider integrating psychiatric rehabilitation knowledge and skills, as well as other technologies and psychotherapies, for intervening with SMD, not only into mainstream psychology literature but, more importantly, into the curriculum and training experiences of graduate programs. Within the public sector, policymakers on both the state and federal levels have been calling for psychology's involvement by providing incentives for training programs willing to integrate curriculum and training in working with seriously mentally ill populations (Hanley, 1990; Hargrove, 1990a, 1990b; Hyde, 1988; Stratoudakis, Tomes, Wohlford & Stockdill, chapter 7, this volume). The Ohio Project, described below, is one such effort.

The Ohio Project

Seven faculty members from two different universities (University of Cincinnati and Xavier University [XU]), representing four different disciplines (psychiatric nursing, psychology, psychiatry, and social work) and five different departments (two different psychology departments, one doctoral program at UC, and one masters' program at XU), began meeting regularly with a community planning specialist. A grant proposal was developed by the two-university group for a multidisciplinary training program to prepare the four core mental health professionals to work with the seriously mentally disabled population and their families. A modest planning grant of $30,000 from the Ohio Department of Mental Health (ODMH) enabled us to continue working together for the academic year of 1986–1987. We called ourselves the Academic Steering Committee and have become known as a part of "the Ohio project." Since then, we have been awarded five major grants from ODMH with the mission to train graduate students and psychiatric residents in the four core disciplines at the two universities in multidisciplinary collaboration skills and successful intervention skills with the seriously mentally disabled population. Additionally, our mission is to positively influence the attitudes and skills of mental health educators, students, and professionals toward this client group and their families. To achieve those ends, the program is aimed at improving the curriculum and training of the four core mental health professionals.

From the beginning, we considered it most important to include the opinions of relevant community members who work and live with the SMD population. We therefore formed a Community Advisory Committee, comprised of university faculty (ourselves), community mental health administrators, providers, consumers, and their family members. Input regarding perceived training needs was obtained from the community members via surveys and group meetings. Our original plans included developing multidisciplinary course modules to be cross-listed across departments and universities and to be made available for students from any of the disciplines. It soon became apparent that a multitude of practical considerations (e.g., semester vs. quarter systems, different accreditation requirements, etc.) made the approach unwieldy. As a result, our curriculum planning and development objectives have evolved as follows: (a) to encourage each discipline at each university to review existing courses and program experiences in an effort to identify training gaps and to incorporate appropriate knowledge and skill experiences about the SMD patients and their families, (b) to encourage each discipline to develop new courses while also integrating a knowledge and skill base into more traditional courses and training experiences, (c) to develop a multidisciplinary series of seminars on the seriously mentally disabled population for selected students and psychiatric residents presented at an approved training site, and (d) to teach and promote collaboration skills to graduate students and psychiatric residents for working in gaining an interdisciplinary training experience.

In order to develop our own faculty expertise, a working grant was successfully obtained from the Boston University team funded by NIMH and headed by Bill Anthony and Marianne Farkas. The grant provided faculty training and consultation to meet our curriculum and training objectives, especially by incorporating state-of-the-art psychiatric rehabilitation knowledge and skills into our programs. The Boston experience was not only extremely valuable in that our faculty learned a particular model and set of technologies in psychiatric rehabilitation, but it also opened some of our eyes as to how the psychiatric rehabilitation technology can merge with some of the more traditional clinical interventions with the seriously mentally disabled population. On a more basic level, the Boston experience infused an even greater atmosphere of optimism in our group for working successfully with this population.

In preparing for the first year of implementation (1987–1988), we invited mental health agencies of the Greater Cincinnati area to submit a proposal for collaborating with us as a clinical training site. Due to our objective to develop multidisciplinary team experiences for both staff and students, health agencies submitting proposals were required, among other criteria, to be willing to form interdisciplinary teams in working with the seriously mentally disabled patients and their families. Three clinical training sites were selected by the Academic Steering Committee: (a) a state extended-care hospital that serves adults, (b) a university-based clinic, and (c) a comprehensive community mental health center. Since the first year, we have expanded the clinical training sites to agencies that do not include all four disciplines. In reality, the interdisciplinary team experiences over this first year taught us that it was unrealistic in all cases to define *team* in a way that mandates participation from all four core disciplines simultaneously. Although considered ideal, such a team composition does not reflect the staffing patterns found in all sites in the real world.

The impact of our joint efforts has been significant within the training experiences of all five academic departments as well as within mental health agencies in the Greater Cincinnati area. It was critical to develop good training experiences provided by clinical staff in community support agencies (e.g., hospitals, community mental health centers (CMHC), case management agencies, rehabilitation agencies, etc.). The level of training experience provided at the University and at the clinical sites where students are placed for traineeships, practica, and so forth, are frequently at different levels of development. It has been our experience that clinical social workers and psychiatric nurses working in clinical sites are more acquainted with state-of-the-art rehabilitation knowledge and skills than are staff psychologists and psychiatrists. Consequently, some of our efforts and strategies have been directed at developing a mechanism for providing continuing education programs to train clinical staff already employed in community agencies. The Community Advisory Committee is currently playing a major role in our development of continuing education programs aimed at improving agency staff attitudes, and their knowledge base and skills are helping in working with the seriously mentally disabled population.

Xavier University Masters Psychology Program

Since 1961, Xavier University has been offering a masters program in psychology with concentrations in the clinical, counseling, industrial/organizational, or experimental areas. The concentration in clinical psychology has always maintained a liaison with two state hospitals in the Cincinnati area, one for student placements in a hospital for adults and geriatric seriously mentally disabled patients, and one for student placements that service seriously mentally disabled children and adolescent patients.

As part of a curriculum review process within the Department of Psychology coupled with the work of the ODMH grant, it became possible to integrate two new courses specifically focused on the seriously mentally disabled patients and their families. Drawing from the Boston University curriculum, a course called "Clinical and Research Issues: Working With the SMD Patients" was first introduced in 1988 and was designed with a knowledge-based objective (i.e., exposure-level). The second course was introduced in 1990 with a skill-based objective (i.e., experience-level) and was titled "Interventions With the SMD Population." Among other topics and technologies, these courses introduced the students to clinical issues related to rehabilitation diagnosis, rehabilitation planning, and rehabilitation intervention skills. Both of these courses are available to graduate students who are concentrating in either clinical or counseling psychology, whereas the former course is also open to advanced undergraduate students in multiple disciplines. Additionally, several of our traditional clinical and counseling courses (e.g., "Psychopathology" and "Psychological Testing") were reviewed and updated with state-of-the-art information about the seriously mentally disabled population. Other faculty members who were not involved in the training grant also had their professional consciousness raised by bringing in outside speakers to present at departmental colloquia on the topic of seriously mentally disabled patients and their families. Twenty-two of our graduate students over the past 5 years have been selected for their interest and desire to undertake working with the seriously mentally disabled population (expertise-level) via training grants in hospitals, community mental health centers, and most recently, a community case management agency. In addition to their clinical training experiences in these agencies, the selected students have also had the opportunity to attend specially designed seminars in which the academic steering committee members and outside specialists presented topics related to the seriously mentally disabled population. The format for the seminars included bringing together not only the graduate students from our program at Xavier, but also the nursing, psychology, and social work graduate students and psychiatric residents from the University of Cincinnati. In practice, it has been primarily the psychology and social work graduate students that have participated in these seminars. Unfortunately, it has been difficult to attract as many nurses and psychiatric residents into this part of the program. Nursing has been limited because of the limited number of nurses accepted into the program each year, and the psychiatric residents are all currently funded by different training monies in other agencies. In contrast, all psychology and social work graduate students are funded strictly through the ODMH grant. The Academic Steering Committee is looking at possible incentives for attracting more nurses and psychiatric residents into the seminar series.

The graduate students in all disciplines who were funded by the ODMH grant were placed in an approved clinical site (e.g., state mental hospital) and expected to work a set number of hours a week (e.g., 16 hrs) with the seriously mentally disabled population while also attending relevant supervision sessions, seminars, and university functions. The ODMH grant provided each student with an hourly stipend for approximately 40 weeks a year. In psychology, the graduate students were generally selected during their second year of training from both the masters program and the doctoral program. Within the doctoral program, a number of these students have elected to renew their traineeship for a second year because they reported finding the experience both exciting and fulfilling. In both the masters and doctoral programs, a significant increase in numbers of theses focusing on research issues with the seriously mentally disabled population has occurred. Additionally, a research team specifically dealing with schizophrenic disorders was recently inaugurated.

As a result of the state–university linkage, our masters program in psychology now incorporates a state-of-the-art knowledge base (exposure) relating to the seriously mentally disabled patient and family functioning for all clinical and counseling students, while providing an experience-level of training for a smaller number of students. A select few graduate students each year have the opportunity to develop more expertise-level training through the traineeships funded by ODMH that were described above. By the time these students complete the program, they have gained at least basic skills in (a) interacting with the community mental health agencies; (b) understanding not only the roles of psychologists but also the roles of other professionals and paraprofessionals; (c) understanding the roles and functions of case management; (d) understanding basic theory and practice of psychiatric rehabilitation; (e) understanding basic research and program evaluation techniques; (f) developing a solid foundation in the theory and practice of psychodiagnostics, counseling and psychotherapy; and (g) understanding the basics of chemotherapy as applied to this population.

Teaching the skills did not require major changes in our overall 2-year masters program curriculum for students in the clinical or counseling concentrations. All students, regardless of concentration, still fulfill over 40 semester hours in courses, including a track in general psychology, a research track leading to an empirical research thesis, and selected courses in the track consistent with the student's area of concentration. Historically, a high percentage of our students have continued their graduate training in psychology, earning a doctorate.

Although it is still too early to determine precisely what job roles XU students who do not go on for a doctorate will pursue in the area of working with the seriously mentally disabled population, there does appear to be a growing market for a person with a masters degree in psychology with a concentration in serious mental disability. Apart from more traditional diagnostic and treatment roles in direct service, such students could be suitable for positions as clinical case managers (Kanter, 1989), as well as administrators and members of the counseling staff in community agencies. Detailed job roles for psychologists working with the seriously mentally disabled population have been presented elsewhere (Bond, Hellkamp, Dilk, & Eberlein, 1993). Of the 22 students at XU who have been or are being funded by the ODMH grant, 9 are still completing their masters degree with us, 5 others are currently enrolled in doctoral programs in clinical psychology at other universities, and half of the remaining former students are working in agencies that serve the seriously mentally disabled population. In all but two instances, the students have expressed a strong interest in the seriously mentally disabled population and plan to continue involvement in their future professional lives. A similar attitude is also being expressed by the graduate students in the doctoral psychology program at the University of Cincinnati.

As a final observation, I would like to make some comments about the differences in competencies between the masters student in psychology and the doctoral student in psychology, both of whom are exposed to specialized training with the seriously mentally disabled population. The graduate students in both training programs are very bright, enthusiastic men and women. When students enter the masters program at XU, the majority expect to continue to complete a doctorate in psychology. Over the past decade, fewer students in the masters program have actually continued their studies for a doctorate after completing the masters. This is probably due to geographical limitations related to an increased percentage of nontraditional students with family responsibilities. It is my opinion that the students who elect to enter the job market with a masters who have been trained in working with the seriously mentally disabled population are reasonably well grounded and would be excellent providers of service. Unfortunately, as licensing requirements in psychology have become more doctorally defined, the masters graduates find themselves without a "professional identity." The licensing laws keep them from being able to call themselves psychologists in most instances, and yet, they are different from counselors and social workers. Unfortunately, administrators in public agencies are usually not aware of the skills these masters students bring with them for working with the seriously mentally disabled patients. It has been my experience that many of these administrators still associate a student with a masters in psychology as being trained in very traditional, office practice clinical skills that they do not see as being useful for their job needs. Consequently, efforts at educating the administrators to the marketability of the masters student is necessary. The Council of Applied Master's Programs in Psychology sponsored the first national conference addressing such issues in detail (see Lowe, 1990).

Conclusion

Preparing psychologists to work effectively in the public sector with the seriously mentally disabled population and their families is a complicated and necessary undertaking. Currently, many barriers need to be overcome to gain the attention of graduate students and faculty about training programs for working with the seriously mentally disabled (e.g., the masters vs. doctoral degree issue, increased incentives [salaries] for public sector employment). Nevertheless, effective treatment requires well-trained psychologists who have developed a broad range of state-of-the-art attitudes, knowledge, and skills in working with the seriously mentally disabled population, their families, and the community support systems. Setting up a graduate program that draws students into working with the seriously mentally disabled population requires more than changing the curriculum within the department, whether on a masters or doctoral level. It also requires role models among faculty in order to develop student interest in working with the seriously mentally disabled population. Unfortunately, the zeitgeist still draws the majority of graduate students in psychology to the office practice model of service delivery in the private sector. Although we are attracting more graduate students into considering a future in the public sector, it is my opinion that the public sector policymakers must continue working at providing greater incentives for psychology students, both on a masters and doctoral level.

Current clinical training programs in psychology that elect to get involved will likely need to hire core faculty with expertise in working with the seriously mentally disabled, review and change aspects of their curriculum, consider faculty development programs, and work together to develop linkages with state, federal, and community agencies to improve research and training opportunities for their students. In our case, traineeship funding through ODMH has been critical for the evolution of our training program for working with the seriously mentally disabled. Without it, our efforts would have been impossible. Last, but not least, effective training will demand that faculty and students listen to and involve consumers and family members in this training process. Networking with the local Alliance of Mentally Ill (AMI) can be productive along those lines. AMI members have played a significant role in our Community Advisory Committee as well as being directly involved in several of our seminars.

References

Anthony, W. A., Cohen, M., & Farkas, M. D. (1988). Professional pre-service training for working with the long-term mentally ill. *Community Mental Health Journal, 24*(4), 258–268.

Anthony, W. A., Cohen, M., & Kennard, W. (1990). Understanding the current facts and principles of mental health systems planning, *American Psychologist, 45*(11), 1249–1252.

Bond, G. R., Hellkamp, D. T., Dilk, M. N., & Eberlein, L. (1993). Psychology and psychiatric rehabilitation. In M. D. Farkas and W. A. Anthony (Eds.), *Psychiatric rehabilitation and community support monograph,* 1 (*1*) (pp. 35–45). Boston: Center for Psychiatric Rehabilitation, Boston University.

Farkas, M. D. (1990). Clinical training with a rehabilitation focus. In H. P. Lefly (Ed.), *Clinical training in serious mental illness.* (DHHS Pub. No. ADM 90-1679). Washington, DC: U.S. Government Printing Office.

Farkas, M. D., & Anthony, W. A. (1989). *Psychiatric rehabilitation programs: Putting theory into practice.* Baltimore: Johns Hopkins University Press.

Halter, C. A., Bond, G. R., & DeGraaf-Kaser, R. (1992). How treatment of persons with serious mental illness is portrayed in undergraduate textbooks. *Community Mental Health Journal,* 28 (*1*), 29–42.

Hanley, J. H. (1990). Master's providers and child, adolescent and family services. In R. Tucker (Ed.), *Sourcebook for the National Conference on Applied Master's Training in Psychology* (p. 45). Norman: University of Oklahoma.

Hargrove, D. S. (1990a). Key issues in training in psychology for service to the seriously mentally ill. In H. P. Lefley (Ed.), *Clinical training in serious mental illness* (pp. 53–63). (DHHS Pub. No. ADM 90-1679). Washington, DC: U.S. Government Printing Office.

Hargrove, D. S. (1990b). Public–academic linkages. In R. Tucker (Ed.), *Sourcebook for the National Conference on Applied Master's Training in Psychology* (pp. 34–35). Norman: University of Oklahoma.

Hellkamp, D. T. (1993). Serious mental disorders. In G. Stricker & S. Gold (Eds.), *Comprehensive handbook of psychotherapy integration* (pp. 385–398). New York: Plenum Press.

Hyde, P. S. (1988, September). *Welcoming speech.* Presented at the Tenth National Human Resources Development Assembly. Columbus, OH:

Kanter, J. (1989). Clinical case management: Definition, principles, components. *Hospital and Community Psychiatry, 40*(4), 361–368.

Lowe, R. H. (1990). *Proceedings of the National Conference on Applied Master's Training in Psychology.* Norman: University of Oklahoma.

CHAPTER

17

Developing the Maryland Training Consortium on Serious Mental Illness

Robert D. Coursey
University of Maryland at College Park

Stanley E. Weinstein
Maryland Mental Hygiene Administration

Lee E. Deckelnick
Maryland Association of Psychiatric Support Services

The concept of linkage is sometimes thought of as a connection between the public service system and the state university. However, the reality—at least in our state—is that systemwide linkages are needed among the mental health centers, rehabilitation services, hospitals, the multiple educational institutions, and the human resource development staffs from the state, county, and private nonprofit organizations. Thus, for example, a single liaison between a graduate psychology department and a community mental health center, while worthwhile, does not have the range of expertise and resources needed to make a significant impact on the needs of educational programs or the needs of staff who work with clients with serious mental illnesses.

Background and History of Linkage Efforts in the State of Maryland

Before we describe the development of the Consortium, three major players in the state need to be described: the Maryland Human Resource Development Division of the Mental Hygiene Administration (MHA), Maryland Association of Psychiatric Support Services (MAPSS), and the relevant University of Maryland departments.

Maryland Human Resource Development Division

Prior to 1979, the state paid little attention to a systematic view of human resources available or necessary to deliver quality services. The state needed to develop the capacity for human resource development and planning. Data on staffing was often not available or reliable, academic linkages had a history of failure, and the state did not grasp the relevant human resource development issues and problems in order for prioritization to occur. Problems in the recruitment, distribution,

We would like to thank all of the members of the Maryland Training Consortium on Serious Mental Illness for developing the material on Appendixes B–E, for their work in developing the Consortium, and for their commitment to education and training.

utilization, and retention of personnel undermined the attempt to provide better services. In 1979 and 1984, Maryland was awarded capacity-building grants from the National Institute of Mental Health (NIMH). As a result of this opportunity, the Human Resource Development Division accomplished many initiatives (see Appendix A, this chapter) that set the stage for later developments.

Maryland Association of Psychiatric Support Services (MAPSS)

MAPSS represents 50 community and residential rehabilitation agencies serving Maryland adults with severe mental illnesses. MAPSS seeks to address the rehabilitation industry's overriding workforce problem: most of its rehabilitation workers need to increase their knowledge, skills, and professional maturity in order to perform their jobs as management describes them.

Two factors account for this lack of adequate knowledge and skills. First, the industry lacks the resources to offer to workers the salary and advancement opportunities they would reasonably require if they were better trained. Second, few such workers can be found because few schools run programs to train them. The need to increase managerial expertise within the industry presents another challenge to increasing workforce competence.

MAPSS concluded that the industry bears the primary responsibility for solving this complex problem. Doing so requires the establishment of intensive industry-based in-service training. It also requires development of a training support system involving all groups that have a stake in the industry's long-term performance, including the Maryland Consortium.

MAPSS created Project Excellence to provide on-site technical assistance to agencies whose managers commit themselves to increasing their workforce's competence systematically and continuously. To do this, it uses a two-step method. First, it encourages and assists management in planning and implementing new or revised service programs. This process leads to a definition of new in-service training needs. Then, Project Excellence assists managers in making plans to meet these needs, and it advises them during the training and program implementation phases about such matters as evaluation. Through this process, Project Excellence seeks to help managers learn techniques and skills that they can use to develop their organizations and staff more effectively in their subsequent management practices.

Project Excellence also works to develop a statewide support network that links the growing number of industry staff who have major responsibility for human resources development and training. Called "The Network," this group seeks to produce and distribute to its members useful training products and other information. The Network also fosters its members' professional development and provides them with opportunities for mutual support.

Project Excellence represents just one example of the Consortium's potential as a constructive change agent. In fact, it resulted from a collaboration of two Consortium partners, MAPSS and the MHA, whose grant to MAPSS established Project Excellence. One should note that MHA obtained a human resource development (HRD) grant from the NIMH (now Center for Mental Health Services [CMHS]) for this work, nicely illustrating the potential benefits of creating such federal, state, and local partnerships. One creative aspect of Project Excellence was the barter system developed to share skills and resources among various rehabilitation programs.

MAPSS believes that the Maryland Consortium represents at least one possible model for meeting the critical workforce needs of an emergent public–private mental health system. It enables all members to play a role based on their unique strengths and perspectives. Consumers and family representatives can drive the mental health service industry to provide high-quality services that empower and liberate consumers and families in the process.

Colleges and universities can support the industry by conducting research and disseminating the results through publication and provision of technical assistance. Local educational institutions can also make very useful contributions by helping to teach trainers to work in the industry and by designing preservice and continuing education programs that ease the training burden of service organizations.

The state agency can continue to give guidance, funding, and other supports to the industry while holding it accountable for the quality of its services through the project management and regulatory process. It can also take the lead in securing resources to provide adequate pay and career opportunities for the workforce, an imperative because fixed depressed salaries and dead-end jobs make maintenance of a competent workforce extremely difficult over the long term.

The entire mental health provider industry must take steps to help its organizations gain better control of their management and delivery processes, which is essential to achieving continuous improvement in the quality of services.

Finally, all these stakeholders can work to form among themselves the bonds of collaboration needed to make a new human service system. MAPSS believes strongly that the Consortium can help create a workforce development system based in industry, driven by empowered consumers, and supported actively by families, government, educators, professionals, and community leaders.

University Programs

A number of educational departments and schools (e.g., social work and nursing) have created linkage programs with state and local mental health departments. The graduate clinical/community psychology program (Tyler & Gatz, 1976) at the University of Maryland at College Park has attempted, both in its coursework and in other structures, to relate to the public mental health system. Students are required to complete a didactic practicum at a systems level of understanding, which often involves them in codeveloping and evaluating programs around such issues as drug abuse in the school system, services for street kids, multicultural integration among high school students, evaluation of mental health programs, and so forth. An early notion in the clinical/community program was an outreach "field station" staffed by a faculty member who carried a reduced course load. This field station was primarily a commitment to work in the community on a variety of projects such as consultation and evaluation services for the Model Neighborhood Mental Health Center. The clinical/community program also invited psychologists from both the state and the university to a biannual conference that examined topics of joint interest (e.g., crisis intervention, mental health program evaluation, and consultation). The papers from these conferences were subsequently published (e.g., Coursey, Specter, Murrell, & Hunt, 1978). In the late 1970s, another effort at increasing the interaction of the faculty with psychologists in the public mental health system was set up. The Psychology Training Advisory Board, consisting of elected psychologists from the university and the mental health system, had as its goals to provide consultation to the state about training psychologists and to solicit, evaluate, and find state funding for innovative year-long psychology externships. These externships had to be proposed by both faculty and a psychologist administrator working within the mental health delivery system. Externships ranged from providing transitional oversight to patients being deinstitutionalized, to psychoeducational programs for family caretakers, to developing job analyses of actual tasks that state psychologists performed, to assisting the State Mental Health Association's lobbying efforts for mental health legislation. The Training Advisory Board also set up a day-long conference for about 60 psychologists from the state mental health delivery system and the university to seek out ways to develop further relationships and to inform one another of their respective assets and needs.

The psychiatry department at the University of Maryland Medical School has had a long-standing interest in community psychiatry and a relationship to the state MHA. The psychiatry department helped the state hospitals achieve accreditation from the Joint Commission for the Accreditation of Hospitals (JCAH); took over the Maryland Psychiatric Research Center, which is located on the grounds of one of the state hospitals; and, in general, provided frequent consultation to the state, primarily through the Center for Mental Health Services Research (Dr. Howard Goldman) and the Center for Psychiatric Rehabilitation (Dr. Anthony Lehman). The state has also provided grant funds to the psychiatry department to do needs assessments for preservice and in-service training for staffs of both psychosocial rehabilitation and mental health centers. Other grants have provided funds both for developing training packages and coordinating funding for human resource development consultants to psychosocial rehabilitation agencies. State funding for the "Maryland Plan" resulted in an integrated psychiatric residency training program. Residents rotated through state psychiatric hospitals and were encouraged to work in public sector output and outpatient programs.

Other organizations in the state that are active in seeking improved education and training for the staff who serve people with serious mental illnesses include the International Association of Psychosocial Rehabilitation Services (IAPSRS[1]); On Our Own, a consumer advocacy group that has a number of local centers; and the Alliance for

[1] IAPSRS. Ruth Hughes, PhD, Director; 10025 Governor Warfield Parkway, Suite 301; Columbia, MD 21044-3357.

the Mentally Ill (AMI) of Maryland and its local affiliates. IAPSRS is more focused on national and international issues, but its recommendations about training and its yearly meetings have some impact on training in some of the rehabilitation centers. Both On Our Own and AMI have actively sought increased training for staff and increased funding for programs and agencies that serve people with serious mental illness. In light of chronic underfunding and a need for building coalitions, all of these agencies and departments are quite open to forming alliances with other agencies and professionals.

As can be seen even in the short history of the development and dissolution of linkages in the state of Maryland, there are a variety of ways to create linkages between academic institutions and the public service sector. In the current chapter, we shall focus on a different type of structure in which interested people from a broad range of academic departments and schools meet with consumers, family members, and interested staff from a cross section of service delivery agencies and relevant government offices, in order to address the training and educational needs of those who serve people with serious mental illnesses. The participants represent a cross section of organizations, ranging from a high school teacher to several directors of rehabilitation centers, from a social work staff member at a state hospital to a "psychiatric survivor" from a private mental hospital, from a psychiatrist to a graduate student, and so forth. These are people who are drawn together by their common interests and commitment to training people to work with serious mental illness.

We shall describe the steps we took in developing the Maryland Training Consortium on Serious Mental Illness so that others might have a sense of how to proceed. One of the advantages of our process was that it did not require the active initiation and participation by people at the top of academia or the mental health delivery system, nor has it required much in the way of resources to run it.

Finally, we shall describe a proposed statewide training program that the Maryland Consortium developed for the Center for Mental Health Services as a model of local, state, and federal cooperation.

Developing the Maryland Training Consortium

Finding One Another and Developing a Network

Like the beginnings of most organizations, ours began in an informal fashion. Agnes Hatfield, PhD, from the Human Development program at the University of Maryland at College Park and long active in the National Alliance for the Mentally Ill (NAMI); Anthony Lehman, MD, from the Psychiatric Rehabilitation section of the Department of Psychiatry at the University of Maryland Medical School; Phil Holmes, the executive director of MAPSS, and Robert D. Coursey, PhD, met at various state lectures, workshops, and mutual projects. Inevitably, we would begin talking about the lack of training for people working with individuals who had serious mental illnesses. This also included checking out what other people around the state were doing. All of us had also been involved in education projects for staff, students, and family members, and all of us had worked on training or human resource development grants from the state. However, except for Phil Holmes, we had worked rather independently of one another.

Forming a Core Group

We kept talking about getting together in a more formal way to discuss training and educational issues and we finally did. We invited a small group together that included three people from various parts of the University of Maryland, several advocates for families and consumers, several practitioners interested in education, and Stanley Weinstein, PhD, from the state government. The informal conversation centered around the educational needs in the state, what could be done, and what were the next steps. We finally addressed the critical questions: Did we want to have an ongoing group? Who would we want to have on it? Who would organize the first meeting, and who would be responsible for running it?

Inviting a Larger Group to a Preliminary Meeting

Because we wanted key people involved in the Consortium, we tried to choose people who were in charge of continuing education, were directors of agencies that did training very well, or were active in teaching and training. Both before this initial meeting and during it, we tried to find interested representatives from the mental health centers; rehabilitation centers; university departments such as social work, nursing, psychology, psychiatry, and rehabilitation counseling; and community and 4-year colleges. We found Sandra Sundeen, MS, RN, Chief of the State Division of Human Resource Development; however, we needed directors of umbrella organizations that represent relevant service delivery agencies, staff from state hospitals, people from consumer groups, and family members from AMI. (Currently, NAMI is attempting to set up training committees in all 50 states.[2]) Whoever knew a relevant person was asked to invite him or her. Twenty-two people came to the first meeting. We then attempted to obtain people from missing areas as well as accepted other people who wanted to join. Currently, we have approximately 40 members. We know that all of these people have busy schedules and will not always be interested in the current issues we are dealing with, but we feel that their support and input is critical, especially when it comes to looking at final recommendations and advocacy efforts. As our work proceeds, we are also seeking out other people who may not be active participants but who are people we need to keep informed of our work (e.g., a key legislator, the assistant director of mental health, etc.).

In our early meetings, we attempted to find out about similar groups in other states. We learned about some of the linkages reported in this book and about the work of the mental health program of the Western Interstate Commission for Higher Education,[3] Matrix,[4] and Thresholds Research and Training Center.[5] However, we could find no one who had created anything similar to the consortium that we were trying to develop.

Developing a Working, Trusting Group

In a group that has strong family advocates, activist consumers, service providers, and academics, there is a strong need to develop a working group in which the members really know each other's position and trust that they will not be undermined by the process. This allows for a process in which smaller work groups can be trusted to complete specific projects and return to the larger group for feedback and direction. To create such an environment, one of our members who also does organizational development work, Diane Greyerbiehl, PhD, led us through a series of structured exercises that helped us both with this process of group development and with relevant goal-setting for our Consortium. Two of the tasks were really quite easy and straightforward but also allowed the group to achieve a sense of united purpose and direction. The two tasks involved developing consensus statements about (a) the needs in the state for education and training for people who provide services to clients with serious mental illnesses (see Appendix B, this chapter, for our list) and (b) trends in the mental health field, politics and regulations, economics, and education and training that were relevant to our goals. For each of these areas, we had to identify which were the opportunities and which were the threats for our goals.

A third task was much more difficult because there were some very strongly held differences as well as a surprisingly strong consensus overall. This third task involved developing a statement of the Consortium's values. We spent a long time on this topic and developed value statements in four areas: (a) values about the educational process, (b) values about consumers and their families, (c) values of service providers, and (d) values that programs and the larger service delivery system should exemplify. These can be seen in Appendix C at the end of this chapter.

The fourth task involved developing a mission statement for the Consortium (see Appendix D, this chapter), and the fifth involved developing a set of overall goals based on the results from the other four tasks (see Appendix E, this chapter).

The Consortium then decided that there would be four work groups, or committees, for the first four goals listed in Appendix E and that the fifth goal would be the function of the whole Consortium. These committees were the Resource Development Committee (goal 1), the Curriculum Development Committee (goal 2), the Training Advocacy Committee (goal 3), and the Educational Standards Committee (goal 4).

Introducing the Consortium to a Larger Constituency

While the committees began their work, we felt that it was important to let the wider audience (staff of agencies that serve people with serious mental illness, consumers, and their families) know of our existence. We did this by providing

[2] The names of NAMI members on these state committees can be obtained by calling the Curriculum and Training Committee at NAMI, 703-524-7600.

[3] Western Interstate Commission for Higher Education. PO Drawer P; Boulder, CO 80301.

[4] Matrix. Rick Baron, Director; 2979 School House Lane; Philadelphia, PA 19144.

[5] Thresholds Research and Training Center. Judith Cook, PhD, Director; 561 W. Diversey, Suite 204; Chicago, IL 60614.

These and similar programs are described in *Community Support Network News,* 7(2), December 1990. Write to the Center for Psychiatric Rehabilitation; Boston University; 730 Commonwealth Ave.; Boston, MA 02215.

three free lectures by three nationally known speakers who live in Maryland and who gave their talks for free (William Carpenter, MD; Anthony Lehman, MD; and David Pickar, MD). Before each lecture, we introduced the Consortium and its mission. Notices were put in various newsletters and were also sent to all of the relevant agencies.

Setting Specific Objectives

The four committees of the Consortium began work. Because of the members' extremely busy lives, we substituted committee meetings for the general meetings. All of the committees did some initial work, and several of the committees (the Curriculum Development Committee and the Educational Standards Committee) advanced on projects more quickly. However, we found that serious issues arose: Our goals were too global for committees to keep focused on a specific project (they even had difficulty choosing a single project), each project needed input from other committees in order to proceed, and the larger Consortium was in danger of losing its sense of cohesion and continuity because the work was being done in four smaller committees with little feedback to the larger Consortium. Finally, the workload was clearly too much for the members who were already overworked in their own organizations.

In order to counteract these problems, the whole Consortium met again and we focused our goals into one specific short-term objective. We used five criteria in selecting our objective: (a) We acknowledged that there are a large number of possible, worthy, and important objectives but that the members only have a limited amount of time and energy to contribute. Therefore, the choice of one specific objective now should not be seen as a statement about the importance of other issues or that we would not work on them later. (b) We wanted an objective that would capture the energy and commitment of most of the more active Consortium members. (c) We wanted to focus on something that would have long-term consequences and not just respond to emergencies or plug holes in a leaky dam. The underlying structural issue here was whether the training consortium would itself provide (some of) the education and training or whether we would be an organization to identify needs, develop policy, foster development of training programs, provide oversight, and do advocacy. We decided not to directly provide education and training ourselves, except on a very limited basis, but rather to provide indirect services such as policy development and consultation to the state and to organizations seeking our expertise, standard-setting guidelines, and so forth. (d) Finally, we wanted to set an objective that we could make visible progress on in a relatively short period of time; in other words, we needed some timely positive reinforcement for our work.

The objective we chose was to develop a statewide preservice educational policy for all community service providers who work with people who have serious mental illnesses. To do this, we examined the certification processes in the state for other types of service providers (e.g. alcohol and drug counselors, child care workers, etc.). We narrowed the proposal down to two alternatives and consulted with other significant organizations in the state (e.g., MAPSS and IAPSRS). We were also aware that the state was rewriting the regulations for community agencies that provide services to people with serious mental illness. We decided to push either regulations or legislation mandating minimal educational requirements for staff, even though we knew there was some opposition to such requirements. We sent initial drafts of our proposal to MAPSS for their input. Within 2 weeks, the state Department of Human Resource Development offered a grant to MAPSS to complete their preservice training package and set it up at 25 of its member rehabilitation agencies (see Project Excellence above). Members on the Consortium who also served on the MAPSS Education and Training Committee then requested that we delay our attempt at changing the regulations until MAPSS had time to implement the training program. Believing that it was an excellent first step, the Consortium agreed and turned to a second pressing agenda—education about serious mental illnesses in colleges and professional schools in Maryland. A committee of faculty and students from community colleges, 4-year colleges, a high school, and relevant graduate schools began meeting and sharing information with one another about the current status of educating their students about serious mental illness, what they needed, and what they could offer one another. Although some of the requests were unique to each setting (e.g., a delegation from the Consortium requested approaching a department chairperson about needed changes in the curriculum; a request for a letter to the state education board asking them to withdraw their proposed requirements for high school students that would have indirectly eliminated high school psychology courses), a number of common themes also arose.

Most faculty mentioned the need for a list of outside speakers who would be willing to provide a lecture to their classes and the need for suggestions about syllabi, references, textbooks, placements, and so forth. Responses to all of these are either now being done or are being planned.

As a result of these contacts, encouragements, and consultations, a new graduate course on serious mental illness is now required by the Rehabilitation Counseling program. A jointly sponsored minimester course is being planned for graduate and undergraduate students in social work and psychology. A request is being sent out to all of the rehabilitation programs in the state asking them to send job announcements to several faculty who teach about serious mental illness at the undergraduate and graduate levels. The Consortium has also surveyed all two and four year colleges in the state about any education they provide on serious mental illness, the specific content that is taught, and any interest the colleges may have in further training and resources. This information was then used as a basis for obtaining a grant that will develop educational resources and a continuing education program for undergraduate faculty.

Supplemental Benefits From the Consortium

Although the Maryland Training Consortium has been in existence for only 2 years and is just now turning to some of the major training issues in Maryland, it has provided opportunities for faculty and some service providers to become well-known to each other. Concretely, this has resulted in numerous joint activities outside of the Consortium such as graduate students doing research in psychiatric rehabilitation centers, staff in rehabilitation centers training both graduate and undergraduate students, graduate students providing psychoeducational programs to clients, and faculty and students making presentations on various topics to rehabilitation agencies and to providers at local workshops and conventions. In addition, members of the Consortium have provided mutual support and encouragement for grant applications from the state, from other agencies, and from some of the faculty in the Consortium. In general, everyone has become better informed about each other's realities, and a mutually supportive network is growing.

Discussion

Future Directions in Linkages

Nationwide, NAMI has been active in attempting to create linkages with service providers, administrators, professional schools, and professional organizations. Over the past several years, the Curriculum and Training Committee of NAMI has provided training for state and local AMI members to set up their own curriculum and training committees to join with professional schools in improving their training about serious mental illnesses and to promote preservice and in-service training for service providers. Of course, different states have different levels of effectiveness and assertiveness. In California, AMI has made a dramatic impact on state-supported social work training. After repeated attempts to get the schools to include more material on serious mental illnesses, they decided to go to the state legislature, at which point the schools joined them in designing some curricular materials on serious mental illnesses. California AMI has also joined the Harbor–University of California—Los Angeles Medical Center to design a new rehabilitation center. In Pennsylvania, AMI joined the Pennsylvania Psychological Association in presenting a 2-day conference titled "New Directions in the Psychological Treatment of Serious Mental Illness." This was supported in part by the American Psychological Association's Practice Directorate. Prior to this, a conference coalition was established in Texas and included the Texas AMI, the Texas Mental Health Consumers Organizations, the directors of all university psychology training programs, and the Texas Department of Mental Health/Mental Retardation. The Curriculum and Training Committee of NAMI also arranged to bring faculty and their students from nearby universities to the national NAMI convention for 1 day.

In Maryland, there are several other recent groups that are attempting to develop linkages that will benefit people with serious mental illnesses. The Maryland Psychological Association (MPA) has created a committee co-chaired by Dr. Faith Dickerson from Sheppard Pratt Hospital and Dr. Robert Coursey. After surveying the members of MPA, it was clear that there are many obstacles that prevent the members (who are predominantly private practitioners) from working with people with serious mental illnesses or their families. Consequently, the committee looked beyond just the members to all of the psychologists in Maryland and developed a day-long continuing education program on the treatment of people with schizophrenia. With the support of the state's Mental Hygiene Administration and NIMH, it was offered at little or no cost to the psychologists in the state. The purpose of low cost was to attract psychologists who might not otherwise attend.

In addition, the Center for Mental Health Services Research at the University of Maryland Medical School, in conjunction with the director of Maryland's Mental Hygiene Administration, set up a policy forum that addresses in detail a variety of policy issues facing the state of Maryland as it tries to improve its services to children and adults with serious mental illnesses. It uses a steering committee composed of service providers and faculty to focus and pilot specific topics. The people invited to participate in the forums vary according to the topic but are widely representative of the various stakeholders and experts in the area.

Statewide Training Program on Serious Mental Illness

As the national Center for Mental Health Services struggled to rethink the future of training grants, the Maryland Training Consortium proposed a new model of federal support.

The overall goal. The goal would be to create a training structure that will lead to well-trained service providers in agencies that have a clear notion of what quality service is and see the need for staff training to meet their quality goals. Too many training projects have had very little impact because the training was not intensive or long enough for the person to put new skills into practice, or the new views and skills were not supported by his or her agency. The idea for this structure is to create training that has a significant impact.

Retraining the workforce. This goal has a number of implications about the ideal training program. It means that the focus should be on retraining people already in the field. Preservice training is important, but if the agency and personnel do not support the new ideas and skills, the preservice training is quickly eroded. Moreover, there has to be a critical mass supporting the introduction of people with specific skills in the agency. Focusing on people already in the field can be both a reward and an opening for advancement for them, which in turn will encourage them to remain in the field for some time. Furthermore, such retraining fits with President Clinton's goals of retooling the workforce.

In this plan, the people who will receive further training would be both the staff from agencies as well as faculty interested in training students with relevant skills for the current public mental health market. Because there will be limited funds, for maximum impact, the focus would be on present and future leaders. An example of this type of endeavor is the community leadership training program in Baltimore. A small group of young adults who already show outstanding potential for being future civic leaders are chosen for this program. The group meets with current civic leaders in training sessions designed to foster an indepth understanding of the city's problems, resources, and change methods, and to increase leadership the individuals' leadership skills.

Technical support for agencies and schools. Technical support would need to be given to the agency or school while training is given to selected staff. Project Excellence of the Maryland Association of Psychiatric Support Services is an example of helping agencies define their service goals and consequent training needs. The state would need to provide the technical support component of the overall training plan. For example, the technical assistance could come from other highly skilled providers and administrators within the state.

A second option would be to provide the training at the time when a new program is being started up. A good example of this occurred when Stein and Test (1980) retrained hospital staff for their Assertive Community Treatment program in Wisconsin.

The start-up process. Important groundwork needs to precede the implementation of such a training program. The first project is to develop a consortium of all of the stakeholders (e.g., educators, service providers, consumers, etc.) concerned about the service delivery system. This takes time, energy, and some small financial support. Second, the Consortium needs to develop or review training needs of the state and to develop a consensually supported, coordinated plan that allows the participation of various training components (e.g., preservice training in the colleges and university, continuing education by professional groups, the role of the state HRD, etc.).

The need for seed money. In order to encourage this and make it possible, seed money needs to be available to the states prior to receiving the main training grant. Additionally, there must be some assurance on the part of the Center for Mental Health Services (CMHS) that the grant requirements will not change during the planning period and that the long-term prospects of getting a grant are worth the investment of time and effort.

A basic training program example. The proposed grant from CMHS would support a very small state training center (a director and secretary) that would plan, coordinate, and implement the grant; provide stipends for the fellows; develop a library of training materials; and raise and distribute money for consultants and trainers. The Maryland Training Consortium or its equivalent would then function as its board and steering committee. The center needs to be housed on neutral ground but have credibility and staying power. Various options for this would need to be considered.

The training center would offer weekly classes that would provide common core information for everyone and a weekly support and discussion group. The core curriculum would be covered by a core faculty. Specific skill development would depend on the unique needs of the individuals and their programs. Training would take place both through the training center and elsewhere (even out of state) depending on the needs and ability of the state's training resources. Different years could focus on different themes (e.g., psychosocial rehabilitation or children with serious mental illness).

The training fellows would be a small group (e.g., 8–10) who would represent a diversity of professions and services. The fellows would make a commitment to remain in the service system, preferably in the agency that supported them, for a specified time period, and they would provide supervision to other staff. The agencies would be expected to define quality of service and develop specific training strategies for their staff to achieve them.

Applications to the program would be jointly made by the agency and potential fellows for both individual training and program change.

Federal grant support for model programs. To make such a coordinated training program actually work, the annual grant needs to be adequately funded. To achieve a smoothly working training program and make a long-term impact on the quality of the service delivery staff, faculty, and services, the grant would need to be for a 5-year period.

New initiative is not a replacement for other types of training grants. Currently, graduate and undergraduate schools are not adequately training their students in the skills they will need to provide service in the public mental health system (e.g., working with adults with serious mental illnesses). There is a desperate need to recruit new professionals with postgraduation commitments to enter the field. An excellent way to recruit these new professionals is by supporting their education on institutional clinical training grants. These grants have also helped to improve the quality of professional training programs both through the training proposals that were funded as well as through the feedback given to all grant proposals. Higher annual support levels per grant would generate considerable interest and create a long-term change in professional training programs. In addition to the payback through service by the students, CMHS might consider requesting some specific types of commitments from the recipient programs to continue the basics of the program set up by the grant.

There is also a continuing need for HRD grants to states for specific innovative training projects.

The Fundamental Principle

The basic principle underlying all of these successful linkages requires that there be mutual benefit to all of the parties involved. This then presumes that all of the parties have some interest, expertise, needs, and resources, and that these needs and resources are seen to be complementary across members. Therefore, it is in the members' best interest to share information about their own needs and resources. However, such an exchange also presumes a degree of trust and mutual respect as well as a dedication to the common good. Hopefully, what emerges out of this matrix are ongoing personal relationships and knowledge about each other's continually changing systems and resources and a willingness to contribute to one another. It has been our experience in building the Maryland Training Consortium that there is a large pool of people with the interest, expertise, resources, and goodwill to create these "mutual self-help groups." All that is needed is someone to light the fire and help organize it. The forms that linkages may then take are probably limited only by the creativity of the participants.

Reference

Coursey, R., Specter, G., Murrell, S., & Hunt, B. (Eds.). (1978). *Program evaluation for mental health: Methods, strategies, and participants.* New York: Grune & Stratton.

Stein, L. I., & Test, M. A. (1980). Alternatives to mental hospital treatment. I. Conceptual model, treatment program, and clinical evaluation. *Archives of General Psychiatry, 31,* 393–397.

Tyler, F. B., & Gatz, M. A. (1976). If community psychology is so great, why don't we try it? *Professional Psychology, 7,* 185–194.

APPENDIX A

Maryland State Programs Supported by Previous NIMH Human Resource Development Grants

- Utilization studies of core discipline personnel.
- Academic linkages with graduate, professional, undergraduate, and paraprofessional colleges and universities.
- A fellowship in administrative psychiatry.
- A direct care worker curriculum.
- Curricula in psychosocial rehabilitation training, consumers' rights and empowerment, and training to work collaboratively with families of people with serious mental illness.
- A curriculum for correctional officers.
- Job satisfaction survey related to recruitment and retention of social workers.
- The "Maryland Plan," which recruited over 200 university-trained psychiatrists into Maryland's public mental health system.
- An Advocacy Committee/Board Training Manual project for consumers who participate on various state, local, and private/nonprofit boards.
- Two training institute libraries: one for consumer organizations and one for the staff of psychosocial rehabilitation organizations.

APPENDIX B

Needs That the Training Consortium Intends to Address

- Training and education for community and hospital mental health providers who work with people suffering from serious mental illnesses.
- Further development of graduate and undergraduate curricula for providers of direct care as well as for providers of indirect services such as management.
- Resources to do the training.
- Promotion of more collaboration among rehabilitation and mental health providers, consumers, their families, and educational organizations.
- Education of policymakers and program managers about the importance and necessity of training and education of service providers.
- Heightened awareness and interest in serious mental illnesses among people in educational systems, mental health, and rehabilitation fields.
- Appropriate education and training standards for service providers who work with people who have serious mental illnesses.

APPENDIX C

General Values of the Maryland Training Consortium

Goals of the Educational Process

- Education should provide a full range of options, understandings, and viewpoints about the problems and solutions in the field.
- The process must include both training (of specific skills) and education (exploratory learning and reflection).
- Education of service providers needs to provide a balance between scientific and clinical

knowledge and the human experience of the disorder.

• Students should be trained to think critically, to respect data and evaluation, and to stay current in the scientific and applied aspects of their work.

• Future service providers should receive training as a systems change agent.

• Service providers should have a wide range of knowledge and skills relative to helping individuals with disabilities.

• Service providers should respect and use the diverse skills provided by other disciplines and seek to develop transdisciplinary relationships.

• For each field of mental health providers, there should be a minimally required knowledge base and skills competency in working with people with serious mental illnesses.

Values Concerning Consumers, Their Families, and Service Providers

Respect for and empowerment of clients and their families should be an underlying value. Examples of its realization would include:

• Individuals receiving services, and their families, are potential teachers about coping with the challenges of serious mental disorders. Service providers can and should learn from those receiving services and from their families.

• Students and staff should be aware of the power dimension in staff–consumer relationships and should be taught how to avoid abusing it.

• Consumers and family members need to be involved in all decisions concerning themselves. To the extent possible, all forms of coercion and physical force should be avoided.

• Service providers need to be respectful of the consumer's and the family's experiences, perceptions, and values that are brought to the relationship.

• Service providers need to respect the choices of people with serious mental illnesses. As much as possible, success must be formulated in each individual's personal terms.

• Students must see people with serious mental illness as fellow human beings, be able to enter their frame of reference, and understand their cultural and ethnic background. This is also true in working with families.

• Service providers should value the role of families in the care and support of their mentally ill relatives.

• Service providers should understand the value of the consumer and family movements and other forms of self-help groups.

• Service providers should seek client feedback on their procedures.

Values Concerning Service Organizations, Programs, and Larger Systems That Affect Service

• Community integration is a mandate for the service system and the community, while preserving the consumer's right to make choices about his or her living arrangements. This assumes a proactive stance on the part of service providers to educate the community and to build the necessary bridges for people with serious mental illnesses.

• Education should help students to understand the impact of larger socioeconomic, legal, and administrative systems on service provision and on clients.

• Staff should be aware of how economic arrangements provide incentives and disincentives for particular types of behaviors, programs, and systems.

• Staff need to work to diminish the fragmentation of the service delivery system.

• Staff need to be trained to develop programs and interventions that fit the diverse nature of the population rather than expecting people to fit existing programs.

• The value of respect and empowerment should also apply to direct service staff. For example, input from direct service staff needs to be solicited in designing and running programs.

APPENDIX D

Mission Statement of the Maryland Training Consortium on Serious Mental Illness

The Maryland Training Consortium on Serious Mental Illness is a training, resource, and advocacy consortium consisting of individuals from the various components of the mental health service system, people with serious mental illnesses, advocates, families, and training institutions. The Consortium is primarily concerned with developing an educated, informed, and experienced workforce who provide mental health services to children, adolescents, and adults with serious mental illnesses. Services will include disseminating information, developing resources, determining educational and training needs, and developing curriculum and training proposals as well as educational standards for this field. Basic values integral to the functioning of the organization include:

- Citizens with long-term serious mental illnesses and their families deserve high-quality services by well-trained service providers.
- Maryland should become a model for the nation in its education and training programs for service providers who work with serious mentally ill people.
- Education, training, and services should be based on scientific, experiential, collaborative, and multidisciplinary approaches to these serious mental disorders.
- Education and training should inculcate a respect for and empowerment of clients, their families, and the staff who serve them.
- Education should include consideration of the larger economic, political, cultural, and organizational contexts that affect clients, staff, and service programs.

APPENDIX E

Overall Goals of the Maryland Training Consortium on Serious Mental Illness

- Identify resources that will provide Maryland access to training materials and information from within the state and across the nation. Also identify people in the state who have expertise in relevant areas and who would be available for educational programs.
- Promote and develop education and training for people across disciplines and all experience levels who work with people of all ages with serious mental illnesses. Further develop graduate and undergraduate curricula for these careers.
- Advocate for resources for training. Provide an annual report on the state of training in Maryland for those working with people who have serious mental illnesses.
- Promote educational and training standards for personnel who work with people who have serious mental illnesses.
- Provide input to the state about its mental health training. This would involve developing collaborative relationships with relevant state systems such as the Mental Hygiene Administration, especially the Human Resource Development Division, Department of Vocational Rehabilitation, and the Department of Education.

CHAPTER

18

Creating a Competent Workforce in Vermont: Promoting Public–Academic Linkages and Human Resource Development

Annamarie T. Cioffari, John D. Burchard, and Paul J. Carling
University of Vermont

Rodney E. Copeland
Vermont Department of Mental Health and Mental Retardation

Vermont has had a long history of both public–academic collaboration and human resource development related to its mental health workforce. However, in the past, as in most other state systems, program and services development and reallocation of resources from institutional to community programs has proceeded without the necessary systematic attention to the long-term human resources development capacities critical to successful outcomes for consumers and their families. The Vermont Department of Mental Health and Mental Retardation, Division of Mental Health (DMH), is in the process of fundamentally restructuring its service system to implement state-of-the-art community services for its two primary mental health client target populations: children and adolescents experiencing a severe emotional disturbance and adults with psychiatric disabilities. In both areas, Vermont is seen as a national leader, both in the development of innovative services as well as in developing processes to foster fundamental systems change.

In this chapter, we present a brief description of the history of public–academic linkages in Vermont and of current efforts to expand those linkages in order to better meet the ongoing needs of the Vermont mental health workforce.

History of Public–Academic Linkages in Vermont

Training

Much of the public–academic collaboration in Vermont, in the area of community-based services for adults with psychiatric disabilities and children and adolescents experiencing severe emotional disturbances, has occurred between the Department of Psychology at the University of Vermont (UVM) and the Vermont Department of Mental Health and Mental Retardation, Division of Mental Health (DMH). For example, in the 1980s, DMH funded a psychosocial rehabilitation (PSR) project through the Department of Psychology. This project developed training for mental health staff working with adults with psychiatric disabilities as the Vermont State Hospital was downsizing and new support services were being developed in local communities. The emphasis of this training was on statewide conferences, workshops, and seminars, often led by out-of-state consultants, that introduced staff to emerging and innovative service models. This type of training model worked well to build consensus about service approaches as Vermont moved toward a community-based system of care. It built service providers' awareness of new models and presented an opportunity for information sharing and networking. In addition, statewide workshops often were followed by individual technical assistance to local mental health agencies.

In children's mental health, as in the adult system, training development and collaboration with higher education occurred in the context of systems change. For example, in the mid 1980s, simultaneously with statewide systems planning through the National Institute of Mental Health's (NIMH) Children's and Adolescent's Services System Project (CASSP), a series of training events were planned and implemented. These events again enabled the system to embrace new technologies and were helpful in allowing debate and ultimately bringing about consensus in Vermont on the system of care for children and adolescents experiencing severe emotional disturbances. The training that occurred was particularly successful in generating improved interagency collaboration between the mental health and child welfare and special education systems and in establishing new relationships with individual faculty within higher education (Burchard, Clarke, Hamilton, & Fox, 1990; Burchard & Schaefer, 1992).

From the beginning, attention was paid to involving current consumers, ex-patients, and family members in training initiatives. For example, as new systems of care were being planned for children, parents were included at all levels. This involvement led to significant awareness building between professionals and parents. Much of the awareness revolved around the dissatisfaction parents expressed about professional practice and training. This consumer feedback has proved invaluable as Vermont has attempted to develop a more relevant and responsive system of care and more relevant professional training programs. The recommendations from parents involved in these collaborative trainings apply directly to academic training for clinical psychologists and are summarized, along with recommendations from other advocacy and professional groups, under the description of the current Public–Academic Linkage/Human Resource Development (PAL/HRD) initiative in Vermont.

The PSR project involved consumers, ex-patients, and families through both workshops developed specifically with and for them and by designing statewide conferences to include consumers, families, and providers. One particularly successful event was a seminar series held at the University of Vermont (Cioffari, Blanch, Wilson, Carling, & Pierce, 1988), which served as a forum for public education and discussion as DMH began its current regionalization project, an effort to complete the community system of care for adults. Presenters included a cross section of national experts on rehabilitation and community support. The seminar series drew an audience from around the state, was well attended by consumers, ex-patients, families, and providers, and began to attract university students and faculty from other disciplines. Several clinical psychology graduate students participated in the seminar and pursued community clinical internships based on that experience.

The PSR project and other training initiatives taught us that, as we move from a facility-based to a community-based system of care, the mental health workforce becomes the key to successful services and supports for people with psychiatric disabilities. Staff need recognition and support for the essential work that they do. Also, a community-based system of care only works well when consumers, ex-patients, and family members are integrally involved in service planning, development, delivery, and evaluation.

It became obvious that Vermont needed an ongoing capacity to train staff that retained the flexibility of the PSR project and the training events offered in children's services but that also had the ability to provide more comprehensive, in-depth training. As community programs became better established, they began to look for training that could address staff skills as well as knowledge and awareness. They also began to look to Vermont's academic programs to better prepare new graduates to work with people with serious emotional disabilities in community settings.

Internships

The primary way in which students have been exposed to public mental health issues in the past has been through internships developed jointly with DMH. The Department of Psychology has a long history of placing graduate students in internships in the public mental health system. Starting in the 1980s, DMH was particularly successful in developing social policy internships for doctoral-level psychology students in the area of community integration and community-based treatment for children, adolescents, and adults with serious emotional disabilities. Doctoral students have been involved, in adult services, in conducting needs assessments and evaluations of supported employment programs and in working with self-help and support groups and various other community support programs at the local and state levels. With the advent of the CASSP program being funded in Vermont, a number of the social policy interns placed at DMH through the Department of Psychology began focusing on children's mental health issues. A series of needs assessments, white papers, and program development activities were carried out. As a consequence, the accomplishments of the doctoral interns played a major role in bringing about systems change in the Vermont public mental health system for both adults with psychiatric disabilities and children and adolescents experiencing serious emotional disturbances (Carling, 1988a, 1988b).

In spite of this close collaboration between the psychology department and DMH in systems change efforts and the involvement of graduate students in those efforts, most of the clinical internships offered students were in more traditional settings. For example, all of the clinical internships that provided students an opportunity to work with adults with psychiatric disabilities were in Vermont State Hospital. Although there were a few internships in community mental health centers (CMHC), these were not necessarily focused on the Vermont system's priority populations, and over time, they tended to either be eliminated or moved to the Outpatient Counseling section of the agencies. As a consequence, few students were leaving the psychology department with a sense of the types of supports needed for adults with psychiatric disabilities in the community or having had the opportunity to talk with consumers, ex-patients, and their families about the types of supports they desired.

Similarly, children's internships provided excellent training for the provision of traditional services delivered in outpatient settings. However, the vast majority of families who have children with a serious emotional disturbance do not access those services. Another goal of the current PAL/HRD initiative and related projects, therefore, was to design internships that reflected the changes occurring in Vermont's mental health system.

The Current PAL/HRD Initiative

In order to eliminate the gap in human resource development capacity on a statewide basis, the Vermont DMH and the Center for Community Change through Housing and Support, which is part of the UVM Department of Psychology, jointly proposed an NIMH PAL/HRD initiative. The current changes in the Vermont mental health system, as well as changes occurring at UVM, made this initiative particularly timely. For example, there is a new masters in social work program at UVM, the counseling department has been revising and expanding its community counseling program, and the nursing program has proposed developing a new masters in psychiatric nursing program. In addition, the Department of Psychiatry and DMH have begun a joint appointment program, which has recently brought a new faculty member to UVM to develop community psychiatry training and residencies. This faculty person also serves as the state-level medical director at DMH. The purpose of the PAL/HRD initiative was to fundamentally restructure the long-term relationship between the public mental health system and higher education, beginning with UVM, Vermont's only university, and expanding to the state college system and interested private colleges. The goals were that preservice training, which directly prepares students to work in public mental health with people with serious emotional disabilities, and training for current staff, linked to academic credit and continuing education, would be routinely available.

The PAL/HRD Task Force

The first step undertaken was to establish a PAL/HRD task force at UVM. There was excellent support for this initiative from the start. The chairs of all six human service departments at UVM (Psychology, Psychiatry, Social Work, Counseling, Nursing, and Special Education) agreed to serve on the task force. The task force also included consumer, ex-patient, family, and service provider representatives, along with representatives from DMH, the Vermont Department of Social and Rehabilitative Services (SRS), and the Department of Education. In the first 18 months of the project, the task force attempted to address the following questions: What are the competencies (attitudes, knowledge, and skills) needed by people who work with children and adolescents experiencing a serious emotional disturbance and adults with psychiatric disabilities in the community? What do we currently offer (courses, internships) that addresses those competencies? Are there ways we can collaborate to better address those competencies and the needs of Vermont's, and hopefully other states, mental health workforce?

Child Adolescent, and Adult Work Groups

Two work groups, one on child and adolescent issues and one on adults, were formed. They consisted largely of service providers recognized as excellent in the state mental health system and consumers, ex-patients, and family members, with additional representation from state agencies and academia. The work groups developed a preliminary list of basic competencies for people working in the Vermont mental health system and for people working with children within related systems (SRS, Department of Education).

At the task force's request, the work groups held several training and information-sharing days for the UVM faculty in order to develop a consensus on the workforce competencies. The work groups also made several broad recommendations, which follow, on the type of training that should be available for people planning to or currently working in mental health. These apply generally, across disciplines, but are very relevant to the types of clinical psychology training necessary to prepare students to work in public mental health, in community-based services, and with people with serious emotional disabilities.

Recommendations for Training From the Work Groups

Recommendations from the work groups for training are listed below.

1. As much as possible, training in this field should be multidisciplinary in nature. Service providers reported that they have not found the disciplines in which their staff were trained to be particularly relevant, beyond the need for good medical coverage, in community services. Much more important were a good grounding in public mental health, flexibility, an openness to change, and a willingness to "do what needed to be done," whether or not it matched expected roles in service delivery.

2. All training, preservice, and in-service should involve consumers, ex-patients, and families in an integral way. Academia has a responsibility to introduce students in the human service disciplines to the importance of choice and empowerment in the recovery process. Students need to understand that there is much to learn from the subjective experience of mental illness and to respect consumers and families as the experts in this area. One important way to make training more relevant is to begin to involve consumers, ex-patients, and family members in curriculum development, instruction, field supervision, and program and student evaluations.

3. Effective community services and supports are based on a collaborative service delivery model. Therefore, the best training will model that collaboration and will develop the skills for working collaboratively: across disciplines, among agencies, and with families, consumers, and ex-patients.

4. Curricula should include good, basic information on psychiatric disability and severe emotional disturbance. Perhaps even more importantly, curricula should be grounded in the philosophy of community integration. It is critical that human service programs begin to graduate students who can provide services on an outreach basis and who are comfortable working with people in their homes, in school settings, on the job, and in other community settings. It takes experience and skill to provide outreach-oriented services and to support natural-support networks (e.g., family, friends, neighbors, landlords, employers, etc.). From the work groups' perspectives, it

seems that these "out-of-office" skills are the most often missing in new graduates in the field. In addition, the experience of working in community settings and with innovative services is critical to the recruitment of new graduates to the field.

5. Finally, in both in-service and in preservice and academic training, attention needs to be paid to making programs accessible to consumers, ex-patients, and family members. Many are providing services now; services can only benefit from the further involvement of people who have experience, directly or secondarily, with the mental health system. Academia will also benefit from the direct involvement of consumers and families in its programs. A commitment to diversity means addressing some of the barriers (e.g., tuition, lack of on-campus supports, etc.) that prevent consumers and families from matriculating in training programs.

Initial Outcomes of the PAL/HRD Initiative

The PAL/HRD initiative had an almost immediate impact on the current human service programs at UVM. In the past 2 years, consumers, ex-patients, family members, service providers, and state agency representatives have begun to be included as instructors, on a regular basis, in introductory and advanced human service courses across the campus. Several new courses have been developed. The Department of Psychology is offering two new or adapted courses in the 1991–1992 year, one focusing on children and adolescents and one on adults with serious psychiatric disabilities. Although psychology has a tradition of involving people from the field in its courses, these courses are particularly designed in a collaborative training model. Service providers, consumers, ex-patients, and family members are serving as co-instructors. Graduate students and current mental health workers are participating as students. Students from a wide variety of disciplines are involved. A UVM Instructional Incentive grant has been received to update instructional materials and make them available across campus, and efforts are being made to find ongoing funding for the faculty salaries involved in offering these courses so that tuition reductions can be offered to current practitioners wishing to participate.

With consultation and, in some instances, co-teaching with staff from the Center for Community Change Through Housing and Support (CCC), the Department of Counseling has developed a new community counseling course, and the Department of Social Work has revised its basic mental health course. All graduate students in these departments are required to take these courses. Also, as noted earlier, the new faculty person in the community psychiatry department is developing new course work and community mental health center residencies for the psychiatry department.

The DMH also has begun to fund a multidisciplinary package of public mental health internships. Three psychology doctoral students are placed on assertive community treatment teams, working with adults with psychiatric disabilities in community mental health centers and a homeless health project. As a result of a similar PAL project in children's services, clinical psychology trainees worked on Project Wraparound, a 3-year demonstration project designed to maintain children experiencing severe behavioral and emotional disabilities in less restrictive mainstream settings through the provision of intensive services in the home, school, and community (Burchard & Clarke, 1990; Clarke, Schaefer, Burchard, & Welkowitz, 1992). Also, with respect to children's services, two clinical psychology trainees serve as research assistants on the Vermont System for Tracking Client Progress, a university project designed to monitor the outcomes for children and families who are receiving case-managed, wraparound services in the community (Burchard & Schaefer, 1992).

Ongoing social policy internships, often involving joint projects between the DMH, the Department of Psychology, and CCC, also are part of this multidisciplinary internship program. Doctoral psychology students continue to be involved with planning and evaluation activities, as described earlier, at DMH. In addition, School of Social Work interns have worked at DMH and CCC over the past year in the areas of mental illness and substance abuse and with women with psychiatric disabilities who are parents. A counseling intern has been working in the area of social integration, developing a policy paper for CCC, and in a support program at a local mental health agency. Finally, the visibility of the PAL/HRD effort has encouraged several community mental health centers to begin to expand linkages with human service programs in their local areas on their own.

The task force was less successful in addressing structural change at UVM. For example, the task force considered developing a new multidisciplinary masters specialization in public mental health. However, the beginning of this planning, and the planning for the proposed masters in psychiatric nursing, raised several similar questions. It was not clear what the market in Vermont was for existing, as well as new, degrees. Seventy-six percent of the Vermont mental health workforce has less than a masters degree, and paraprofessional staff seem to be the fastest growing group. In addition, salary levels, and lack of other supports for staff, make it difficult to attract and retain more highly credentialed staff. It also became clear that a UVM-based strategy was not enough to address the ongoing training needs of current practitioners on a statewide basis.

The task force agreed to continue at UVM, perhaps on the model of a similar Multidisciplinary Task Force on Aging. The Task Force on Aging plans yearly events to keep issues important to elders visible and integrated into the campus community. In addition, the Task Force agreed to continue updating information, as needed, on courses, continuing education events, and so forth, in their own departments, which could be shared in order to enrich the education available to students on public mental health and on people with serious emotional disabilities.

Next Steps

In response largely to the work of the Task Force, the final year of the PAL/HRD initiative in Vermont has focused on a much more broad-based initiative to create a competent workforce in the state (Cioffari & Carling, 1992). With the support of the Agency of Human Services, DMH and CCC have brought together a group of providers, consumers, ex-patients, families, state agency representatives, advocacy organizations, and academics to participate in a planning process to develop comprehensive ongoing training and statewide public–academic linkages that will ensure competence throughout Vermont's mental health workforce. Many of the original UVM Task Force members have been key participants in this planning process. The representation from academia has been greatly expanded to include other state colleges, the Community College of Vermont, and several private higher education institutions that have particular expertise in adult education and education in public mental health and community integration for people with disabilities.

The outcome of this planning process will be a report to the Agency of Human Services and the Vermont legislature on the training, education, and support needs of Vermont's mental health practitioners. The report will be used to plan for the resources needed for an ongoing, comprehensive PAL/HRD system in Vermont. The planning group already has produced several key recommendations (Cioffari & Carling, 1992). For example, starting with the competencies initially developed by the child, adolescent, and adult work groups, the planning group has recommended a core set of trainings that should occur on an annual basis for all practice staff in the mental health workforce. The recommendations include a standardized curricula for introductory-level staff; a curricula covering emerging models and innovations and introductory management training for advanced-level staff; ongoing management training available, some through a standardized curriculum and some through special topics workshops, planned annually; and, similar to the PSR project, four–six annual events that cover emerging issues and allow for staff recognition, networking, and information sharing around the state. It was recommended that all training events be linked, whenever possible, to academic credit, continuing education units, or a certificate series designed to recognize staff interested in nondegree training options.

The planning group also recommended that the competencies be used to develop a set of standards for all staff. The DMH and local agencies would then develop training and supervision guidelines to ensure that all staff meet these standards within a given time period.

To create a closer link between the planning for training of current practitioners and degree programs, it has been recommended that a Vermont Mental Health Training Institute be developed, with DMH having a lead role and involving consumers, families, service providers, and higher education programs. The Institute would serve to ensure that the recommended in-service training occurred and that it was linked to academic credit. The Training Institute would also serve as a clearinghouse identifying training needs for academic programs and directing practitioners to programs that provided training that met the basic competencies.

A variety of needs for new academic programs, or programs that added specializations or tracks in working with children and adolescents experiencing a severe emotional disturbance and adults with psychiatric disabilities, were identified, including associate's, bachelor's and masters degree programs with an emphasis on public mental health, a psychiatric nursing program at the masters level, and community psychology and psychiatry training. The planning group currently is looking at strategies for increasing academic coordination across the state so that staff who start an associate's degree program at the community college could, for example, transfer at least the course work specific to mental health to a bachelor's human services program at one of the state colleges. This type of coordination is another activity that could be undertaken by a statewide institute.

The planning group also has taken on the task of developing strategies to meet the other HRD needs of the Vermont mental health workforce: increasing salaries and benefits to make mental health careers more attractive, offering scholarships and other incentives to encourage staff development, and developing organizational and state systems that support staff. Finally, the planning group has made a commitment to identifying what is needed to make training programs accessible to consumers, ex-patients, and family members who want to be part of the professional workforce.

The ongoing participation and level of commitment shown by all the planning group members has been phenomenal. It is very clear that the PAL/HRD initiative has been successful because of the types of collaboration that are fundamental and valued in Vermont. The recommendations of the planning group have emphasized the value of consumer, ex-patient, family, provider, and higher education collaboration. The result, for the PAL initiative, has been that we are truly on the road to having a state mental health system and a statewide academic system that work in concert to produce a well-trained, skilled workforce on an ongoing basis.

References

Burchard, J. D., & Clarke, R. T. (1990). The role of individualized care in a service delivery system for children and adolescents with severely maladjusted behavior. *Journal of Mental Health Administration, 17,* 48–60.

Burchard, J. D., Clarke, R. T., Hamilton, R. I., & Fox, W. L. (1990). Project Wraparound: A state–university partnership in training clinical psychologists to serve severely emotionally disturbed children. In P. Magrab & P. Wohlford (Eds.), *Improving psychological services for children and adolescents with severe mental disorders: Clinical training in psychology* (pp. 179–184). Washington, DC: American Psychological Association.

Burchard, J. D., & Schaefer, M. C. (1992). Public mental health services for children and families and graduate training in psychology: Bridging the gap. In M. Kessler, S. Goldston, & J. Joffe (Eds.), *Essays in honor of George Albee* (pp. 138–154). Newbury Park, CA: Sage.

Burchard, J. D., & Schaefer, M. C. (1992). Improving accountability in a service delivery system in children's mental health. *Clinical Psychology Review, 12,* 867–882.

Carling, P. J. (1988a, April). *Principles for promoting community integration of people with psychiatric disabilities: The challenge to the academic psychology community.* Paper presented at the National Conference on Clinical Training in Psychology, Houston, TX.

Carling, P. J. (1988b, April). *Strategic attempts of a psychology department to promote community integration: The University of Vermont experience.* Paper presented at the National Conference on Clinical Training in Psychology, Houston, TX.

Cioffari, A. T., Blanch, A. K., Wilson, S. F., Carling, P. J., & Pierce, J. E. (1988). *Building a vision of community support: A collaborative colloquium series* [Monograph on state–higher education collaboration]. Boulder, CO: Western Interstate Commission on Higher Education.

Cioffari, A. T., & Carling, P. J. (1992). *Creating a competent mental health workforce for the 21st century.* Burlington, VT: Trinity College, Center for Community Change Through Housing and Support.

Clarke, R. T., Schaefer, M. C., Burchard, J. D., & Welkowitz, J. W. (1992). Wrapping community-based mental health services around children with a severe behavioral disorder: An evaluation of Project Wraparound. *Journal of Child and Family Studies, 1,* 241–261.

CHAPTER

19

The Colorado Postdoctoral Training Consortium: An Innovative Postdoctoral Program in Public Psychology

Carl N. Zimet and Courtenay Harding
University of Colorado School of Medicine

Community psychology formally began in the late 1960s with former President Johnson's signing of the Mental Health Centers Act. It reached its zenith with the President's Commission on Mental Health (1978) during the Carter administration, which recommended significant expansion of community mental health programs and facilities. It was not long before the denouement of community mental health programs, which came in the early 1980s with the emphasis on state block grants and the privatization of health care.

The period prior to the community mental health era was notable by an emphasis on the private practice of psychotherapy and psychoanalysis in psychiatry and, to a lesser degree, clinical psychology. If we go back further, to the 1950s, psychology was primarily an academic discipline, with much of clinical training in psychology taking place within the Veterans Administration medical centers. This situation led to a hospital-based clinical focus with a heavy medical component. Treatment was primarily for men; therefore, whole segments of the population (e.g., women, children, elderly, and adolescents) were unfamiliar to the budding clinicians. The focus was on psychodiagnostics rather than psychotherapy, although that rapidly changed and reversed itself (Albee, 1964).

Clinical psychologists began to move in directions other than solely toward the halls of academia. That was not altogether surprising since the Boulder Conference, which set the course for clinical psychology, defined the clinical model of training and practice (Raimy, 1950). Psychologists began to take a variety of positions in a broad range of mental health settings. One thin stream moved toward the private practice of clinical psychology, which in succeeding years became much more significant. Simultaneously, there was a significant focus on prevention (Albee, 1959; Bower, 1963). The prevention direction was toward delinquency, teenage motherhood, school difficulties, obstacles of the aged, marital and family dilemmas, the impact of cultural and ethnic tensions, and other problems that might cause mental health problems (Combs, Fisk, Fine, Zimet, Wiberley, & Nesbitt, 1954). The Joint Commission of Mental Health and Mental Illness in its report "Action for Mental Health" (1961), as well as the 1965 Conference on the Professional Preparation of Clinical Psychologists (Hoch, Ross, & Winder, 1966), all reshaped and broadened the targets and service delivery mechanisms (Albee, 1959). The classroom, the neighborhood, and the workplace became the new home base for community psychologists as clinicians, consultants, and prevention engineers (Albee & Joffe, 1977; Brown, 1965; Caplan, 1964; White & Harris, 1961). The most seriously ill patients were still behind locked doors. Community mental health centers became the major setting for psychologists to practice primary prevention. However, the winds of change have come again for both psychiatry and psychology.

Public Psychology

With deinstitutionalization taking place in the 1970s and 1980s, we have ended up with over 2 million very seriously mentally ill patients in the community needing secondary and often tertiary care within a community setting (Turner & Ten Hoor, 1978). The model of community psychology needs to change to that of "public psychology." Public psychology is based on a public health model (McMahon & Pugh, 1970); a model that presupposes an epidemiological base of incidence and prevalence rates of mortality and morbidity (e.g., Robbins & Regier, 1991). Programs are geared to target those populations that are shown to be highest at risk. Community mental health centers with their limited funding streams are now required by Public Law 99-660 to serve the most seriously mentally ill. Suddenly, the field is waking up to find that the training that psychology graduate students receive is outmoded for the wide-ranging needs of these multiply disabled patients (Davis, Moore, & Sanchez, 1990). Psychosocial rehabilitation strategies, understanding of psychopharmacological effects and side effects, case management techniques, accessing of entitlement monies and residential alternatives, spanning boundaries of multiple systems of care, involvement of clients and their families, community offerings of natural supports, shaping of policy, planning of programs, and administrative management are all part of the new public psychology curriculum (see Appendix, this chapter).

The preeminent fields of psychology and psychiatry have played relatively minimal roles in the care of such patients until recently (Torrey, 1973). For both psychiatrists and psychologists, the status of working in a state institution, with some exceptions, has been quite low in these two professions. Members of both professions, psychologists more recently than psychiatrists, have viewed private practice with upper-middle-class individuals as the ideal. There appears to be no systematized training at the graduate or postdoctoral levels in public psychology. University-based clinical psychology programs have mostly side-stepped the issue of serious mental illness with very little academic clinical focus being placed on this area. Currently, almost all psychologists working in the public sector with this population have received their training on the job "by the seat of their pants" and most have never had exposure to possible career paths and options within the mental health system. However, it is clear that individuals with severe mental illness need more extensive public care than has been available to them.

In 1990, within the context of the above situation, the National Institute of Mental Health (NIMH) and Georgetown University sponsored the National Conference on Implementing Public–Academic Linkages for Clinical Training in Psychology (Linkages Conference), which is reported in this book. The Linkages Conference occurred simultaneously with the development of the Colorado Program for Public Psychology.

Colorado Program for Public Psychology

The program's evolution was spurred on by the Linkages Conference, thus creating a new program of four postdoctoral fellowships in this area. This new program has become a part of the ongoing training programs of the Division of Clinical Psychology of the University of Colorado Health Sciences Center. A rough blueprint for such an undertaking existed, because the Department of Psychiatry, of which the Division of Clinical Psychology is a part, had already initiated an innovative Program in Public Psychiatry several years ago (Neligh et al., 1991). One person, a member of the psychology faculty and the Associate Director of Programs for Public Psychiatry had many contacts in the public sector and was working within an established public–academic linkage system. She, together with the Head of the Division of Clinical Psychology, began work to bring this training process to reality. We convened a working task force consisting of 22 psychologists who represented the Colorado Public Mental Health System to evaluate the possibility of putting together and funding a postdoctoral program in public psychology.

There existed serious and persistent technological gaps and a lack of psychologists specifically trained to provide care, to design and implement policies and programs, and to conduct meaningful research in the area of serious mental illness. The task force was enthusiastic about such an endeavor and began to proceed conjointly in the effort to develop such a program. This collaborative effort was directly congruent with the mission and goals of the NIMH public–academic linkages initiative.

The initial meeting involved psychologists from the Colorado Division of Mental Health, the Colorado Mental Health Institute of Pueblo (formerly the Colorado State Hospital), the Colorado Department of Corrections, the Mental Health Corporation of Denver (the umbrella organization for the community mental health care delivered in Denver) and the Mental Health Program of the Western Interstate Commission for Higher Education (WICHE). The idea of several postdoctoral fellowships, funded and located primarily within these settings, was discussed, with the Division of Clinical Psychology serving as the organizing entity.

Members of that group met frequently during the following 12 months to work out the training modules and curriculum and to identify the responsible training supervisors in each of these settings. Although discussions of the content of the training were in the forefront, the issue of the financing of this venture was not far behind. As might be expected, it was money that created the largest stumbling block. In the relative absence of current NIMH training funds as incentives for collaborative ventures, the Health Sciences Center representatives proposed that each of the community settings would need to provide the entire full-time equivalent of $29,510 for each postdoctoral fellow in the first year (1992–1993), even though agency funding streams have been severely cut. The breakdown of that amount is as follows: Stipend—$20,000; health and malpractice insurance—$3,657; supervision, training, and administration of the program—$5,853.

Each of the institutional representatives discussed this proposal within their own organization. The following five agencies eventually agreed to participate and to serve as training sites: Site 1—Forensic Unit of the Colorado Mental Health Institute of Pueblo, one position; Site 2—Colorado Department of Corrections at the Denver Reception and Diagnostic Center, one position; Site 3—Mental Health Corporation of Denver, one position; Site 4—Colorado Division of Mental Health (DMH), .5 position; and Site 5—Mental Health Program of WICHE, .5 position.

There will be one fellow who will split his or her time between Sites 4 and 5. Forensic fellows at Sites 1 and 2 will rotate through the two agencies for 2 days a week in each throughout the year. Site 3 fellow will be full-time (i.e., 4 days a week) at that community mental health agency. For 1 day a week, all fellows will participate in the seminar series of the Program for Public Psychiatry as well as in a psychology case conference. They will also receive additional supervision at the university. The primary supervision, however, will be on-site with the psychology director and other training staff. In each placement site, opportunities for administrative (i.e., policy planning, budget making, and programming) as well as research training exist. In all but Sites 4 and 5, clinical training is also one of the central activities. Each program will be tailor-made by mutual assent so that both the needs and interests of each agency as well as those of each fellow are taken into consideration. The program will then be approved by the faculty.

Because the program at Sites 1, 2, and 3 involves clinical training in addition to research and administrative training, appointments will be limited to those who have completed a doctorate and an internship from the American Psychological Association (APA) accredited programs. Sites 4 and 5 differ from the others in that only research, policy making, program planning, curriculum building, and administration are part of the program. Thus, graduates from programs in areas other than clinical and counseling psychology have been invited to apply.

Our progress in getting the program up and running has not been as swift as we would have liked. In fact, we had to postpone the program for a year due to several factors impinging on the process. We were delayed in advertising in the APA *Monitor* (April 1992) because one agency was late with brochure information and one was late with advertising money. Thus, our candidate pool was significantly reduced. Second, we found that agencies were unwilling to sign contracts until Congress voted on the block grants to states in 1992. This event happened in July. Furthermore, we failed to appreciate the layers of bureaucracy through which the contract signing had to go. By that point, we had lost the few good candidates we had found. In addition, when we presented this program at the annual meeting of the American Psychiatric Association's Institute on Hospital and Community Psychiatry in October, we discovered that representatives from the fields of psychology, nursing, psychiatry, and social work had no conception of what modern-day public psychology was. We brainstormed in that session and renamed the concept "public/community psychology."

Having learned from our adventures, we had the agency contracts signed early, and we advertised in January 1993. Of interest to us is the fact that applicants appeared before the advertising because of word of mouth. We have narrowed the focus to 2 or 3 fellows in the DMH/WICHE combination and in forensics. The advertising has focused on offering "new skills for career advancement in public administration, policy-making, program planning and evaluation as well as forensic/clinical experience." We are optimistic that we can now go forward with this fellowship opportunity and, in fact, have accepted our first fellow.

We believe that the Colorado Program for Public Psychology Postdoctoral Training represents an exciting opportunity to fill the vacuum existing in the United States. We expect to entice, train, and retain cadres of psychologists well versed in public mental strategies to make policy, design programs, provide administrative leadership, develop curricula, conduct meaningful research, and provide state-of-the-art service delivery for the targeted population, which is in desperate need of continuity, excellence, and innovation.

In conclusion, we would like to add a statement that we think provides an appropriate final note to this chapter. It was made during our problem-planning sessions by Frank McGuirk, PhD (one of our supervisors and Director of the Mental Health Program of the Western Interstate Commission for Higher Education), who said: "The public sector needs more conceptual leadership. Psychologists have the most training in theoretical constructs and in cause/effect analyses of serious mental illness. Psychologists should be articulating the relationships and transmitting them to line staff on a daily basis. They should take their hypothesis-testing skills and convert them to day-to-day skill building and assess whether or not strategies are consistent with constructs. Psychologists do not have to be pigeon-holed as specialists (e.g., neuropsychologists, projective testers, etc.), but possess concepts, theories, and experience in solving problems with a crisp clean manner. Models and research findings could and should drive policy making and program building more than it does" (F. McGuirk, personal communication, April 16, 1993; see also Demler, Moore, McGuirk, & Sanchez, 1992).

It is indeed time for psychologists to remarket and reinsert their special expertise into a broadened presence across the public sector currently overwhelmed by massive service delivery problems in treating the seriously mentally ill population in the United States.

References

Albee, G. (1959). Mental health power trends; a report to the staff director, Jack R. Ewalt. (Joint Commission on Mental Illness and Health, Monograph series no. 3). New York: Basic Books.

Albee, G. (1964). A declaration of independence for psychology. *Ohio Psychologist, 11,* 2–4.

Albee, G., & Joffe, J. M. (1977). *Primary prevention of psychopathology: Vol. 1: The issues.* Hanover, NH: University Press of New England.

Bower, E. M. (1963). Primary prevention of mental and emotional disorders: A conceptual framework and action possibilities. *American Journal of Orthopsychiatry, 33,* 832–848.

Brown, M. (1965). Form follows function—psychologists in broadening roles. *Comprehensive Psychiatry, 6,* 274–281.

Caplan, G. (1964). *Principles of preventive psychiatry.* New York: Basic Books.

Combs, A. W., Fisk, R. S., Fine, H. J., Zimet, C. N., Wiberley, A., & Nesbitt, D. A. (1954). The Syracuse studies. *Journal of Social Issues, 10*(2), 5–8.

Davis, M., Moore, D., & Sanchez, M. (Eds.). (1990). *Strengthening linkages between state mental health systems and higher education in the west.* Boulder, CO: Western Interstate Commission for Higher Education.

Demler, J., Moore, D., McGuirk, F., & Sanchez, A. M. (1992). *Training needs of a changing mental health system: Exploring relationships with two-year colleges* (Publication No. 3B74). Boulder, CO: Western Interstate Commission for Higher Education.

Hoch, E. L., Ross, A. O., & Winder, C. L. (1966). *Professional preparation of clinical psychologists.* Washington, DC: American Psychological Association.

Joint Commission of Mental Illness and Health (1961). *Final report: Action for mental health.* New York: Basic Books.

McMahon, B., & Pugh, T. F. (1970). *Epidemiology: Principles and methods.* Boston: Little, Brown.

National conference on implementing public–academic linkages for clinical training in psychology (1990, December). Sponsored jointly by NIMH and Georgetown University Child Development Center, Washington, DC.

Neligh, G. N., Shore, J. H., Scully, J., Kort, H., Willett, B., Harding, C. M., & Kawamura, G. (1991). The program for public psychiatry: State–university collaboration in Colorado. *Hospital and Community Psychiatry, 42*(1), 44–48.

President's Commission on Mental Health (1978). *Report to the President* (Vol. 1). Washington, DC: U.S. Government Printing Office.

Raimy, V. (Ed.). (1950). *Training in clinical psychology.* New York: Prentice-Hall.

Robbins, L. N. & Regier, D. A. (Eds.). (1991). *Psychiatric disorders in America: Epidemiologic catchment area study.* New York: Free Press.

Torrey, F. (1973). *The death of psychiatry.* New York: Chilton Press.

Turner, J. C., & Ten Hoor, W. J. (1978). The NIMH community support program: Pilot approach to a needed social reform. *Schizophrenia Bulletin, 4,* 319–348.

White, M. A., & Harris, M. W. (1961). *The school psychologist.* New York: Harper.

APPENDIX

Curriculum on Public Psychiatry and Psychology Department of Psychiatry and Division of Psychology, University of Colorado School of Medicine 1993–1994 Academic Calendar

Survival Skills for the Professional in the Public Sector

- Course Overview and Review of Educational Objectives
- Role of Multidisciplinary Team Members: Part 1
- Building and Participating in a Multidisciplinary Team
- Medical Psychiatric Assessment
- Assessment of Functional Status
- Psychopharmacology and Therapeutic Relationships
- Comprehensive Treatment Planning
- Ethical and Legal Issues Unique to the Public Sector
- Emergency and Crisis Care

Overview of Public Mental Health and Mental Illness

- History of Public Mental Health Systems in the United States and Abroad
- Schizophrenia: Old Mythologies and New Evidence
- Working With Families
- Working With Consumer Groups
- Schizophrenia, Affective Disorder, Panic Disorder, and Organic Syndromes
- Impact Upon Society and the Economy
- Substance Abuse and Mental Illness
- Epidemiology I: Historical Studies, Epidemiological Catchment Area (ECA), and Record Linkage
- Patterns of Service Delivery
- Epidemiology 2: Children

Service Delivery

- Prevention (Primary, Secondary, and Tertiary): The Debate
- Role of Multidisciplinary Team Members: Part 2
- Psychosocial Rehabilitation
- Case Management Models
- Residential Options
- Overflow Systems
- Research Issues

Designing Systems in Public Mental Health

- Basic System Architecture
- Role of Multidisciplinary Team Members: Part 3
- Public Information and Involvement
- Funding Public Systems
- Political Systems and Relationships
- The Mentally Ill and the Legal System
- Public–Academic Linkages

Running Systems

- Minimal versus Optimal Care
- Introduction to Administrative Psychiatry and Psychology

- Administrative Strategies
- Employee Motivation, Recruitment, and Retention
- The Impaired Employee
- Total Quality Management
- Hospital Psychiatry and Psychology in Managed Care Systems
- Total Quality Management
- Staff Training and Education
- Research and Evaluation in Public Mental Health

Developmental Disabilities (DD) System/Mental Health (MH) Structure of DD

- Behavior Management in Psychiatry and Psychology
- Habilitation With Team Approach
- Working With Nonverbal Clients
- Training in Working With People With DD
- Research Issues in DD Patients and Service Delivery
- Assessment by Participants in Program and Service Delivery

PART IV

Ensuring Quality and Competence in Training for Mental Health Services

CHAPTER

20

Using Research and Evaluation to Develop a Competent Workforce for Mental Health Services

Paul Wohlford and Ronald W. Manderscheid
Center for Mental Health Services

Introduction

More than two dollars of every three dollars spent by mental health organizations in 1988 was spent on their workforce (Sunshine, Witkin, Atay, & Manderschied, 1991). However, very little is known about this workforce. This is a very serious state of affairs if we wish to plan and improve service delivery programs and modify future clinical training practices.

We begin with a basic assumption that quality clinical training in mental health depends on a foundation of quality mental health services, an assumption that is widely shared by the authors of other chapters in this volume (e.g., chapters 2, 3, 4, & 5). This chapter discusses three contexts for improvement of the mental health workforce: the prevalence and treatment of mental illness and the lack of availability of providers; research and evaluation to improve mental health services, training programs, and competencies of individual service providers; and knowledge translation and transfer of research findings by trainers and faculty to mental health service providers. The purpose of this chapter is to provide a conceptual framework for these topics, to outline current progress, and to indicate future directions.

Mental Health Needs

One of Out Four Americans Have Mental or Addictive Disorders

Over 28% of our population, or 52 million adult Americans, have mental or addictive disorders as of 1990, according to the best available estimate based on the Epidemiologic Catchment Area (ECA) study (Regier et al., 1993). Of this total, about 41 million have mental disorders, almost 18 million have substance abuse disorders; these figures include about 6 million who have mental disorders with comorbid substance abuse (Regier et al., 1993).

In the ECA study, of those with mental disorders, over 23 million had anxiety disorders, and almost 18 million had affective disorders, including 2 million with bipolar depression and over 9 million with major unipolar depression. Finally, 2

The opinions expressed in this chapter are those of the authors and do not necessarily reflect the official policy or position of the Center for Mental Health Services. The authors wish to thank Carol T. Bush for her contribution to the section on mental health needs, and Frank J. Sullivan for his comments on the whole chapter.

million had schizophrenic disorders, and 5 million had severe cognitive impairment (Regier et al., 1993).

In a separate analysis, from the perspective of functional impairment, the total number of adults with a severe mental illness[1] was about 5 million (Barker, Manderscheid, Hendershot, Jack, & Schoenborn, 1992). Most of these people are currently limited in one or more functional areas so that they are unable to work, are limited in their capacity to cope with day-to-day stress, have difficulty making and keeping friends, and/or cannot concentrate long enough to complete tasks. Half of the severely mentally ill population live in households, but 200,000 are homeless on any given day; 1.1 million are residents of nursing homes; 60,000 are patients in mental hospitals; and 50,000 are inmates of state prisons (Barker et al., 1992).

Approximately 7.5 million children and adolescents have mental disorders; half of these children and youth have serious emotional disturbances that compromise their current functioning, imperil their development, and jeopardize their future (National Advisory Mental Health Council [NAMHC], 1990).

Most People Receive No Treatment

Of those 52 million with mental or addictive disorders, only a limited number receive any treatment at all, and an even smaller number get adequate treatment. Only 28% of the adults who have mental or addictive disorders receive any treatment at all; about 22% receive treatment from health or mental health care system providers; and only about 13% are seen in specialty mental or addictive health service settings (Regier et al., 1993). Less than 1.5 million children receive mental health treatment in organized systems (NAMHC, 1990). The capacity of the system is very small in comparison with the breadth of the need. Additional evidence of this includes the growth of the mentally ill population in prisons and among the homeless. Mental disorders were found in more than 55% of prisoners (Regier et al., 1990) and more than one third of homeless people (Manderschied & Rosenstein, 1992). The vast majority of these people require some treatment for mental illness.

If national health care reform ultimately includes mental and addictive disorders, it will enhance demand for these services. Of the 37 million Americans who currently have no health insurance, about 10 million are estimated to have mental or addictive disorders, based on the current prevalence rate (Regier et al., 1993). Using the current rates of use, up to 2.9 million of these people may seek services (Regier et al.), and it can be assumed that some proportion of these would be new service recipients. In addition, a large number of Americans who currently have some health insurance have limits that exclude or severely restrict treatment for mental and addictive disorders. Therefore, the total demand on mental health services is expected to increase if national health care reform includes these disorders.

Providers Are Not Available to Meet the Potential Demand

In 1990, about 531,000 full time equivalent staff worked in organized mental health settings (Redick, Witkin, Aray, & Manderschied, 1993). About 25% were administrative and support staff, and another 25% had not received college degrees. Included in this group were licensed practical and vocational nurses, aides, orderlies, and assistants. The remaining 50% were classed as professionals, including psychiatrists, psychologists, social workers, registered nurses, and other mental health workers with a bachelor of arts or higher degree. In short, about 248,000 professionals work in organized mental health settings (Redick et al., 1993). An additional 56,000 mental health professionals were in private practice (Dial et al., 1990). Therefore, the current total of mental health professionals, even broadly defined, who are in organized settings or private practice is only about 304,000.

Considering the 48 million American adults and children who have mental disorders, the current mental health service providers are spread very thinly. There is potentially only one provider per 145 people with mental disorders. Therefore, the relatively small number of mental health providers, their uneven geographical distribution, and the fact that many were trained 20 or more years ago (Dial et al., 1990), causes concerns about immediate and future mental health care. For

[1] Persons with a *severe mental illness* have a diagnosed mental disorder and have experienced substantial functional impairment for at least one year. They constitute a subset of the larger group of persons with *serious mental illness* who also have a diagnosed mental disorder and at least one substantial functional impairment, but with no criterion of duration of the impairment.

example, the Council on Graduate Medical Education (1993) reported a shortage of physicians in the specialties of child and adult psychiatry and an overall scarcity of minority physicians.

Framework for Improving Training of Mental Health Professionals

Historically, the field of mental health has had three primary functions: service, research, and training (see Figure 1). The interrelationships among these functions need to be considered. Ideally, the latest scientific advances in mental health research would be conveyed to service providers. A likely avenue for this to occur is through clinical training programs with expert faculty or trainers who would serve as intermediaries between clinical and service researchers and service providers.

The proposed model of this process would begin with current services to priority populations (bottom circle in Figure 1). Next, clinical and services research knowledge would be developed through an interactive process between services and research (note overlap of Services and Research in Figure 1). Through another interactive process of researchers and faculty, research knowledge would be translated and transferred to training faculty (note overlap of Research and Training in Figure 1). Then, clinical training faculty would share their knowledge with students in academic education and training (Training in Figure 1). The students would then apply what they learned, providing services to actual clients, under supervision in field training sites or internships (note overlap of Training and Services in Figure 1). Finally, students who completed their training would complete the cycle by practicing as credentialed professionals in regular service settings (Services in Figure 1). In principle, this circle that unites services, research, and training, could be repeated throughout service providers' careers in the form of continuing education for regular updating of skills and methods with the latest scientific knowledge. (The model in Figure 1 is elaborated more fully and applied to priority populations in Figures 1 through 4 in Chapter 26 of this volume).

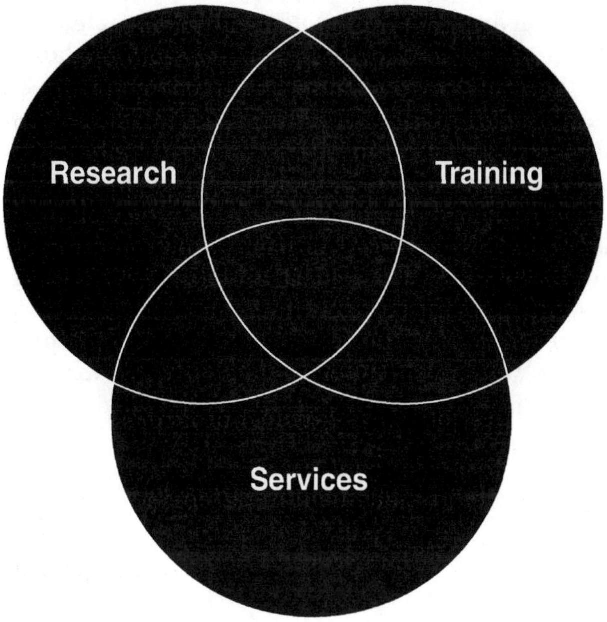

Figure 1. Model of the Interrelated Nature of Mental Health Functions

The services–research–training model may be used to develop a comprehensive conceptual framework for the overall goal of improving mental health services. Research and evaluation in three interrelated areas are needed to improve mental health service systems for individual clients and patients, training programs and faculty performance, and competencies of service providers. Research and evaluation activity in each of these three areas can be considered at four levels: national, state, program and system, and individual, generating the 12-cell matrix shown in Table 1. The activity level in the 12 cells ranges greatly from an extensive formal research literature, to occasional evaluation studies, to virtually nothing. The purpose of presenting this table is to identify the most important issues for each of the 12 topics, including areas of knowledge and areas that will require attention in the future. Space permits only a brief review of each topic.

Research and Evaluation to Improve Mental Health Service Systems

National Level

The quality of mental health services for clients and patients is partly addressed by national accreditation programs of hospitals by the Joint Commission on the Accreditation of Hospital Organizations (JCAHO) and of mental health service systems by the International Association of Psychosocial Rehabilitation Services (IASPRS).

The quality of mental health services is also addressed by the national evaluation of mental

Table 1. Overview of Research and Evaluation to Improve Mental Health Services, Training Programs, and Competencies of Individual Service Providers

Level	Services delivery system for individual clients	Training programs	Competencies of individual service providers
National	National evaluation of hospitals and service programs for accreditation (JCAHO, IASPRS) National evaluation of service grants	National evaluation of training programs for accreditation and for training grants Surveys of training programs Impact studies Comprehensive evaluation of training programs	Mental health workforce studies National board examinations for professionals Projection of future personnel needs
State	State evaluation of service programs	State evaluation of training programs	State licensing of professionals
Programs/Systems	Services research to improve services systems: Quality of care, cost, and access issues.	Evaluation of training programs	Evaluation of individual staff by service programs and systems
Individual	Clinical research to improve quality of care for individual clients and patients	Evaluation of individual faculty	Evaluation of competencies of individual service providers

Note. JCAHO = Joint Commission on Accreditation of Hospital Organizations; IASPRS = International Association of Psychosocial Rehabilitation Services.

health service programs. The federal government, through the Center for Mental Health Services (CMHS) directly supports certain services demonstration programs. The Community Support Program (CSP) and the Child and Adolescent Service System Program (CASSP) are service demonstration programs for seriously mentally ill adults and seriously emotionally disturbed children and adolescents, respectively, as mentioned in Chapters 8 and 9. These programs, plus the new child mental health services program, undergo national review in competition for service grants and generally undergo broadbased evaluations. Also CMHS reviews and evaluates the plans and programs for the state block grants for mental health services, as discussed below.

State Level

As state mental health agencies have assumed more responsibilities for public mental health services, many states have contracted with providers for these services. These states generally assess performance of the mental health service contracts on an annual basis as part of the implementation of their overall state mental health plans.

Within this context, a potentially powerful avenue for improvement of services lies in the state mental health planning process linked to the CMHS block grant. Because the states, local mental health agencies, consumers, and family members are mandated to participate in this process, the potential exists to significantly change service systems to improve the quality of services provided to individual clients and patients. This process is more fully described in Chapter 7 and in Appendix C.

Program and Systems Level

Services research is frequently oriented to the program level to improve mental health service systems, addressing issues such as quality of care, financing of services, and accessibility of services to various populations such as children, elderly, ethnic minorities, rural, and so on. Though these issues have been the subject of study and evaluation for several decades or even for centuries (White, 1993), the emergence of services research as a scientific discipline is much more recent.

Individual Level

Clinical research is oriented to the level of the individual client or patient to examine the etiology, diagnosis, course, treatment, and prevention of mental disorders. Clinical research has had a long history that includes critical efficacy studies about which treatments work and which do not. National health care reform is likely to focus renewed attention on efficacy studies to ensure that limited health-care resources are spent wisely. One of the greatest challenges is to translate and transfer knowledge based on such research findings to service providers. This transfer process needs to occur more effectively, as discussed in the Mental Health Knowledge Translation and Transfer section later in this chapter.

One fundamental though understudied component of clinical research is a careful description of successful treatments of particular disorders with particular groups of clients and patients to use as a recognized standard of care. Using this approach, the Agency for Health Care Policy and Research (AHCPR) has begun to systematically sum up research findings for treatment of specific disorders developing what they term *clinical protocols*. AHCPR has completed its clinical protocol on depression in primary care (AHCPR, 1993a, 1993b, 1993c, 1993d) and is now preparing one on schizophrenia. Having generally recognized standards of care for particular disorders, or clinical protocols, would prepare one to make some judgments about the clinical competencies of the provider. Establishing what constitutes quality services may be a most daunting task, although it is being taken up by the Task Group on Defining Clinical Competencies and Establishing Standards of Care, which is discussed in Chapter 26.

Research and Evaluation to Improve Training Programs and Faculty Performance

National Level

Evaluations of clinical training programs may rely on data from three sources: Self-reports of training program directors and faculty, students, and outside observers (site visitors). Wohlford (1990) proposed a model in which these three domains of data are partly overlapping: Each of the three perspectives shares some of its "reality" with the two others but also has its unique view. A comprehensive evaluation must take all three perspectives into account.

Three types of national-level evaluations of training programs include training program review for accreditation by national professional accrediting bodies, competitive training program review for clinical training grant awards, and other studies including surveys of training programs and comprehensive evaluations of training programs.

Accreditation review. The evaluation of training programs for the purpose of national accreditation is an important quality assurance mechanism for each mental health discipline, including psychology. Each discipline establishes its own standards and permits training institutions to set their own goals and objectives in the context of societal needs for quality services, disciplinary standards, and unique circumstances of each institution. For actual evaluations, programs undergo extensive self-studies followed by site visits, and finally committee review. This process is discussed in Chapter 23.

Clinical training grant review. From 1986 to 1992, about 1,500 clinical training grant applications were reviewed by NIMH, and about 300 new grants were awarded. Such national competition seems to result in the identification and correction of potential problems in training programs and, finally, improvement of training practices.

Other studies. To determine what training is provided for services to seriously mentally ill adults, Johnson (this volume) surveyed directors of clinical psychology training programs. He found that although nearly all programs included some material on serious mental illness, less than one tenth had tracks on serious mental illness.

The most important single piece of evaluation data for training programs is outcome. One type of outcome of clinical training was recently reported to Congress regarding clinical trainees who incurred a payback service obligation. Of the 6,072 trainees who incurred a payback obligation and completed their training, 93% completed their payback service requirement. Of those who completed their payback service, 80% are continuing to work in public or private nonprofit mental health service (CMHS, 1993b).

State Level

The state evaluation of training programs should not be overlooked. Indeed, the level of state support for clinical training appears to be quite extensive, over $45 million in 1990, according to the National Association of State Mental Health Program Directors (S. Broad, personal communication, February 9, 1992). Yet, in states that presently support clinical training, one would expect some review of the training programs.

Program/Systems Level

As discussed earlier under national accreditation, extensive self-evaluation is the first step of the accreditation review. Theoretically, it is possible to expand this self-evaluation of training programs to include other similar local programs, which could then comprise a quality review circle. An example of this is available. To prepare for future national accreditation, the postdoctoral clinical neuropsychology programs in the north central States formed an informal quality review circle in which participant programs prepared self-study documents and had mock site visits (M. Meier, personal communication, July 14, 1993).

Individual Level

This section focuses on the performance of the individual faculty member or trainer. With the explosion of knowledge and the inevitable specialization of practice and research, keeping up with any general clinical area requires special efforts. Because of the conceptual and operational difficulties of evaluating individual faculty members, little is currently known in this area. Efforts to review this should be made in the future. Regardless of what is done to evaluate the performance of individual faculty members, there should be, at minimum, systematic faculty development programs and national clearinghouses for the latest information and curricula on the various priority populations, as discussed in the final section of this chapter.

Research and Evaluation to Improve Competencies of Service Providers

National Level

National surveys of the mental health workforce. The major professional associations are collaborating on a long-term project to improve the comparability of human resource data. Several phases of work are being undertaken:

1. Dial and colleagues (1990) collected and reported statistical information for each of the four historical core disciplines (i.e., psychiatry, psychology, social work, and psychiatric nursing). Making use of data available through surveys already done in the four disciplines, they reported demographic data, training characteristics, and professional activities of providers.

2. Subsequently, Dial and colleagues (1992) added the three developing practice areas of marriage and family therapy, clinical mental health counseling, and psychosocial rehabilitation to the other four disciplines in a statistical report on trainees. Besides presenting information about training, practice, licensure, and certification, they presented available demographic data on students and trainees and trends in the disciplines.

3. The areas in which the seven professional associations will collect comparable data or human resources will be expanded in future surveys. The objective is to attain uniform data about human resources across all relevant mental health disciplines. A minimum data set has been developed for use by all disciplines, and planning is underway for a joint survey to be conducted in the future so that comparable data are available for all disciplines at the same time.

One can be cautiously optimistic that the data situation with respect to human resources will improve in the future. Clearly, the first step in this process has been the recognition that considerable improvement is needed in a database that is key to the future of the mental health field.

Projection of future personnel needs. CMHS is currently undertaking an effort to project human resources for the public sector through the year 2000, based on past trends. It is anticipated that the results of this work will be available in 1994.

A major policy study is needed to determine shortages of mental health personnel, particularly in light of national health care reform. For example, the Council on Graduate Medical Education (1993) states that currently a shortage of psychiatrists exists. A careful databased study should take into account the general concern that in the near future absolute shortages may occur in public mental health personnel across all disciplines.

From the results, any immediate mental health personnel shortages should be identifiable, as well as any anticipated shortages in the intermediate-term future (Goldsmith, Witkin, Sacks, & Manderscheid, 1993).

National examinations of proficiencies and competencies in the mental health professions. The mental health professions have national board examinations for individual professionals to achieve certification of a high proficiency level. Examples include the American Board of Psychiatry, the American Board of Child and Adolescent Psychiatry, the American Board of Professional Psychology (an umbrella organization now covering eight specialty boards), the American Nurses' Association certification of clinical specialists, and the Academy of Certified Social Workers, among others.

Having a provider who passed national board exams is one important quality control for consumers, relative to the state of the art in that specialty, as reflected by the acknowledged leaders who give the exam. The provider who is "boarded" is more likely than a nonboarded provider to be thoroughly familiar with the field, more acquainted with relevant literature, and better able to apply this knowledge with a variety of populations, including seriously mentally ill adults, severely emotionally disturbed children, and so on.

State Level

Competencies of individual mental health services professionals are assessed at the state level by licensing or certification examinations and procedures. State licensing of professionals is the oldest and most important formal mechanism for safeguarding the public welfare by attempting to ensure some (even minimal) level of professional competency. Because of the public's other need, that of an adequate supply of providers, the level of the licensing standards probably constitutes a floor rather than a desired level for professional practice. This issue is discussed in more detail in Chapter 22 of this volume.

Program/Systems Level

Assessment of staff competencies has not been examined in a systematic way, due in part to the lack of methodology for assessing the clinical competencies of individual providers, which is discussed in the next section.

Much informal evaluation does occur in training settings and in institutional settings in the form of supervision of the provider. The problem is that this supervision process is idiosyncratic and perhaps subjective. Like the clinical competencies of the provider, the supervisory process has no easily codified, recognized standards other than the credentials of the supervisor. In service settings that are also formal training field settings for internships and residencies, the amount and intensity of supervision is much greater than in ordinary service programs in which actual supervision may vary from regular to nonexistent.

Individual Level

The clinical competency of the individual service provider is the cornerstone on which the entire service system stands. However, curiously, little systematic research or evaluation has been conducted to examine competencies. Sechrest and Scott discuss this critical issue in Chapter 21 of this volume. Initially they expected that competencies would fall into three categories: knowledge, attitudes, and practices (e.g., skills). Whereas some competencies might be trainable, others might not be and might require that selection into the field be made for these (e.g., personal qualities). They divided competencies into personal qualities, knowledge, clinical skills, job-related knowledge, entry-level skills, and updating skills. Clearly, much work is needed in this area.

Linkages Among Services, Training, and Competencies

Some very important evaluation questions arise at the interface of some cells in the 12-cell matrix. One example is the interface between the quality of service at the program level and the competencies of individual providers, taking into account preservice and in-service training experiences. In a recent conference on improving the mental health workforce (CMHS, 1993a), it was noted that one of the missing pieces of vital information for developing competent mental health teams is to know what makes a successful team work. One needs to explore the characteristics of teams that are highly successful in enhancing the quality of life of the persons they serve. In addition, what is the structure of the provider staff, what preservice training have individual providers had, and what in-service training is offered? What other factors, such as morale, contribute to service outcome?

In an initial study, mental health administrators, providers, and consumers identified 180 service programs they judged were truly excellent for providing service to a priority population (Coursey & Wohlford, 1993). Next, these excellent service programs will be contacted to determine their provider staff structure, preservice and in-service training of providers, and other factors that result in their excellent reputation.

The critical interface between services research and the improvement of clinical training should also be systematically examined.

Mental Health Knowledge Translation and Transfer

As Arons and Goodwin point out in the Foreword to this volume, "A major challenge in clinical training is to minimize the discrepancies between the state of science, the state of clinical training, and the typical state of practice." In short, the latest scientific knowledge needs to be translated into mental health services practice through preservice and in-service training.

The highly differentiated service needs of consumers, specifically seriously mentally ill adults, seriously emotionally disturbed children, elderly people and ethnic minorities with mental disorders, individuals diagnosed with dual disorders, and mentally ill people in rural areas, have generated highly differentiated research projects yielding rich and complex findings. The need to translate and transfer the latest research findings from these studies applies to both the interface between services and training and the interface between training and service providers. This is a three-part challenge composed of research, translation, and transfer.

- First, research: to conduct the actual research that is relevant to services issues.

- Second, translation: to identify, out of hundreds and thousands of research reports, the solid new research findings that may be applied to clinical situations. To render these research findings usable by faculty and trainers requires systematic translation, including the critical analysis of conflicting findings and synthesis in an understandable summary. The 1991 National Institute of Health Consensus Conference on Treatment of Depression in the Elderly is a good example of translation of research findings.

- Third, transfer: to give these findings to faculty and trainers. This is a separate process, and systematic faculty development, including a national clearinghouse for curricula materials, and Regional Centers of Excellence for Mental Health Services, Training, and Research, has been recommended (see Appendix A). The transfer process also includes the dissemination of this translated knowledge on a large scale to a broad range of training settings in universities and field training sites. The transfer of the latest research knowledge from faculty and trainers to new providers occurs in preservice education programs. Although that continues to be important, much more attention must be given to systematic and continual in-service training and continuing education as part of a career-long effort to keep individual providers informed and up-to-date in their specialties.

Conclusion

Never before has the contribution of research and evaluation been so clearly an integral part of the overall goal of improving health services. In this chapter, a functional model was proposed to illustrate the interconnectedness of mental health services–research–training systems. The logic of this model was then used to develop a conceptual framework for examining the role of research and evaluation in the three domains of service delivery, training programs, and competencies of individual service providers, each at the national, state, program, and individual levels. The model and framework are useful conceptually to illustrate the interrelationships of different subsystems within the overall mental health system. They are useful heuristically to identify gaps in knowledge. Finally, the knowledge translation and transfer strategy is critical to the ultimate success of achieving the overarching goal of improving mental health services.

References

Agency for Health Care Policy and Research (AHCPR). (1993a). *Depression in Primary Care: Detection, Diagnosis, and Treatment. Quick Reference Guide for Clinicians.* Clinical Practice Guideline Number 5

(DHHS, Publication No. AHCPR 93-0552). Washington, DC: U.S. Government Printing Office.

Agency for Health Care Policy and Research (AHCPR). (1993b). *Depression in Primary Care: Vol. 1. Detection and Diagnosis.* Clinical practice guideline number 5 (DHHS Publication No. AHCPR 93-0550). Washington, DC: U.S. Government Printing Office.

Agency for Health Care Policy and Research (AHCPR). (1993c). *Depression in Primary Care: Vol. 2. Treatment of Major Depression.* Clinical practice guideline number 5 (DHHS Publication No. AHCPR 93-0551). Washington, DC: U.S. Government Printing Office.

Agency for Health Care Policy and Research (AHCPR). (1993d). *Depression is a Treatable Illness: A Patient's Guide.* Clinical guideline (DHHS Publication No. AHCPR 93-0553). Washington, DC: U.S. Government Printing Office.

Barker, P. R., Manderscheid, R. W., Hendershot, G. E., Jack, S. S., & Schoenborn, C. A. (1992). Serious mental illness and disability in the adult household population: United States, 1989. In R. W. Manderscheid, & M. A. Sonnenschein (Eds.), *Mental health, United States, 1992.* (DHHS Publication No. SMA 92-1942, pp. 225–268). Washington, DC: U.S. Government Printing Office.

Center for Mental Health Services (CMHS). (1993a, February). *National conference on building a competent mental health workforce for the 21st century,* Washington, DC.

Center for Mental Health Services (CMHS). (1993b). *Report to the United States Congress: Evaluation of the mental health clinical training program payback requirement.* Rockville, MD: Department of Health and Human Services.

Council on Graduate Medical Education (COGME) (1993). *Improving access to health care through physician manpower reform: Directions for 21st century. Highlights of the third report of COGME.* Washington, DC: Author.

Coursey, R. D., & Wohlford, P. (1993). *Excellent service programs for seriously mentally ill adults, children with seriously emotional disturbances and other underserved groups: A preliminary study of staff structure and training.* Unpublished manuscript.

Dial, T. H., Pion, G. M., Cooney, B., Kohout, J., Kaplan, K. O., Ginsberg, L., Merwin, E. I., Fox, J. C., Ginsberb, M., Staton, J., Clawson, T. W., Wildermuth, V. A., Blankertz, L., & Hughers, R. (1992). Training of mental health providers. In R. W. Manderscheid & M. A. Sonnenschein (Eds.), *Mental health, United States, 1992, Center for Mental Health Services and National Institute of Mental Health* (DHHS Publication No. SMA 92-1942, pp. 142–162). Washington, DC: U.S. Government Printing Office.

Dial, T. H., Tebutt, R., Pion, G. M., Kohout, J., VandenBos, G., Johnson, M., Schervish, P. H., Whiting, L., Fox, J. C., & Merwin, E. I. (1990). Human resources in mental health. In R. W. Manderscheid & M. A. Sonnenschein (Eds.), *Mental health, United States, 1990* (DHHS Publication No. ADM 90-1708, pp. 196–215). Washington, DC: U.S. Government Printing Office.

Goldsmith, H. F., Witkin, M. J., Sacks, A. J., & Manderscheid, R. W. (1993). *Estimates and projections of staffing categories of state and county mental hospitals and Veterans Administration medical centers: United States 1970 to 1995.* Manuscript submitted for publication.

Manderscheid, R. W., & Rosenstein, M. J. (1992). Homeless persons with mental illness and alcohol or other drug abuse: Current research, policy, and projects. *Current Opinion in Psychiatry, 5,* 273–278.

National Advisory Mental Health Council. (1990). *National plan for research on child and adolescent mental disorders* (DHHS Publication No. ADM 90–1683). Washington, DC: U.S. Government Printing Office.

Redick, R. W., Witkin, M. J., Atay, J. E., and Manderscheid, R. W. (1993). Staffing of mental health organizations, United States, 1988. *Mental Health Statistical Note No. 206* (DHHS Publication No. SMA 93-1992). Washington DC: U.S. Government Printing Office.

Regier, D. A., Farmer, M. E., Rae, D. S., Locke, B. Z., Keith, S. J., Judd, L., & Goodwin, F. K. (1990). Comorbidity of mental disorders with alcohol and other drug abuse: Results from the Epidemiologic Catchment Area (ECA) Study. *Journal of the American Medical Association, 264,* 2511–2518.

Regier, D. A., Narrow, W. E., Rae, D. S., Manderscheid, R. W., Locke, B. Z., & Goodwin, F. K. (1993). The de facto U.S. mental and addictive disorders service system: Epidemiologic catchment area prospective 1-year prevalence rates of disorders and services. *The Archives of General Psychiatry, 50,* 85–94.

Sunshine, J. H., Witkin, M. J., Atay, J. E., and Manderscheid, R. W. (1991). Expenditures and sources of funds for mental health organizations: United States and each state, 1988. *Mental Health Statistical Note No. 199.* (DHHS Publ. No. ADM 91-1829). Washington, DC: U.S. Government Printing Office.

White, K. L. (1993, summer). Health care research: Old wine in new bottles. *Pharos,* 12–16.

Wohlford, P. (1990). National responsibilities to improve training for psychological services for children, youth, and families in the 1990s. In P. R. Magrab & P. Wohlford (Eds.), *Improving psychological services for children and adolescents with severe mental disorders: Clinical training in psychology* (pp. 11–34). Washington, DC: American Psychological Association.

CHAPTER

21

Assessing the Competencies of Clinical Psychologists

Lee Sechrest and Anne Scott
University of Arizona

Evaluating the competency of clinical psychologists is both timely and necessary, particularly if the field is to maintain a professional status with the public and the health services field. Although assessment of an area as complex and nebulous as clinical psychology may seem overwhelming and replete with problems, this chapter aims to focus on specific assessment issues relevant to the profession, address drawbacks and limitations, and offer some preliminary findings and possible strategies for assessment procedures.

Beginning in 1987, we undertook a series of pilot studies, supported by the National Institute of Mental Health (NIMH), aimed at identifying clinical competencies, especially those involved in working with the seriously mentally ill, and at exploring approaches to assessment of those competencies. We thought it likely, but not a foregone conclusion, that the competencies desirable for working with the seriously mentally ill might not be coterminous with those required for working with other types of disorders and problems. In general, we expected that competencies would fall into the three rather general categories of knowledge, attitudes, and practices (i.e., skills). We suspected, too, that not all competencies are likely to be trainable (i.e., some of them, particularly in the area of attitudes, but also some skills, might represent dimensions of temperament and personality not very amenable to specific training efforts).

Our efforts to pilot test methods of assessing competencies were fairly broad in scope, and we did not restrict ourselves to those methods that would be easy and inexpensive to administer. As will be clear from this chapter, the reasons for wanting to assess competencies are diverse and not all of them reflect a prime concern for expediency. Thus, we tried some paper-and-pencil measures, but we also tried an approach that required use of a trained actor being interviewed by clinicians who believed him to be a bona fide mental patient. We were restricted to pilot testing of methods and could never offer any firm conclusions or very directly interpretable results, but our general position now is that, as in so many endeavors, you get what you pay for. Cheap and easy methods are not very satisfactory. Any serious interest in assessing clinical competencies will have to be in the context of serious effort, including a lot of developmental work, and serious funding.

Assessment of competencies for dealing with patients who are seriously mentally ill has received almost no attention. Perhaps it might be thought that such competencies are not much different from those involved in dealing with psychological and mental illness problems more generally, but that is doubtful. Certainly more knowledge of a biological and biomedical nature would be useful, including more extensive knowledge of psychopharmacology. Seriously mentally ill people probably require more caution and sensitivity to symptom exacerbation on the part of clinicians. More knowledge and skill in working with community agencies, including police and legal services, is also required. In any case, the questions that might be raised about the need for specialized competencies for working with the seriously mentally ill are empirical in nature, and they have not been addressed as yet.

We suspect that a distinct bifurcation in career paths and in modes of practice exists between clinicians who offer their services to the general public and those who work with the seriously mentally ill. In a current study we are doing of telephone yellow pages advertising of mental health services (Sechrest & Smith, in press), several thousand listings of psychologists and psychotherapists reveal not one instance of any specific mention of services for the seriously mentally ill nor any mention of any "serious" disorder such as schizophrenia, bipolar disorder, or psychosis, let alone any claim to specialize in such problems. The reason, undoubtedly, is that services for the seriously mentally ill have, with the possible exception of some private inpatient facilities, been driven out of the private and into the public sector. Services to the seriously mentally ill in the public sector depend heavily on subdoctoral (often only baccalaureate) level personnel (Mechanic & Aiken, 1987). These personnel may never have undergone any formal competency assessments at all (e.g., such as they might have gotten in formal training programs). In the meantime, private sector practitioners are likely to avoid seriously mentally ill patients, even if they happen to come into contact with them. Seriously mentally ill patients very often have no financial resources, and they often spell clinical trouble; they are likely to be referred elsewhere.

Reasons for Assessing Clinical Competencies

Before addressing assessment design issues, it is important to acknowledge the many reasons one might want to assess competencies in clinical psychologists. Depending on which reason one might have for assessment, different approaches would be needed in order to arrive at an adequate answer. For example, one reason for assessment might be to provide for better decision-making in hiring, assigning, and compensating workers. Another reason might be to enhance quality assurance in service delivery (i.e., to determine whether staff are actually competent to deliver a high level of services to the clientele being served). Sometimes this competency may be thought of as meeting a required standard for an individual clinician, but competency may also be assessed for the program as a whole. The supervisor might also want to monitor services delivery in order to determine whether the upgrading of personnel, training for current personnel, or increased supervision might be necessary. Occasionally, assessment of a specific aspect of clinical services may be of interest (e.g., an agency might want to determine whether a new approach to case management is effective). The assessment during training of competencies of trainees by their supervisors is another potential interest. Assessing training programs might be at issue either because the quality of a specific program is of interest or because the program may represent a generic type or approach. For example, one might want to assess a specific case manager program in an agency, but one might also want to assess case manager programs generically as approaches to dealing with some types of problems in mental illness. Some of the concerns for competency have to do with the education and training of clinicians, whereas others are relevant to clinicians already in practice, whether they are in individual practice or in a group setting.

The reasons cited for assessing competencies affect an array of concerns and decisions related to specific approaches to and methods of assessment. One needs to be concerned about which specific competencies are being assessed, whether competencies must be assessed under highly standardized conditions, whether a 100% sample is required rather than a partial sample, how quickly assessment results may be obtained, and what the cost of the assessment process will be. Assessment for purposes of individual personnel decision-making requires that critical, but not necessarily all, competencies be assessed, that assessments be standardized, that all personnel in a relevant category be assessed, that results be available very quickly (especially for hiring decisions), and that the cost of assessment be low. Evaluating training programs, by contrast, may not require assessment of a wide range of competencies and may not require more than a sample of the eligible participants. Moreover, evaluation of training programs may not require that results be immediately available, and more expensive assessment procedures may be justified. In fact, for purposes of evaluating model generic programs, expense of the assessment may, within limits, not be of much concern at all.

Establishing a Theory of Competency in Clinical Psychology

Before trying to design an assessment strategy, it must first be established what is meant by a "competent clinician." Clinical psychology itself has never been adequately defined, which makes development of an evaluation approach problematic. Although some of the paths to the clinical practice of psychology lack official sanction, those who take them often gain professional acceptance from third-party payers, referral sources, and other clinical psychologists of repute. Obviously, when one cannot even determine for sure just who is a clinical psychologist or how a person became one, it is not an easy task to say just what would constitute competency.

The actual, detailed activities of clinical psychologists are extremely diverse and not well-known. Clinical psychologists practice under widely varying conditions and engage in a wide range of professional services from neuropsychological assessment to industrial/organizational consultation. Some practice in near isolation in small rural communities; others practice in urban group practices with scores of other health professionals. Until the specific kinds of activities clinical psychologists perform and the amount of time spent on each are known, it will be difficult to know how to best train and then assess clinicians. Although the diversity of clinical psychology is one of its greatest strengths, that very diversity will make it difficult to evaluate the training and education of clinical psychologists.

Some information has been documented; for example, the 1983 report *Job Analysis of Licensed Psychologists in the United States and Canada* (Rosenfeld, Shimberg, & Thornton, 1983) provided considerable detailed, although unfortunately superficial, information about what clinical psychologists do. An "intervention" item, for example, was to "provide assistance to individuals regarding personal and organizational problems" (Tables V-22 and B-3, Rosenberg et al., 1983). The report showed that nearly all clinical psychologists engage in that activity, but the category is so broad as to be virtually meaningless. One needs to know whether some clients were suicidal, whether they came from lower- or middle-class backgrounds, how many were children, whether some had legal problems, and so on. Planning effective educational and training programs and their evaluation is likely to be beyond us without much better knowledge about practice.

Career Patterns of Practicing Clinicians

One approach to a better understanding of what is a competent clinician may be to examine the career patterns of professional psychologists in order to design better evaluation strategies. For example, how do clinicians end up in independent practice—do they usually begin their careers in another clinical setting? We are currently looking at data we have collected on over 100 local (Arizona) practitioners and have found that most practicing clinicians who specialize in various areas (which in our city is by far the majority of clinicians) did not start out in that specialty area. This finding means that they probably acquired the skills and knowledge necessary for that specialty outside of their educational program. We need to know more about how they obtained the knowledge and skills necessary for that field. We do know from our own study that more practitioners believe that experience (90%) is very important to being a competent clinician as opposed to education (71%) or even training with an expert (73%). What exactly does this "experience" mean to these clinicians? Experience could be construed simply in terms of time in practice or number of cases seen, or it could represent intensive processing of cognitive and affective material related to cases.[1] We should also determine the proportion of professional psychologists who are in part-time private practice and what activities they engage in during the rest of their working day. Answers to these questions are prerequisites for a clear conception of entry-level professional skills and for a sense as to which additional skills should later be developed and how long all of this should take.

Professional Activities of Practicing Clinicians

Another approach might be to determine the actual activities that clinical psychologists engage in, the frequency of the activities, and their clientele. This would help to evaluate the relevance of education and training to the demands of the profession. Who are their clients and what is the nature of these contacts, their hours, and conditions of work? In what other types of professional activities do they engage? From our own study, we have found that clinicians spend most of their time

[1] One of our mentors, George A. Kelly, used to relate from time to time the story of a man who had had "one year of experience repeated thirteen times."

providing therapy, consultations, and interventions for clients. Very few of the clinicians sampled for our study attended workshops or lectures (10%). Thirty-seven percent of the respondents claimed to spend 5–20 hours a week reading journal articles and books in their own specialty area.[2] Information from self-report surveys could be biased and provide only limited information of what clinicians do, whereas activity logs have been demonstrated to be a feasible route to describing the practices of physicians (Mendenhall & Abrahamson, 1973) and could be easily kept by a sample of psychologists recruited, and perhaps compensated, especially for this purpose.

Data on how professional psychologists know and define the boundaries of their competence could be useful in developing a program to evaluate education and training. Guideline 1.6 of the specialty guidelines for clinical psychology (Committee on Professional Standards, 1981) states that "clinical psychologists limit their practice to their demonstrated areas of professional competence" (p. 7). The text goes on to establish the basis for competence as verifiable training and experience and the extension of services beyond the range of their usual practice. No such guideline can be very specific, but it seems important to know how clinicians and other psychologists come to identify their competencies and define the boundaries of those competencies. For example, a psychologist could have had ample training and experience with a particular problem, yet still sense a deficiency in his or her personal competence on other grounds. How much training and experience is sufficient surely differs from one professional to the next, and some would undoubtedly be bolder than others in generalizing the effects of their training and experience across age groups, problems, modalities, and so forth. Data on how psychologists define their competencies could be useful in developing a program to evaluate education and training. We know of no such data.

Based on feedback from practicing clinicians, it might be decided that adequate assessment of the competencies of clinicians does not necessarily involve testing in all areas in which a person could be knowledgeable and competent. Perhaps almost all clinicians are fairly competent on some set of basic skills, and therefore the focus should be on critical aspects of what a clinician does that distinguishes a competent one from an incompetent one. It might be helpful to identify critical incidents in the practices of professional psychologists in which education and training play a role. One useful approach to evaluation might be to determine whether psychologists have experienced critical incidents (Flanagan, 1954; McDermott, McGuire, & Berner, 1976) that influenced their education and training. For example, a clinician might report an ethical dilemma for which he or she was well prepared because of a seminar in ethical considerations in professional psychology. Another might have treated a case in a particular way because of similarities to a case handled during an internship. Standard critical incident methodology could be used with samples of professional psychologists of different types to produce the data. Similar data could be obtained from supervisors of students and interns. Although incidents reflecting directly on the value of training may be rare, they may also be greatly informative. The threat to quality of service may lie not so much in routine mediocrity as in occasional but highly damaging blunders.

More information is also needed about the extent to which skills can become obsolete. If competence depends much more on judgment and problem-solving ability than on specific knowledge and skills, it may be that the "half-life" of competence in professional psychology is much longer than is the case for professions more dependent on technique. On the other hand, emerging service needs may present problems for psychologists not trained to meet these needs (Jenson, 1979). How to sustain competence and develop skills to meet new needs are questions of fundamental importance to the task of evaluating and demonstrating professional competencies.

Types of Competence

Although the competencies that we need to think about assessing are not very well known or agreed on, a wide array of nominated competencies were obtained from a small study of experts in the field (Sechrest, 1990). The details of the study have never been published because it was in the nature of a pilot study, but it did inquire into competencies specifically for working with the seriously mentally ill. In general, the areas of competency that

[2] That finding is considerably discrepant from reports obtained by other investigators, which generally suggest that practicing psychologists spend very little time reading journals and other professional materials (Cohen, Sargent, & Sechrest, 1986). Once, during an American Psychological Association panel discussion considering the kinds of publications that might be needed by practitioners, an insistent plea was made for brief, abstract-type reports because clinicians were said to have very little time for reading (L. Sechrest, personal communication, August 1983).

need to be considered in assessing mental health workers include personal qualities, knowledge, and clinical skills.

Personal Qualities

Qualities such as intelligence, problem-solving ability, flexibility, tolerance, and compassion are often named as requisites for working with the seriously mentally ill. Some of these qualities are obviously difficult to measure (e.g., compassion) and may be difficult to train. If certain critical competencies are believed to be unlikely to respond to training or experience, then we should select our clinical students based on assessment of these skills before they enter a program. For example, interpersonal skills are important for working in this field and yet they can be very difficult to improve. In 1979, Daniel Hogan, a lawyer and social psychologist, published a four-volume study called *The Regulation of Psychotherapists,* in which he concluded that "the effectiveness of therapists is determined more by the presence or absence of certain personality characteristics and interpersonal skills than technical abilities and theoretical knowledge" (cited in Fallows, 1985, p. 65). Hogan's conclusions that the skills that make a good psychotherapist are mainly commonsense human skills and that advanced technical training is irrelevant to positive therapeutic outcome illustrate the extreme, yet increasingly held view of education and training in the mental health professions in general and clinical psychology in particular–psychologists are on the defensive. We note here that the experts we surveyed (Sechrest, 1990) agreed, too, that many personal qualities required for working with the seriously mentally ill are not likely to be very responsive to training.

Knowledge

Knowledge of the general principles of psychology and how they relate to behavior and psychopathology are also important competencies that we might expect. Certainly this kind of knowledge appears to be trainable, and it should not be especially difficult to assess, although its translation into practice may not be so easily determined.

Peterson (1976) argues that psychologists should have a comprehensive educational background because they need to deal with the psychological functioning of individuals and how they interact in groups and social organizations. This comprehensive education would include biological psychology, the various psychological approaches to therapy, and group and social theories. Although psychologists may and usually do choose to specialize later during their careers, this comprehensive educational background is crucial, Peterson claims, in order to be a professional. Others also agree that a set of basic skills and an outlook common to clinical psychology as a professional specialty should be imparted in any educational and training program (Committee on Professional Standards, 1981). Virtually all other professions are characterized by initial training of a general nature, culminating in a professional degree, with any specialization and concomitant recognition achieved later. To date, clinical psychology has followed this model, and education and training should be evaluated from that perspective.

In some ways, what experts seem to have in mind with respect to general knowledge is more like a theory or outlook on human behavior and problems than specific knowledge. This theory must extend to the understanding of services, what they are, and how they work. Mental health workers must have a good understanding of why they are doing what they do if their own behavior is to be kept on course. For example, we had one instance in a local project of case managers believing that they had engaged in "collaborative participation" with families when they called the family in and explained what they were going to do.

One serious limitation to the evaluation of education and training of clinical psychologists is that, in addition to the other deficiencies in information, there is not a good understanding of what actually happens in clinical training. The American Psychological Association (APA) has an accreditation procedure devised to produce some uniformity in clinical training, but it is in actuality only a verification that programs meet a minimum education and training standard. Otherwise, useful documentation of the training of clinical psychologists is scarce and may exist only at the level of the graduate school transcript for both the program and the individual. The fact that courses are required does not guarantee that they will be taken, let alone that they will have their intended effects, and usual experiences are not universal. The outcome of the accreditation process is simply a binary conclusion of accredited or not accredited. Dumke (1986) makes the provocative suggestion that training programs should be graded according to their quality. Is clinical psychology ready to admit that it has some "B" and "C" programs?

Clinical Skills

We also need to be concerned about fairly specific skills, which seem to fall into two categories. One of these is general interpersonal skills, related to the personal qualities mentioned previously, and the other is clinical skills. General interpersonal skills have to do with knowing how to relate effectively to people, how to engage others in conversation, how to explain things, how to persuade others to join in an effort, and so on. Clinical skills have to do with the ability to conduct an interview and get needed information efficiently, how to deal with an uncooperative patient, what to say to a patient who is hallucinating, and so on. These skills, both general and clinical, are probably trainable to some extent, but clinical skills may have to be acquired largely on the job through practica and internships.

The outcome of education and training in a profession is not simply an array of practices based on complex, disciplined knowledge. Training must inculcate a set of beliefs, attitudes, and values that are conducive to a high level of personal and professional responsibility. Part of the definition of a professional has to do with the capability of that person to practice independently, a capability that must have as its basis a firm ethical sense, respect for clients, commitment to maintaining competence, and so on. Whether or not it can be taught, judgment is a fundamental capacity of the professional (Klemp, 1977). Knowing what to do, how, and when (as well as knowing when not to) are all critical aspects of competence. These aspects of professional outlook and practice demand careful consideration in planning an evaluation of education and training. Moreover, the responsible, well-trained professional knows the limits of personal competence and accepts them.

Job-related knowledge. Experience in various aspects of clinical practice will result in a wide array of knowledge. For example, mental health workers working in the community learn about other services available to their clients. They also know how to access these services and how different organizations within the community work. In our work we attempted to develop brief objective measures of knowledge about psychopharmacology and about epidemiology, but neither measure proved very interesting in terms of internal consistency nor in probable relationships to other measures. Obviously, any measure of knowledge about local services and agencies and so on would have to be developed at each site, because the information would be site-specific. It is possible that some general principles for constructing such measures could be devised.

Because there is such a close relationship between the training program and the internship, it is difficult to evaluate either in isolation. Most academic programs are planned with some assumptions about the internship experiences their graduates will have, and internship agencies in turn tend to select students with academic backgrounds that meet their needs. Therefore, a training program may neglect some aspects of clinical training because the internship is supposed to provide the experience, whereas another program has a completely different emphasis. The potential for gaps in training on one side or the other is evident, and the evaluation of any student or program would depend heavily on whether it was carried out pre- or postinternship. One interesting possibility to get around this would be to compare graduates of regular programs with graduates of those programs with "captive" internships (i.e., programs that provide internship experiences that complement their academic programs). Perhaps the result would be that clinical psychologists from captive programs would prove to be more thoroughly trained, suggesting the possibility of a national revamping of the relationship between academic graduate programs and internship agencies. Certainly reason exists to believe that internship experiences may often be less than satisfactory (Tucker, 1970; Tucker & James, 1971).

Entry-level skills. An attempt should be made to determine expected and desired entry-level skills of professional psychologists. A useful evaluation requires better understanding of what the newly trained psychologist should be expected to think, know, and be able to do. Again, surveys could help determine this, with respondents selected so as to represent potentially diverse views. As an example, Dana, Gilliam, and Dana (1976) attempted to determine what skills are expected and desired of psychology interns at the time of entry into internship programs. Expectations differed from one setting to another, but assessment skills were generally regarded as more critical than others. This type of job analysis for the entry-level psychologist should not focus exclusively on specific skills and knowledge but should also attempt to determine the crucial attitudes and judgment capabilities required for competent functioning. It should pay attention to the hazards of professional practice and those factors that help to avoid them. Ferguson (1976) believes that students should be prepared to accept the limitations of psychology, imbued with "regretful self-acceptance" as a basis for using those skills that can be taught.

After entry-level knowledge, attitudes, and skills have been described, more structured plans could be developed for their assessment. Entry-level skills may be more important than they seem initially. It appears that professionals do what they were trained to do and perpetuate these practices not only throughout their own careers but in their supervision of neophytes, making initial acquisition of the right skills and attitudes even more imperative. Among the most important of these may be a readiness for change and continuing professional development, balanced by a steadiness of view and judgment that discourages indulgence in professional fads and other inadequately tested practices.

Self-assessment and updating of skills. Fallows (1985) noted the fallibility of the processes that lead to the award of credentials and the presumption of once-and-for-all competence that underlies their acceptance. He suggested, for example, that the licensed physician, however competent at the time of licensing, does not necessarily remain competent (see Inspector General of Health and Human Services, 1986). Skills erode, and the knowledge base changes. Fallows presented as an alternative model for professional certification the case of commercial airline pilot training and certification. The Federal Aviation Administration does not assume that pilots, once trained, remain skillful for the remainder of their careers. In order to maintain their licenses, they must undergo regular competency checks. When they are to undertake a new assignment such as piloting a new aircraft or landing at an airfield they have not used before, they must go through a set of specified procedures to check out their skills.

The comparison of pilot certification to that of professional psychologists is interesting and not in our favor. How many psychologists are out there diagnosing Alzheimer's disease without having had any specific training for that task, let alone without having been "checked out" on their ability to do so? How many psychologists will agree to provide therapy for an anorgasmic female client, although they have never had any specific training in sex therapy of that sort? How many psychologists regularly have their work checked out by a senior peer to make sure they are on track?

The American Psychiatric Association has a self-assessment program that permits psychiatrists at least to check on their knowledge of the basic literature and such other testable skills as diagnostic criteria at intervals as they choose, and such self-assessment programs exist in many other medical specialties. The program has been regarded as quite successful and useful (Quick, Robinowitz, & Wilson, 1981).

Methods of Assessing Competencies

Depending on what is being assessed and at what time during their career clinicians are assessed, different strategies might be used. Probably the easiest and most inexpensive (in terms of both time and money) are the self-report and paper-and-pencil tests. Self-report is usually used for assessing personal attitudes, whereas paper-and-pencil tests are used for measuring knowledge and aptitude. Self-report is the most efficient way to obtain a lot of biographical information and is particularly useful for identifying people who are true outliers in their attitudes and practices. Mabe and West (1982) found that self-evaluation relates reasonably well to other measures of performance, within some limits, particularly when (a) raters expect their own evaluations to be compared to other measures, (b) the raters are experienced with self-evaluation, (c) raters are guaranteed anonymity, and (d) instructions emphasize comparison with others. In our ongoing study with local practitioners (Scott & Sechrest, in press), we found that 51% believed that this method, self-assessment, was only somewhat effective in assessing competencies and 26% felt that it was not an effective method.

Exercises and Simulations

The use of simulations (e.g., having people act out cases representing different mental health problems and then recording the responses made) may be an effective alternative. Although this method would be both time-consuming and costly, using audio or video could be a reasonable alternative. We tried using a professional actor trained to portray a seriously mentally ill person and had the actor interviewed by a faculty member and several students, none of whom suspected the ruse. Ratings of videotapes by judges indicated that differences between interviewers were probably observable and dependable. Relatively experienced student clinicians appeared somewhat more skillful (e.g., in specific responses to manifestations of psychopathology). For example, one interviewer picked up on the fact that on the day in question, the putative patient was, while a bit shabby, dressed in color-coordinated clothing and thought that indicative of a relatively good level of functioning. In contrast, an inexperienced clinician became involved in trying to reassure the actor that no microphones were actually concealed in an electrical outlet. The use of an actor proved fascinating because each clinician could be exposed to roughly the same stimulus, and yet, a fair amount of flexibility and spontaneity was possible. On the other hand, the costs of training an actor are substantial, let alone the costs of repeated sessions, and except for specialized research purposes, the method is probably not particularly feasible. The initial cost of developing and producing an audio or video presentation would be substantial, but such presentations could be used many times by many people. Exercises could be developed that would present various situations to clinicians and have them indicate what they would say and do in response. Berven and Scofield (1980a) reviewed the literature on standardized simulations of clinical situations, which have had considerable use across a variety of professions. The "In-Basket Test" (Fredericksen, Saunders, & Wand, 1957) was an early example of a problem-simulation device, developed for assessing managerial skills but adaptable to a variety of problems. Problem simulations have a fairly long history in medicine also. Berven and Scofield (1980b) reported on a computer-based simulation for clinical problem solving. The flexibility of problem simulations makes them highly attractive as potential instruments to evaluate education and training. Although some simulations are not feasible for use with large numbers of people in scattered geographic locations, the paper-and-pencil and computer varieties could be adaptable to almost any purpose.

Stricker (1982) reported on the development of a new measure of interpersonal competence using videotaped stimulus scenes and both tape-recorded and written responses. Responses are scored for effectiveness, originality, and accuracy. The three scores are all judged and have demonstrated internal consistency. Of interest is the fact that psychology majors score higher than other students, and students who had completed even one psychology course scored higher than students who had not.

Assessing Education

The task of evaluating educational and training activities will have to be broken down into relatively small subtasks and decisions made as to which to undertake first. Those decisions will almost certainly reflect a number of diverse factors ranging from strategic to methodological and practical concerns. The most important questions should be addressed first, and the most realistic starting points must be identified. It is critical, however, that a systematic and comprehensive program of research be developed that avoids the risks of triviality and opportunism.

One possibility is to ask the Board of Educational Affairs of APA to develop standard documentation forms for programs and students. Although the reporting requirements might seem formidable, they are not considered unusual by many other professions. Professional photographers, for example, rarely take a picture without recording the conditions, and pilots keep careful logs of each flight. Dentists and physicians record every patient contact, often in considerable detail. If training programs cannot document the detail in which students are exposed to information about biochemical aspects of mental disorder, and if students cannot document the number of hours they have spent in group-therapy training, then the most basic documentation practices are absent.

On-the-Job Observations

Actual experience, whether during school or after, could be assessed through on-the-job observations. Practitioners in our study (Scott & Sechrest, in press) were most likely to cite this method as being an effective method for assessing clinical competency (79% of the respondents believed that this method was effective and only 4% felt this was not effective). Supervisors of clinicians who are in training may make judgments on their trainees but this does not mean that this assessment is adequate. Often, supervisors have very limited contact and may make inconsistent recordings of these judgments. Nonstandardized methods of observation may make their way into the files of students through notes, telephone messages, or other conversations without ever being read or accessed again. Clinical students have been known to advise other newer students not to worry about negative comments recorded by their internship supervisors because "no one really reads those things anyway." Therefore, this entire process needs to be more uniform and systematic if the input is to be of any value. One option would be to systematically assess behavior during classes and training sessions. One case in which this method is used is that of the Minnesota School of Professional Psychology (Olson, 1990), which uses the Goal Attainment Scaling procedure developed by Kiresuk and Sherman in 1968 (Kiresuk & Sherman, 1968). Goal setting involves both the trainee and supervisor after the trainee has started working and has had adequate time to begin establishing relationships with the staff and site. That delay puts trainees and supervisors in better positions to come up with reasonable sets of goals. These goals consist of three–six separate items for each time period (usually 3 months) and consist of a minimum of five levels for each goal. Contents of these goals cover such skills as observational abilities, assessment interview skills, psychological testing—general, objective, and projective—diagnostic skills, presentations, ethical issues, and relationships with clients and colleagues. Ratings do not affect the grades that the trainee receives. This method of assessing clinical training provides feedback to trainees so that they can work on their shortcomings and to the site, permitting the latter to determine whether they do indeed provide adequate training.

Conclusion

The assessment of competency in clinical psychology requires a comprehensive and multifaceted research program. Even to begin would require developing a variety of methodologies because neither the measures nor all the designs and methods of analysis eventually required for such an effort are yet in existence. The process of assessment should be iterative and dynamic, because initial results will be applied to improve subsequent evaluation and to change training programs. The evaluations will require a period of time that is so long that programs will be changing in the meantime anyway. The general evaluation model described by Tharp and Gallimore (1979) as evaluation succession could provide a useful basis for an effective plan for evaluating education and training because it allows for the evolution of a program based on feedback from evaluations.

It is only through the use of effective assessments that the profession can be provided with accountability. Then the effectiveness and worth of clinical psychologists can be clearly shown.

References

Berven, N. L., & Scofield, M. E. (1980a). Evaluation of professional competence through standardized simulations: A review. *Rehabilitation Counseling Bulletin, 23,* 178–202.

Berven, N. L., & Scofield, M. E. (1980b). Evaluation of clinical problem-solving skills through standardized case-management simulations. *Journal of Counseling Psychology, 27,* 199–208.

Cohen, L. H., Sargent, M. M., & Sechrest, L. B. (1986). Use of psychotherapy research by professional psychologists. *American Psychologist, 41*(2), 198–206.

Committee on Professional Standards. (1981). *Specialty guidelines for the delivery of services.* Washington, DC: American Psychological Association.

Dana, R. H., Gilliam, M., & Dana, J. M. (1976). Adequacy of academic–clinical preparation for internships. *Professional Psychology, 7,* 112–116.

Dumke, G. (1986, January 15). Accrediting: The weak link in education reform. *Chronicle of Higher Education, 33,* 5.

Fallows, J. (1985, December). The case against credentialism. *The Atlantic,* 49–67.

Ferguson, K. G. (1976). Graduate training in clinical psychology: A further critical evaluation. *Ontario Psychologist, 8,* 31–33.

Flanagan, J. C. (1954). The critical incident technique. *Psychological Bulletin, 51,* 327–358.

Fredericksen, N., Saunders, D. R., & Wand, B. (1957). The in-basket test. *Psychological Monographs, 71*(9, No. 438).

Inspector General of Health and Human Services (1986). *Report on the training and practice of physicians in the United States.* Washington, DC: Department of Health and Human Services.

Jenson, R. (1979). Competent professional service in psychology: The real issue behind continuing education. *Professional Psychology, 10,* 381–389.

Kiresuk, T. J., and Sherman, R. E. (1968). Goal attainment scaling: A general method for evaluating comprehensive community mental health journals. *Community Mental Health Journal, 4,* 443–453.

Klemp, G. O. (1977). Three factors of success. In D. W. Vermilye (Ed.), *Relating work and education* (pp. 102–109). San Francisco: Jossey-Bass.

Mabe, P. A., III, & West, S. G. (1982). Validity of self-evaluation of ability: A review and metaanalysis. *Journal of Applied Psychology, 67,* 280–296.

McDermott, J. F., McGuire, C. H., & Berner, E. S. (1976). *Roles and functions of child psychiatrists.* Evanston, IL: American Board of Psychiatry and Neurology.

Mechanic, D., & Aiken, L. H. (1987). Improving the care of patients with chronic mental illness. *New England Journal of Medicine, 317,* 1634–1638.

Mendenhall, R. C., & Abrahamson, S. (1973). The practical utility of log-diaries in describing physician activities. In *Proceedings of the Twelfth Annual Conference on Research in Medical Education* (pp. 7–11). Washington, DC: Association of American Medical Colleges.

Olson, R. P. (1990). *Manual for setting, scaling, and scoring assessment and therapy practicum goals: A quality assurance procedure.* Minneapolis: Minnesota School of Professional Psychology.

Peterson, D. R. (1976). Need for the doctor of psychology degree in professional psychology. *American Psychologist,* 792–798.

Quick, S., Robinowitz, C., & Wilson, P. (1981). Results of the 1976 APA Self-Assessment Program. *American Journal of Psychiatry, 138*(12), 1587–1591.

Rosenfeld, M., Shimberg, B., & Thornton, R. F. (1983). *Job analysis of licensed psychologists in the United States and Canada.* Princeton, NJ: Center for Occupational and Professional Assessment, Educational Testing Service.

Scott, A. G., & Sechrest, L. (in press). *Clinical psychologists' views of competencies and specialties.* Tucson: University of Arizona.

Sechrest, L. (1990). *Approaches to assessing competencies of clinicians working with the seriously mentally ill.* Unpublished report. University of Arizona, Tucson.

Sechrest, L., & Smith, B. H. (in press) *Psychology in the yellow pages.* Tucson: University of Arizona.

Stricker, L. J. (1982). Interpersonal competence instrument: Development and preliminary findings. *Applied Psychological Measurement, 6,* 69–81.

Tharp, R. G., & Gallimore, R. (1979). The ecology of program research and evaluation: A model of evaluation succession. In L. Sechrest, S. C. West, M. Phillips, R. Redner, & W. Yeaton (Eds.), *Evaluation studies review annual* (Vol. 4, pp. 39–60). Beverly Hills, CA: Sage.

Tucker, R. C. (1970). Strangers in paradise. *Journal of Consulting and Clinical Psychology, 34,* 140–143.

Tucker, R. C., & James, S. A. (1971). Note on "strangers in paradise," or telling it like it isn't. *Journal of Consulting and Clinical Psychology, 37,* 304.

CHAPTER

22

The Role of the State in Ensuring Quality in Health Care Service Delivery and Its Linkage With the Private and Public Sectors

Judy E. Hall
National Register of Health Service Providers in Psychology

"The public sector now pays for 40% of the U.S. health-care bill—54% of the hospital bills and one third of all physician bills, mostly through Medicare and Medicaid" (Cooper, 1991). State government determines which health-care delivery groups will be licensed for practice and, through freedom-of-choice legislation and other payment standards, which will be eligible to receive direct or indirect payment from third-party, federal, and state insurers. The federal government similarly determines which professionals and services will be reimbursed under the various federal programs that pay for mental health and substance abuse services. Clearly, the public sector plays a major role in determining the level of standards of care in health care.

Although the defining concept in licensure is minimal competence, in health-care delivery the focus has been on quality assurance; more recently, with a focus on outcome measurement and correction, the emerging sentinel phrase is (total) quality management. The concepts and the implementation may be slightly different, but the concerns are the same. Providers, payers, regulators, employers, and consumers are all marching with a vengeance on a quest for quality at the best price.

Although space limitations do not permit an in-depth analysis of those trends, this chapter will illustrate some of the collaborative partnerships possible between the public sector, primarily state licensure, and the private sector in relation to quality assurance. (See Stricker & Rodriguez, 1988, for a more complete discussion of this chapter's topic.) The preventive measures are those leading to licensure: education, experience, and assessment of education and experience. The corrective measures that enhance adherence to standards primarily relate to those mechanisms that occur after licensure. As will be apparent, entry to licensure and maintenance of licensure reflect a partnership among the public sector, the private sector, and the academic sector, with the realization that those three spheres are not, should not, and cannot be mutually exclusive areas of activity.

Becoming a quality provider begins with education, generally. Although controversial, a goal or outcome of the education process is education for licensure, either directly or indirectly. The state's role historically begins after the prospective provider has completed the professionally defined sequence of steps necessary for independent practice. A priori, education and training, including experience, have been defined as essential for practice of the profession of psychology. The licensure examination, by definition and implementation an independent evaluation of the knowledge, skills, and abilities acquired in that educational process, is administered by the state. In the case of professional psychology, the profession has identified the necessary elements by measured consensus, not by experimental methodology. However, the programs training for professional practice are evaluated by members of the profession, as well as by the public, according to criteria established by the profession. Similar, but not necessarily identical, criteria are used in the evaluation of individuals applying for licensure. These criteria are those previously established by both national and state bodies, another instance of the collaborative partnership between the public sector and the professional and academic worlds.

In that sense, the licensure examination, which is composed of a national multiple-choice exam and a state-developed oral, essay, and/or jurisprudence exam, is both a product of as well as an input to assuring quality—albeit minimal quality. The Examination for Professional Practice in Psychology (EPPP) is constructed by subject matter experts according to an outline (domains, roles, and responsibilities) that is a product of a series of research projects focused on information deemed essential to practice (Myers & Rosen, 1986). Two critical research initiatives defining those essentials, the role delineation study (Richman, 1982) and the job analysis of psychology (Rosenfeld, Shimberg, & Thornton, 1984), did not define needs based on input from the private or public service sector. To do so would bring a very different need to the surface—the need for service as opposed to the entry-level knowledge needed for practice: "[American Psychological Association] APA accreditation criteria should reflect attention to curricula content responsive to the [service needs of priority populations], as should state licensing examinations in their test items and skills evaluation." (Appendix A of this volume on policy recommendations in regard to curriculum development). The state complementary exam may address certain needs, such as detection of child abuse, but typically does not address how to serve the seriously mentally ill or any other of the priority populations. More often, the intended area of practice for the individual professional provides the focus for the individually administered oral examination, and because many practitioners do not intend to serve the priority populations, assessment of those skills is not guaranteed. Moreover, because many, if not all, of those individuals employed by the state as psychologists for those populations do not need to be licensed (because of the state employment exemption), they may not be examined at all on their credentials, knowledge, or skills. Therein lies an absence of a needed partnership.

It is important to reiterate that the licensure process is not intended to assure quality, only minimal competence; but when combined with quality assurance activities in the private sector and with a redefinition of what is necessary knowledge, the inputs to the licensure process could be a powerful tool in moving the profession in the direction of quality. For instance, over time, the requirements for licensure have been increased from minimal criteria being met in the "grandparent waiver period" in which eligibility for licensure was met by affirming education and/or experience only, to the implementation of the first set of standards; this was followed by requirements for additional or more appropriate experience, for evidence of continuing education, and eventually for mandated continuing education for renewal of licensure. In comparison to knowledge acquisition in doctoral training, measures to evaluate either experience or continuing education have been notoriously lacking. As we will see, more effort has been placed on evaluating the educational component through accreditation, designation, and performance of graduates on the EPPP (Association of State and Provincial Psychology Boards [ASPPB], 1992). Not meaning to be pejorative, it is clear that education, experience, and the examination are restrictive procedures used in the licensure process, to a greater or lesser degree depending on the profession, the jurisdiction, and the timing of the application for licensure (Hall, 1987).

These following mechanisms serve as inputs to direct health service regulation: (a) approval of education and training programs; (b) experience, such as on-the-job experience, that could be documented or actually supervised, or a program of training such as an internship or other organized health service training program, occurring either at the pre- and/or postdoctoral level; (c) examination procedures, assembled and unassembled; and (d) determination of acceptable moral character or adherence to ethical standards. The inputs following licensure include (a) continuing education or competence; (b) requiring relicensure; and (c) monitoring and sanctioning of professional discipline or misconduct. In addition to evaluating each for its effectiveness as an input variable, each can be viewed as an outcome of one of the other variables (e.g., knowledge acquisition in the educational and training programs can be ascertained partly by the performance on the licensure examination of the graduates). These last three inputs also constitute regulation by the state of the profession of psychology, with almost all of it a partnership, whether welcomed or not, between the public and the private and academic sectors and the state government and the public.

In the section to follow, we shall briefly examine each of these inputs to licensure.

State Regulation Before Licensure

Education—Definition of the Requisite Knowledge, Skills, and Abilities

Extensive literature and many conference proceedings define the practice of psychology. However, the first attempt to independently and methodologically evaluate the impact of education on knowledge acquisition originated with efforts by the American Association of State Psychology Boards (AASPB), now called the Association of State & Provincial Psychology Boards (ASPPB). Since the early 1960s, ASPPB has produced the multiple-choice exam now used by all jurisdictions as part of the requirements for licensure. Not content with simply developing the examination, the organization funded a series of studies to define and empirically validate the entry-level knowledge necessary for the practice of psychology. By virtue of the research conducted on the EPPP (summarized in Myers & Rosen, 1986), most notably the Role Delineation Study (Richman, 1982), the Job Analysis conducted in the United States and Canada (Rosenfeld, Shimberg, & Thornton, 1984), and the EPPP Test Specifications Revision Project (Rosen & Mirone, 1986), the EPPP is considered by experts to be a content-valid examination (Anastasi, 1988).

Because a license is a generic passport to practice, providing flexibility in career development as the individual and the profession mature, the proper role for private certification and credentialing organizations should be in the identification of specialists. Especially for psychology, identification of those qualified to deliver health-care services amidst all of the licensed psychologists was especially necessary for psychology. To meet that need, a certification procedure was established in the early 1970s that involved a review according to established educational and experiential criteria of those licensed psychologists who seek recognition as a health service provider. The national organization established for that purpose, the Council for the National Register of Health Service Providers in Psychology, is the most successful certification organization in psychology in terms of numbers listed (over 16,000). Several states have initiated a similar mechanism, typically referring to listing in the National Register as a substitute for their own review. The title *Health Service Provider* is not a specialty but a subset of the generic practice arena designed for purposes of identification for insurance reimbursement purposes of qualified health-care providers in psychology (Council for the National Register of Health Service Providers in Psychology, 1992).

A private certification organization that established criteria for the recognition of specialists in psychology is the American Board of Professional Psychology (ABPP). Using criteria for education and experience, both generic and specialized, the individuals responsible for the review determine candidates' eligibility for examination as a specialist in one of the eight areas recognized by ABPP.

Because specialty and health service certification mechanisms are available but not required for entry into practice, they are labeled voluntary. The absence of either certification typically says nothing about qualifications, only aboutapplication. However, those two types of mechanisms—public (licensure) and private (credentialing)—help to maintain, if not raise, standards for the profession.

Education—Approval of Programs

In relating quality assurance in a profession to evaluation of education and training of professionals, Sechrest and Chatel (1987) affirm that quality assurance begins with the selection of students and the faculty that teach them. Furthermore, the tremendous variability in output among training programs might be attributed to the variance in input due primarily to those selection procedures. That assertion has not been evaluated empirically.

More often, the evaluative focus is on the program. However, even there the review is voluntary.

Programs within the specialty areas of clinical, counseling, and school psychology may apply for accreditation as professional psychology programs by APA. In contrast, programs within any area of psychology may apply for designation by the Joint Designation Project of the National Register of Health Service Providers in Psychology and ASPPB. Although the criteria for defining a doctoral degree in psychology are essentially the same in both designation and accreditation, APA's accreditation process is intended to be more qualitative and attempts to ensure quality, as opposed to designation's goal of meeting minimal standards for definition of a doctoral program for credentialing purposes.

As a result of no mandatory accreditation mechanism, there is no guarantee that graduates of psychology programs will meet the educational criteria established for licensure. Until the designation process was initiated, licensure boards, most of which now use the criteria established at the 1977 Education and Credentialing Conference for defining a doctoral program in psychology (Wellner, 1978), have had to assess individually each applicant's education to determine whether the core educational program requirements have been met. Those criteria were also endorsed by ASPPB (AASPB, 1977), by APA (APA, 1979, 1985) and by the Scientist–Practitioner Conference (Belar & Perry, 1990). Again, the criteria seem reasonable to many as the minimum criteria for definition of a doctoral program in psychology that has among its goals preparation of graduates for licensure and professional practice. However, the direct linkage between the criterion requiring certain curriculum components (Designation Criterion 10) and the content outline of the EPPP has not yet been performed.

The best exemplar of a state mechanism intending to ensure quality in doctoral training programs is that effort carried out by the Doctoral Project of the New York State Education Department. A comprehensive review was recently completed of all psychology training programs offered by any institution, private or public, in New York State. Although much of the review is confidential, one of its products was the definition of criteria for each of the four program paradigms: a research and academic PhD, a scientist–practitioner PhD, a PsyD, and an EdD. That peer review process took place over 5 years, was an in-depth review of the quality of the 103 programs offered in New York State, and encompassed input from three different groups of experts in psychology (a 7-person coordinating committee, a 22-person rating committee, and hundreds of site visitors) from all the specialty areas of psychology. With input and approval from all affected institutions on the criteria, procedures, and individuals chosen, the outcome was the reorganization and reshaping of most programs, closure of several programs, most voluntarily, and invaluable feedback and goals set for each program—all for the purpose of improving the quality of the program offerings. This approach to quality assurance in doctoral education initiated in New York applies to any doctoral degree granting program, whether in an area of a profession or not, and is a responsibility of the state department that also administers the licensure of individuals graduating from those programs. New York State is the only state that houses the academic review function and the licensure review function within the same state department—another example of an important partnership (New York State Doctoral Evaluation Project, 1990).

Experience—A Requirement for Licensure

The profession of psychology has always presumed and generally agreed that to be well educated one must also be well trained. To say otherwise is almost heresy. As a result, almost all of the psychology statutes and regulations require experience prior to approval for independent practice. In the most recent APA Model Act for State Licensure (1987b), the recommendation for 1 year of postdoctoral experience was made very clear. Although there are many among us who would feel more comfortable if there had been an empirical evaluation of the necessity for this year of experience and what it should include, rather than simply consensual agreement (APA, 1992), to date no organization has been willing to fund research to assess the impact of that year on knowledge or on practice, the more ephemeral linkage. A complicating factor in such an evaluation is the wide range of activities and experiences that are accepted in place of, or equivalent to, a planned sequence of training. Only recently did educators, trainers, and others interested in postdoctoral training come together for the purposes of developing policy and standards for postdoctoral training (National Conference on Postdoctoral Training in Professional Psychology, 1993).

Some literature assists us in our belief that experience should be required for entry into the profession of psychology. In 1978, Cathcart and Graff (in Herbsleb, Sales, & Overcast, 1985) developed a model evaluating 30 health professions' need for experience as a prerequisite for licensure. Using seriousness of impact, degree to which practitioners are required to exercise independent judgment, and amount of practical training in the educational program, the authors found physicians and osteopathic physicians needed experience for licensure the most of all the 30 professions. Psychologists received the next highest rating.

Years reported since degree, as one measure of experience, and performance on the licensure examination, shows a curvilinear relationship, with those performing worst with the most (and least) years of experience. However, because the exam is designed for entry-level knowledge with 1 or 2 years of experience and not for someone who may have specialized for 20 years, that finding is not surprising.

Examination

Passing the licensure examination is the major remaining hurdle to becoming an independent practitioner. Jurisdictional boards take this responsibility seriously; and because this is a local matter, even if the examination is developed by a national outside organization, each board is held responsible for the examination. This currently includes determining the pass point for the examination. The member boards of ASPPB have only recently discussed cooperation in setting a national pass point for the EPPP, one of the cherished local decisions that may disadvantage mobil psychologists.

The examination, as indicated above, is a content-valid examination, assessing the generic knowledge and, to a lesser extent, the skills and abilities at the entry level. The domains of intervention, assessment, uses of the literature, ethics, and social systems apply to those practicing in all specialty areas of psychology, to a greater or lesser extent. Although the licensure examination is an input to licensure, performance on the exam is also measurable as an outcome. Since 1988, the cumulative number, mean score, and standard deviation of graduates from each program who take the EPPP has been made available (ASPPB, 1992). Although many state boards perform their own analysis of performance of applicants on the licensure and some provide pass/fail data by program, the Education Reporting Service booklet allows a broader comparison of all candidates by program with all other programs. Examining those data will also tell the reader which programs have graduates that apply for licensure.

As indicated above, almost all jurisdictions complement the EPPP with another examination. Typically, this is an oral examination, but it may also be an essay or an exam on state laws governing practice (jurisprudence). Only recently have efforts focused on validating those components that complement the national licensure examination (Fisher & Hall, 1990a, 1990b). That effort was also the first partnership by a state and the national association of boards in funding of a project—the validation of a complementary examination in the licensure of psychologists.

Moral Character, Character Reference, or Absence of Unethical Determination

Having an ethical code is a defining element of a profession; not surprisingly, evidence of adherence to ethical standards is typically required in the licensure process for psychology. One approach is to ask the applicant to indicate any past violations, such as a felony conviction, that relate to the practice of the profession, broadly construed. This attestation is also required for those licensed in another jurisdiction who apply to a new jurisdiction. Although character references have been used in the review of those seeking admission to the profession, that has not been a meaningful or discriminating measure. More frequently, applicants are asked to affirm that they will abide by the professional conduct code and that they understand that failure to do so will result in the potential loss of a license. For voluntary organizations, the use of attestation forms and automatic reporting makes more sense and places the responsibility on the person who has benefitted from the credential. For licensure boards, such an attestation form may assure the board that the applicant has read the standards of practice for that jurisdiction. Ignorance of the law is no excuse for those brought before licensure boards.

State Regulation After Licensure

The methods used by state governments to regulate the individual practitioner after licensure currently include (a) mandating continuing education, (b) requiring relicensure or reexamination, (c) restricting the licensee to specialty practice, and (d) disciplining the licensee. These inputs are as critical as those prior to licensure but are often least attended to from a quality assurance or quality management approach.

Continuing Education and Competence

Becoming licensed indicates that the practitioner has met the established jurisdictional standards for entry into the profession. The public is thereby assured of minimal competence. How long that competence is maintained is of vital interest to the public and the profession. The answer to that question in psychology may depend on the skills and techniques used by the professional and the population(s) served by that professional. Psychologists licensed 10–15 years ago had very little training in clinical neuropsychological assessment and intervention. The advances in that area of specialized practice are too recent to have been part of the typical entry-level curriculum. For instance, forensic psychology is an area of more recent specialization. Today, there are doctoral programs that prepare psychologists specifically for that area of practice. As the technology and techniques advance, the practitioner cannot maintain competence unless additional training takes place. Realizing that the half life of any profession is getting shorter, not longer, the legislatures who are concerned with the public protection aspects of licensure have called for palliative procedures. The problem has been that the solution has been more cosmetic than real, with efficacy data lacking that would justify the expense of mandating continuing education for all practitioners. However, the absence of proof has not stopped the passage and implementation of continuing professional education (CPE) for most health-care professions.

Sanazaro (1983) reviewed the studies on the effects of continuing medical education on the subsequent performance of physicians. Although most of the studies showed an increase in knowledge and skills, there is no demonstrated impact on the delivery of services to patients. Variables that determined whether there was an improvement in performance included corrective feedback and access to supervision by or consultation with other physicians. Environmental factors that would support behavior change also were important. CPE for medicine—a profession that is so heavily technology-dependent—seems imminently rational a requirement and yet medicine is not convinced of the efficacy of mandated continuing education even though it was one of the first professions to require it for membership in professional associations or for licensure.

What about psychology? In 1985 continuing education was mandated and implemented by 21 states for renewal of licensure by psychologists (Hall, 1987). By 1993 the number had increased to 34, with several more at the proposed stage or with enabling legislation. What has been the impact of those requirements? Do we have any data that would demonstrate the impact of CPE on knowledge or practice? Let's take a look at the only evaluative study of the implementation of a CPE requirement for a profession by a state. This section closes with a brief summary of the only study in clinical psychology that empirically shows the impact of active learning on the practice of certain skills and the necessity for skills assessment prior to entering the continuing educational process.

An Audit of the Accounting Profession

Accountants engaged in public practice in New York State were required by virtue of legislation beginning in 1987 and ending in 1990 to participate in approved continuing professional education. The scientific study of the effects of this requirement included a baseline profile of all licensed practicing accountants, with 50% (10,167) returning the survey form. Respondents and nonrespondents were determined to show no statistical differences on selected variables. That group was asked to report (a) the extent of participation in continuing education in the previous 12 months, (b) the total number of full-time accountants in their firms, and (c) the number of years in practice. A random sample group of 1,750 (from the target sample of 5,740 who had qualified themselves from the initial study respondent sample of 10,167 accountants) was sent self-assessment booklets with 25 test items on taxation, accounting, and auditing. The 633 who completed the self-administered assessment instrument were found not to be different from a target sample that was representative of the population. Another facet of this research was a comparison of the self-administration group and a supervised administration group at three different sites. Again, no difference was found, verifying the self-administered assessment procedure as a valid assessment approach.

The findings show that (a) knowledge proficiency increases with recent (last 12 months) participation in continuing education, (b) knowledge proficiency increases with size (25 accountants) of accounting firm, and (c) knowledge proficiency is nearly constant across categories of years in active practice for those with taxation, accounting, or auditing as the primary area of practice. For general practitioners, knowledge proficiency declines steadily across the same year categories, especially for those with at least 20 years of experience. Accountants with higher levels of participation in approved continuing education courses (more than 48 hours) had higher general knowledge proficiency scores than those with lower levels of participation. Those findings were consistent for different sample groups, for different time periods, and for different assessment instruments. The reports reiterate that the design of this study did not (and could not) address the relationship between participation in CPE and accountancy practice performance, because that is also dependent on "personal and contextual everyday knowledge factors" (Mandatory Continuing Education Committee, 1989, p. 3).

One other outcome related to the findings is the recommendation for delineating and limiting the recognized areas of study and for specifying the amount of concentrated participation in the specific subject areas. In essence, concentrated study in a specific, single area was a more powerful predictor of increased accountancy knowledge than was more general study in a wider range of subject areas.

The final recommendation by the study committee specified continuation of CPE for licensed accountants for another 3 years, with the option of completing a minimum of 40 hours of yearly CPE in recognized areas of study or completing a minimum of 24 hours of yearly CPE concentrating in any one of the three general subject matter areas (Grotelueschen Associates, 1987, 1988, 1989, 1990; Mandatory Continuing Education Study Committee, 1989, 1990). The legislation will serve as a model for other professions that have attempted to convince the legislature of the necessity for continuing education for renewal of licensure.

Although a similar study would need to be repeated for the profession of psychology, especially because the educational requirements for entry to the profession of psychology are quite different from accountancy (doctoral vs. bachelor degree), the model, the concept, and perhaps some of the findings would generalize. Psychology should endorse the yoked requirement for statewide evaluation of the requirement for CPE. It is irresponsible for any legislature and the professional organization to agree to the requirement of expenditure of time and money for those professionals who are deemed competent to practice to complete CPE without assessing how much, when, how, and what.

Another element in this model is sensible—payment for the evaluative study by the affected professionals. New York-licensed accountants were required to pay $35 yearly for the study as part of their licensure renewal fee.

In addition, by examining the next study summarized below, it makes sense to recommend continuing education not as it has been conceptualized, somewhat passive learning in 1–2-day workshops, but as a meaningful sequence of educational activities with mandated evaluation.

Continuing Professional Education for Clinical Psychology

A 5-year research and development project initiated in 1980 and funded by the W. K. Kellogg Foundation had among its goals a fostering of a partnership between the university and the profession so that continuing professional education would be meaningful and would actually impact practice. Practice-oriented CPE was developed and implemented using a seven-phase needs assessment program called the "practice audit model" (see Lindsay, Crowe, & Jacobs, 1987, for an in-depth look at this project). This model assumes that professional competence and continuing education needs assessment are "intimately intertwined," requiring an understanding of what is demanded of a professional in practice before additional education is provided. This philosophy suggests that collaboration among the continuing education professionals, the university faculty members, and the professional associations will produce a better outcome.

In this project, the practice of clinical psychology was first defined through a role delineation study. The outcome of that activity led to a description comprised of 18 responsibilities and 95 tasks representing three major domains (i.e., direct client services, organization, and administration of services and professional activities). A sample of Pennsylvania psychologists rated time spent and importance of each task thereby producing a profile of clinical psychology practice. Because direct delivery of services to clients was ranked the highest on time and importance, the simulation exercises developed in this study focused on the psychologists' interaction with mock clients. Ten global clinical behavior dimensions and 11 specific clinical behaviors were derived from the practice description and were evaluated by trained raters using videotapes of therapy simulation. Other exercises, such as 5 different written client vignettes, 11 different videotaped therapy vignettes developed by the American Board of Professional Psychology, a legal issues test, and a continuing education needs and demands survey, were also included and similarly evaluated in this practice audit.

With 40 participants, the practice audit session produced 411 scorable variables that were then categorized under the practice description responsibilities. A cutoff was established for performance-based learning needs (less than adequate) and self-perceived needs (high). Using summary statistics and percentages of the group achieving a criterion score on each of the variables associated with a responsibility permits inferences about the learning needs of the group. Tables constructed for each of the 18 responsibilities reflected the group scores on the variables used to assess performance. For instance, for responsibility 3, "recognizes own limitations in providing direct client services," 66.7% of the group achieved less than the criterion score established on the client vignette exercise dealing with identification of issues. As a result of these data from (and feedback on) the practice audit session, it was decided that a key area for continuing professional education program development would be that of direct client services.

A workshop was then held to measure participants' clinical skills (as well as to increase sensitivity in making clinical observations, increase the repertoire of available clinical behaviors, and modify individually identified verbal and nonverbal behaviors) in 1984. The 2-day workshop included three types of exercises (live client simulations, written client vignettes, and videotaped client–therapist vignettes) followed by an evaluation using several measures. The results indicate that the simulation exercises were successful in increasing the clinical skills of the participants but that the development costs for the practice audit were high.

The development and administration costs are why there are very few programs for professionals that can be characterized as performance oriented. Most of us recognize that knowledge-oriented programming is characteristic of continuing education. Without cooperation among the university, professional associations, and other groups concerned with professional competence, such as the state regulatory authorities and agencies, programs such as this one will not be available, and practice will more than likely not be affected. It will take money, resolve, and a partnership to change continuing education from passive to active learning.

The challenge for the future is in enhancing the likelihood that such interactive learning takes place based on a clear definition of practice and a needs assessment. As long as criteria established for continuing education programs allow attendance and presentation at professional meetings; typical classroom learning such as seminars, lectures, academic courses, and workshops; and other knowledge-oriented learning to be the norm, it is highly likely that continuing professional education will continue to be perceived as a boondoggle and ineffective. Clearly, except for the few studies indicated above, the concepts of quality assurance have not been applied to mandated continuing professional education. It is important that future legislation mandating CPE as a solution to professional obsolescence require evaluation of the effectiveness of such requirements, if not on practice at least on knowledge acquisition. To repeat or to do otherwise is irresponsible.

Requiring Relicensure, Re-examination, or Recredentialing

As an alternative to mandated continuing education, but with the same goal in mind, legislatures and professional associations have considered but never fully embraced the concept of requiring a re-examination for continuation of licensure. Due to the increasing specialization that takes place after licensure and established practice, the concept of re-examination for licensure has been visited repeatedly but dismissed as unworkable. Using an examination validated for entry-level practice for increasingly specialized practitioners would be an inappropriate and invalid use of the examination. In order to re-examine established practitioners, the examination(s) would have to focus on specialized areas of practice, a common outcome of increasing years of experience. It would be prohibitive to develop enough examinations to evaluate fairly those in specialized practice.

A more popular concept, but not one yet used by state regulatory authorities, is the time-limited certificate given in certain specialized areas of medical practice that expires in a fixed number of years. In order to maintain the specialist title, the licensee must be re-examined by the specialty board by a certain date. In psychology, there is no corollary. The specialty organization in psychology, ABPP, grants the diplomate once in a lifetime. To maintain it, the diplomate must pay a membership fee (since 1983) and not be found guilty of violating ethical practice standards. Time-limited certificates for psychology do not exist as of yet.

Recently, New York State prepared a report on physician recredentialing. Although not implemented, recredentialing is not designed to determine the physician's knowledge of all aspects of medicine but rather to determine whether current practice meets appropriate standards by the use of peer review according to precise protocols on a 9-year cycle. The other two options for recredentialing include achieving specialty certification or recertification within the 9-year period or passing specially developed cognitive and clinical problem-solving tests. This report has recommended a unique approach that is without precedent and currently without approval (New York State Advisory Committee on Physician Recredentialing, 1988).

Restricting Area of Practice to a Specialty

Seeking specialty recognition by a private credentialing body is voluntary and, in most instances, requires an active, unrestricted license in the jurisdiction of practice. Specialty licensure for psychologists is relatively rare. However, for other professions, specialty credentialing has been used to support licensure by substituting for certain requirements. Instances in which completion of specialty certification has been used as a substitute for licensure include the following:

> (i) when a licensed professional is required by statute to have taken the licensure examination within five years of application for licensure, and has not;
>
> (ii) when the license is/can be specialized as opposed to generic, those jurisdictions may accept the specialized examination in place of the generic licensure examination;
>
> (iii) when the licensure examination includes an oral examination, the specialty examination may be substituted;
>
> (iv) when the specialty area is used to limit the license;
>
> (v) when the ability to advertise is tied to the definition and title of the specialty;
>
> (vi) when a question has been raised regarding negligence in professional disciplinary or malpractice hearings, the specialty definition may be used to define the specialty standard used in evaluating negligence;
>
> (vii) rather than using the definition of practice for the profession, the definition of the specialty may be used to define specifically delineated privileges at a hospital or similar facility (Hall & Ames, 1991, p. 2)

Respecialization programs, created for the psychologist wishing to change his or her area of practice, have become relatively popular, especially for those psychologists with increasing years since the doctorate and in general because of changes in the employment climate. However, respecialization programs, although similar, are not considered continuing education. The 2-year sequence of education and experience prepares the psychologist to become a practitioner and to learn a professional specialty. Once an individual has completed the doctoral degree and is qualified for independent practice, any education and training in the use of new procedures, techniques, or knowledge about specific populations constitutes proficiency training and is best addressed through continuing education. Specialty training is best addressed through doctoral training or a formal respecialization program. Training specifically focused on priority populations is proficiency training (Sales, Bricklin & Hall, 1984) if the psychologist is already trained as a professional psychologist.

Professional Discipline

Clearly, mechanisms that sanction practitioners for violation of standards (i.e., ethical, legal, and practice criteria) are an integral part of quality assurance. The difficulty lies in the small numbers affected by this process. No one believes that those not disciplined are adhering to all standards. The psychologists disciplined by state, professional, or federal agencies and organizations are simply representative of all psychologists, to a greater or lesser degree. Since 1980, the ASPPB has collected information on disciplinary actions and included them in a quarterly report known as the Disciplinary Data Report that is sent to licensure boards and credentialing and professional organizations. The numbers listed have clearly increased over the years but are small in comparison to the number licensed (≈200 listed per year out of the ≈50,000 licensed).

The opposite to professional discipline, voluntary adherence to standards of practice, is much more meaningful in terms of assuring quality, but when the profession cannot agree that such standards are necessary and what they are, little progress can be made in assuring quality. When the Standards for Providers of Psychological Services (APA, 1975, 1977) were revised in 1987, they were approved as "aspirational standards," clearly an oxymoron (APA, 1987a). Unless the state adopts the guidelines as state standards or generates their own, the profession has none. The closest set of standards that still exist are the principles contained in the APA Code of Ethics (APA, 1992). The new ethics code has moved beyond being primarily aspirational; it does a much better job of clarifying what is sanctionable and what is general guidance. Even so, psychology is clearly on the fence regarding standards of practice. States have been much more effective, but perhaps also inconsistent from one jurisdiction to another, in the monitoring of practice according to standards.

Conclusion

Psychology has made progress in committing to the development of and adherence to standards that would promote quality assurance in services to the public. Every facet of licensure (i.e., examination, discipline, and requirements for entry) is much more carefully delineated and implemented now than it was 20 years ago. However, the profession has been reluctant to bite the bullet on practice standards and that puts this profession way behind the developments in other health-care professions. Now other individuals are making decisions for psychologists that psychologists would not make. A reluctance to evaluate empirically the standards that exist in education and training has prevented knowing the real impact of those criteria and whether modifications would better serve the profession and the public. Many of the states have mandated continuing education without requiring an assessment of its effectiveness. While psychology is fighting for its position among the established professions in health care, it should use its scientific training to evaluate and refine its own health-care delivery. To do otherwise is to give short shrift to the unique contribution that psychology can make.

References

American Association of State Psychology Boards (AASPB). (1977, August). *Toward a definition of training in professional psychology.* (Available from ASPPB, PO Box 4389, Montgomery, AL 36103)

American Psychological Association. (1975). Standards for providers of psychological services. *American Psychologist, 30,* 685–694.

American Psychological Association. (1977). Standards for providers of psychological services. *American Psychologist, 32,* 495–505.

American Psychological Association. (1979). *Criteria for accreditation of doctoral training programs and internships in professional psychology.* Washington, DC: Author.

American Psychological Association. (1982). *Report of the Board of Educational Affairs Task Force on the evaluation of education, training and service in psychology.* Washington, DC: Author.

American Psychological Association. (1992). Ethical principles of psychologists and code of conduct. *American Psychologist, 47,* 1597–1611.

American Psychological Association. (1987a). *General guidelines for providers of psychological services. American Psychologist, 42,* 712–723.

American Psychological Association. (1987b). Model act for state licensure of psychologists. *American Psychologist, 42,* 696–703.

American Psychological Association, Council of Representatives. (1985, February). Minutes. *American Psychologist, 41,* 633–663.

Anastasi, A. (1988). *Psychological testing.* (6th ed.). New York: MacMillan.

Association of State and Provincial Psychology Boards (ASPPB). (1992). *Educational reporting service: EPPP performance by designated doctoral program in psychology.* (Available from ASPPB, PO Box 4389, Montgomery, AL 36103)

Belar, C. D. & Perry, N. W. (Eds.). (1990). National Conference on Scientist–Practitioner Education and Training for the Professional Practice of Psychology. *American Psychologist, 47,* 71–75.

Cooper, S. K., (1991, July 29). In outcomes we trust. *Healthweek,* pp. 34–38.

Council for the National Register of Health Service Providers in Psychology. (1992). *National register of health service providers in psychology* (Rev. ed.). Washington, DC: Author.

Fisher, C. B., & Hall, J. E. (1990a). *Development and validation of an essay licensure examination: The New York State Board for Psychology Complementary Examination Project.* Unpublished manuscript. (Available from J. E. Hall, 1120 G Street, NW, Suite 330, Washington, DC 20005)

Fisher, C. B., & Hall, J. E. (1990b, September). *Development and validation of complementary licensure or certification examinations: A manual for psychology boards.* (Available from ASPPB, PO Box 4389, Montgomery, AL 36103)

Grotelueschen Associates, Inc. (1987, December). *A profile of practicing accountants in New York state.* (Available from the State Board for Public Accountancy, New York State Education Department, Cultural Education Center, Albany, NY 12230)

Groteluesschen Associates, Inc. (1988, October). *Participation in continuing accountance education and the accountancy knowledge of public-practice accountants.* (Available from the State Board for Public Accountancy, New York State Education Department, Cultural Education Center, Albany, NY 12230)

Groteluesschen Associates, Inc. (1989, March). *Preliminary descriptive findings of the 1988 accountancy assessment.* (Available from the State Board for Public Accountancy, New York State Education Department, Cultural Education Center, Albany, NY 12230)

Groteluesschen Associates, Inc. (1989, July). *An analysis of the effectiveness of mandatory continuing education for licensed accountants in public practice in New York state.* (Available from the State Board for Public Accountancy, New York State Education Department, Cultural Education Center, Albany, NY 12230)

Groteluesschen Associates, Inc. (1990, February). *Preliminary descriptive findings of the 1989 accountancy assessment.* (Available from the State Board for Public Accountancy, New York State Education Department, Cultural Education Center, Albany, NY 12230)

Hall, J. E. (1987). Licensure and certification of psychologists. In B. A. Edelstein & E. S. Berler (Eds.), *Evaluation and accountability in clinical training* (pp. 253–281). New York: Plenum Press.

Hall, J. E., & Ames, E. (1991, February). *The impact of specialty certification on professional licensing efforts.* Presented at the meeting of the Federation of Associations of Regulatory Boards, Albuquerque, NM.

Herbsleb, J. D., Sales, B. D., & Overcast, T. D. (1985). Challenging licensure and certification. *American Psychologist, 40,* 1165–1178.

Lindsay, C. A., Crowe, M. B., & Jacobs, D. F. (1987). Continuing professional education for clinical psychology: A practice-oriented model. In B. A. Edelstein & E. S. Berler (Eds.), *Evaluation and accountability in clinical training* (pp. 331–361). New York: Plenum Press.

Mandatory Continuing Education Study Committee. (1989, August). *Preliminary report on the effectiveness of mandatory continuing education for licensed accountants in public practice in New York state.* (Available from the State Board for Public Accountancy, New York State Education Department, Cultural Education Center, Albany, NY 12230)

Mandatory Continuing Education Study Committee. (1990, April). *Final report: The effectiveness of mandatory continuing education for licensed accountants in public practice in the state of New York.* (Available from the State Board for Public Accountancy, New York State Education Department, Cultural Education Center, Albany, NY 12230)

Myers, R. A., & Rosen, G. A. (1986). *Research digest: The examination for professional practice in psychology.* (Available from ASPPB, PO Box 4389, Montgomery, AL 36103)

National Conference on Postdoctoral Training in Professional Psychology. (1993). *Proceedings.* (Available from the Association of Psychology Postdoctoral and Internship Centers, 733 15th Street, Suite 717, Washington, DC 20005)

New York State Advisory Committee on Physician Recredentialing. (1988). *Report on phase one: General principles, proposed process, recommendation.* (Available from New York Department of Health, Corning Tower, Albany, NY 12237)

New York State Doctoral Evaluation Project (1990). *Doctoral education in psychology.* (Available from Doctoral Evaluation Project, New York State Education Department, Cultural Education Center, Room 5A43, Albany, NY 12230)

Richman, S. (1982). *Final report to the AASPB on the role delineation study for the Examination for professional practice in psychology.* (Available from ASPPB, PO Box 4389, Montgomery, AL 36103)

Rosen G. A., & Mirone, J. A. (1986). *Final report of the test specifications revisions project for the examination for professional practice in psychology.* (Available from the ASPPB, Box 4389, Montgomery, AL 36103)

Rosenfeld, M., Shimberg, B., & Thornton, R. F. (1984). *Job analysis of licensed psychologists in the United States and Canada.* Princeton, NJ: Center for Occupational and Professional Assessment.

Sales, B. D., Bricklin, D., & Hall, J. E. (1984, November). *Specialization in psychology: Principles.* (Available from American Psychological Association, Board of Professional Affairs, 750 First Street, NE, Washington, DC 20002-4242)

Sanazaro, P. J. (1983). Determining physician's performance—Continuing medication education and other interacting variables. *Evaluation and the Health Professions, 6,* 197–210.

Sechrest, L., & Chatel, D. M. (1987). Evaluation and accountability in training for professional psychology: An overview. In B. A. Edelstein & E. S. Berler (Eds.), *Evaluation and accountability in clinical training* (pp. 1–37). New York: Plenum Press.

Stricker, G., & Rodriguez, A. R. (Eds.). (1988). *Handbook of quality assurance in mental health.* New York: Plenum Press.

Wellner, A. M. (Ed.). (1978). *Education and credentialing in psychology.* Washington, DC: Steering Committee of APA, AASPB, and National Register.

CHAPTER

23

Improving the Clinical Training of Psychologists: A Role for Accreditation?

Paul D. Nelson
American Psychological Association

The topic of public–academic linkages for clinical training in psychology is as timely as it is challenging. It is timely in the context of our society's questioning focus on the purposes and outcomes of higher education in general and the professions in particular. The public accountability of our universities and other institutions of higher learning is at issue. Universities are engaged in major self-study, stragically focused on how their missions serve society in a more general sense than their time-honored role as the generators and disseminators of knowledge. Even the meaning of scholarship, the learned institution's historical hallmark, is being re-examined in terms of the relationship between teaching, research, and service to the community (Boyer, 1990). In this chapter, I shall discuss how past conferences on graduate education and training programs in psychology have reflected changing notions of the mission of these programs and recently have led to a growing interest in public–academic linkages. I then address the important question of how education and training strategies can be revised so that both scholarly and societal needs are served, and also discuss the role of accreditation in this process.

Discussion of public–academic linkages is timely in the context of change occurring in our discipline and in the form and substance of its applications to the world about us. The published proceedings of the 1987 National Conference on Graduate Education, titled "Preparing Psychologists for the 21st Century," challenge us to rethink the assumptions we have maintained about our discipline and the paradigms of professional and graduate education with which we have learned to live (Bickman & Ellis, 1990). Serious attention was given at that conference to the changing nature of psychology as a discipline, demographic changes in our student populations, and pedagogical implications of the same. Less attention was given to questions about the impact that societal changes are likely to have on the future practices of psychologists and, consequently, on graduate education and training that preceeds such practice.

Somewhat by contrast, the Boulder Conference on graduate education, held nearly 4 decades earlier (Raimy, 1950), was prompted by the recognition that changes in our society following World War II and the rapidly expanding demand for psychologists, especially those in the clinical field, necessitated the review of those matters in terms of their implication for graduate education and training. Thus, the focus of that conference was on clinical training, a vital part of which was considered to be, and remains to this day, the clinical psychology student's need for field experience in service agencies, to which we refer to currently as practicum and internship training.

The idea of training clinical psychologists in vivo, that is, training in service agency settings under the supervision of psychologists other than faculty and carrying out psychological assessment and intervention procedures with a variety of client or patient populations, had been in effect from the earliest years of clinical training. By conceptualizing such training as an integral part of the academic preparation of clinical psychologists, our profession endorsed a model of public–academic linkages. The Boulder Conference delegates reaffirmed that model as a vital part of doctoral education and training in clinical psychology, a concept that has been reaffirmed in virtually every national conference on professional education and training in psychology since that time.

A Decade of Reflection

Though national conferences have been held on issues of graduate and professional education and training in each decade since the Boulder conference, during no period have there been more of such gatherings than the 1980s. Most have attended to issues of curriculum, models of training, links between education and credentialing of psychologists, and almost invariably accreditation.

It has been largely through National Institute of Mental Health (NIMH) initiatives, however, that we have been prompted once again to think about the quality of professional education and training in our field in terms of how well prepared clinical psychologists are to address the complex health and mental health problems in our society. An example of this is the series of NIMH conferences held in 1988 to address service needs of the seriously mentally ill (Johnson, 1990), of children and adolescents (Magrab & Wohlford, 1990), and of ethnic minority populations (Myers, Wohlford, Guzman, & Echemendia, 1991). These conferences begin with an analysis of the needs in our communities and challenge academic institutions to consider the strategies by which to prepare their students to meet those needs. They pose as one administrative mechanism for creating public–academic linkages. They invite us to re-examine our education, credentialing, and practice structures in the context of change in the social, political, economic, and demographic fabric of our society. They speak, in essence, to interdisciplinary strategies.

How might public–academic linkages be fashioned so as to facilitate innovative, cost-effective responses to societal needs while also preserving the essential scholarly mission of the academy in our society? For psychology, as with other disciplines or professions, we need to rethink our strategies of education and training for practice. Certainly this is not a new plea, as many debates and scholarly writings of the past decade confirm. It is one that will be heeded, I am sure, as the next generation of accreditation policies, procedures, and standards are developed during the next year or 2 for application to graduate programs in professional areas of psychology.

Strategies of Education and Training for Practice

An essential feature of linkages between academic and service institutions is a better integration of research, practice, and public policy in professional education and training. There is also the need for interdisciplinary strategies of education and training, because most significant problems in society are of a complexity that defy solution by a single discipline working alone. I certainly consider that to be true with regard to the problems focused on during the NIMH conferences. They but scratch the surface of problems within our society that implicate human behavior, the subject of psychological science and practice. However, relatively little attention is given currently to this aspect of clinical training in psychology. In contrast, interestingly, it was given more emphasis by our teachers and their colleagues who at mid-century set forth initial guidelines for the accreditation of clinical psychology programs (American Psychological Association [APA] Committee on Training in Clinical Psychology, 1947). In that same period, it was salient among issues of clinical training discussed at the Boulder Conference (Raimy, 1950) and among the priorities established a few years later in Ann Arbor at the first meeting of the new APA board responsible for policies and activities related to education and training in our field (APA Education and Training Board, 1952).

Greater emphasis, I believe, also needs to be placed on public health models of practice in clinical psychology. Given their emphasis on primary, secondary, and tertiary prevention, and their penchant for the integration of research, practice, and public policy, such models are quite meaningful in the context of many behavioral problems in our society. Such a perspective also affords ample reason for the development of public–academic linkages as an integral part of professional training. It argues likewise for more interdepartmental, interdisciplinary training at the graduate level of education.

In the context of these emphases, finally, it is necessary to define the essential competencies that psychologists must have in order to prepare for a lifetime of learning as psychologists and to contribute uniquely as part of interdisciplinary problem-solving teams that are likely to characterize their professional practice. These should be broad, professional, intellectual competencies, based on the foundations of theory and method in the discipline, not thought of as simply those competencies that are narrowly focused technical skills.

It was the psychologists' usefulness as problem solvers in a variety of settings faced with different types of problems, equipped with inquiring intellect and competencies grounded in psychological theory and methods, that resulted in their recognition and demand for their services during and immediately following the years of World War II (Fiske, 1946; Hunt, 1945). One of the outcomes of that demand, indeed, was the rapid expansion of graduate education in psychology after the war, responsive to critical mental health and other needs of society for applications of psychology.

These objectives are not new in psychology. They have undergirded accreditation criteria for more than 4 decades and reflect the thinking of present-day psychologists as well (Stigall et al., 1990). There remains general consensus, I believe, that breadth of education in our discipline remains important as a foundation for psychologists, especially those who intend to offer professional services to the public. The questions open for debate, however, pertain to how breadth is to be defined and how it is to be achieved pedagogically. Beyond that, are there foundational competencies to be expected of all psychologists upon completing their graduate education, and are there additional competencies to be expected of graduates of doctoral programs as a function of the doctoral program's philosophical orientation and goals?

There is an inclination, I sense, for national conferences, interest groups, and even academic institutions to advocate or use what I will refer to as a "curriculum fix" whenever new problems arise or old ones are revisited that pertain to the academic preparation of professional psychologists. By that I refer to the "we'll simply add another course to the required curriculum" approach to graduate education. This approach to curriculum development, I believe, is counterproductive to what we want to achieve in graduate education and training for practice in our discipline, namely to encourage intellectual curiosity and impart learning strategies appropriate to the applications of psychology in addressing human problems.

Peterson (1985) differentiates philosophies of training in preparation for science and practice careers, each of which can be argued to represent an approach to problem solving. Each requires, to some extent, the mastery of a particular knowledge base, an understanding of methodologies, and the development of a set of attitudes and assumptions. Consequently, there is a curriculum appropriate to every graduate student, perhaps more formal and extensive for some than for others. Carried to its extreme, however, the curriculum fix approach to graduate education and training for practice will increase what is already a very expensive process of education, at the risk of compromise to the fundamental objectives of professional education and training. Those objectives have more to do with the development of strategies of inquiry, or what Peterson (1991) refers to as disciplined inquiry, to test current assumptions and to generate the knowledge on which new or modified sets of assumptions can be founded than they do with simply imparting a body of knowledge that has an increasingly diminished half-life of validity.

For graduate departments, professional schools, and programs of professional psychology there are many possible administrative arrangements for public–academic linkages to advance the development of competencies expected. Some may be local to the immediate community in which an academic institution is situated; others may be regional. There may be some that constitute "centers of excellence" by their reputation as referral centers for the more complex, difficult problems, usually characterized by major research and advanced teaching activities as an integral part of the professional services provided. Others may afford a breadth of training experiences at state-of-the-art levels of professional service, program evaluation, and teaching.

Whatever the setting and structure of linkages, the training experience should give students the opportunity to discover firsthand what it means to engage in research-informed practice or policy development and practice or policy-informed research. This requires communication among academic program faculty, agency supervisors, and students about the goals and objectives of their field placements in clinical training.

A Role for Accreditation?

In rethinking our strategies of education and training for professional practice, it seems to many that the way to ensure that public–academic linkages occur is to require their development through the standards or criteria for professional program accreditation. To others, I am sure, such a solution is an anathema to creative, innovative developments that will improve the clinical training of psychologists while also addressing significant health and mental health problems in many communities. These perspectives are based on certain assumptions and expectations about accreditation that need to be examined. I do so briefly below.

Broadly stated, the purpose of accreditation is to assess and facilitate the development of quality in higher education institutions and programs. *Quality* in this context is defined broadly as the extent to which, and manner by which, an institution's or program's goals and objectives are achieved. It also speaks to the public's need for assurance that the institution or the program has the commitment, resources, and procedures to maintain these achievements reasonably well over time. Specialized accreditation, that focused on programs or schools of professional education and training, requires that the goals and objectives of programs accredited be appropriate for the profession, thus allowing the profession some role in defining parameters of what is appropriate to the entry level of independent practice in that profession.

Notice that there is no stipulation about how institutions or programs are to achieve their goals and objectives. That is their business. Rather, there is an assessment of the manner and extent to which their goals and objectives are achieved. This requires, first and foremost, that programs be clear about their education and training goals and objectives, and about the philosophy of training and practice that guides what they do, followed by the acquisition and application of resources to their attainment. How that is done is likely and should vary as a function of many factors, perhaps most important among which are the host academic institution's mission, goals, and resource requirements. How different this seems from the conception held about accreditation by so many in our profession, but how much alike this strategy seems to that set forth by the distinguished psychologists who developed the first accreditation criteria for clinical training in psychology. To wit:

> The general principles which underlie the graduate program appear to us of primary importance—in fact much more important than the details of the program. If clarity in the formulation of goals exists, there should be relatively little difficulty about agreeing on the means for implementing them. . . Our aims are . . . to achieve general agreement on the goals of training and encourage experimentation on methods of achieving these goals and to suggest ways of establishing high standards in a setting of flexibility and reasonable freedom. We also hold that the goals should not be determined by special situations and special demands, but should be oriented toward the question of what is the best training for the clinical psychologist. (APA Committee on Training in Clinical Psychology, 1947, p. 543)

For administrators of professional psychology programs to know whether they are achieving what they set out to accomplish, they need to articulate, among other outcomes, the competencies they expect their students to develop. The profession as a whole should have some idea of fundamental competencies that are expected of professional psychologists. Each graduate program, moreover, with its unique institutional setting and mission, its own focus through the strengths of its faculty, and the career goals of its students, may have its own set of additional expectations about the competencies of its graduates. Are the outcomes of national conferences, such as those sponsored by NIMH, expressed in terms that can be used to develop competency constructs? There is no reason that the future accreditation standards and criteria for clinical training in psychology could not adhere to the philosophy espoused more than 40 years ago while being attentive as well to standards that address the development and assessment of competencies.

Conclusion

Public–academic linkages afford an administrative mechanism for the professional training of psychologists as problem-solvers. Their form and substance should be a matter of choice among the institutions involved, not mandated in any particular way. These linkages should be a natural and rich way for professional academic programs and service agencies to achieve their respective goals and objectives through collaborative effort. There should be some excitement in the air among those so engaged. These programs afford real-life opportunity, moreover, for students of psychology to learn how theory, research, practice, and public policy can be related or unrelated. They also afford opportunity for students of psychology to learn early about the needs for and challenges of interdisciplinary problem solving. Indeed, such linkages with interdisciplinary collaboration may lead to new standards of practice in various problem areas and thus serve, as Nelson and Aletky (1987) suggest, as a frame of reference for future standards of education and training in the profession.

Given that potential, and if the standards and practices of accrediting bodies are to protect the interests of students, benefit the public, and improve the quality of teaching, learning, research, and professional practice (Council on Postsecondary Accreditation, 1990, p. 39), quite clearly there is a role for accreditation in the improvement of clinical training in psychology.[1]

References

APA Committee on Training in Clinical Psychology. (1947). Recommended graduate training program in clinical psychology. *American Psychologist, 2,* 539–558.

APA Education and Training Board. (1952). Educational issues in psychology: A report of the February 1952 Conference of the APA Education and Training Board. *American Psychologist, 7,* 456–460.

Bickman, L., & Ellis, H. (Eds.). (1990). *Preparing psychologists for the 21st century: Proceedings of the national conference on graduate education in psychology.* Hillsdale, NJ: Erlbaum.

Boyer, E. L. (1990). *Scholarship reconsidered: Priorities of the professoriate.* Princeton, NJ: The Carnegie Foundation for the Advancement of Teaching.

Council on Postsecondary Accreditation. (1990). *The COPA handbook.* Washington, DC: Author.

Fiske, D. W. (1946). Naval aviation psychology: The special services group. *American Psychologist,* 1, 544–548.

Hunt, W. A. (1945). Clinical psychology in the Navy. *Journal of Clinical Psychology,* 1, 99–104.

Johnson, D. L. (Ed.). (1990). *Service needs of the seriously mentally ill: Training implications for psychology.* Washington, DC: American Psychological Association.

Magrab, D. H., & Wolford, P. (Eds.). (1990). *Improving psychological services for children and adolescents with severe mental disorders: Clinical training in psychology.* Washington, DC: American Psychological Association.

Myers, H. F., Wohlford, P., Guzman, L. P., & Echemendia, R. J. (Eds.). (1991). *Ethnic minority perspectives on clinical training and services in psychology.* Washington, DC: American Psychological Association.

Nelson, P. D., & Aletky, P. J. (1987). Accreditation: A link between training and practice. In B. A. Edelstein and E. S. Berler (Eds.), *Evaluation and accountability in clinical psychology* (pp. 231–252). New York: Plenum Press.

Peterson, D. R. (1985). Twenty years of practitioner training in psychology. *American Psychologist, 40*(4), 441–451.

Peterson, D. R. (1991). Connection and disconnection of research and practice in the education of professional psychologists. *American Psychologist, 46*(4), 422–429.

Raimy, V. C. (Ed.). (1950). *Training in clinical psychology.* New York: Prentice-Hall.

Stigall, T. T., Bourg, E. F., Bricklin, P. M., Kovacs, A. L., Larsen, K. G., Lorion, R. P., Nelson, P. D., Nurse, A. R., Pugh, R. W., & Wiens, A. N. (Eds.). (1990). *Report of the joint council on professional education in psychology.* Baton Rouge, LA: Land and Land Printers.

[1] The author's remarks are based on his personal experience as Director, Program Consultation and Accreditation, Education Directorate, American Psychological Association. They are not intended as necessarily representing or otherwise reflecting officially the policies or endorsement of the American Psychological Association.

CHAPTER

24

Clinical Training and Research for Children's Services

Robert M. Friedman
University of South Florida

The 1980's were a time of heightened interest in the mental health needs of children, adolescents, and their families. Perhaps even more important, the 1980s was also a time in which major changes were made in basic paradigms for organizing and delivering services to those youngsters with the most serious emotional disturbances and their families. This chapter will briefly describe the role of our Center in these changes, summarize the changes, and discuss the implications of them for service delivery and system of care research in children's mental health in general and for psychologists in particular.

Research and Training Center

The Research and Training Center for Children's Mental Health of the Florida Mental Health Institute, University of South Florida, has had a unique opportunity to both observe and contribute to the changes that are taking place. The Center, funded since 1984 by the National Institute on Disability and Rehabilitation Research of the U.S. Department of Education and the National Institute of Mental Health (NIMH), has three complementary roles related to these changes.

First, the Center is involved in several large-scale research projects dealing with children with serious emotional disturbance who are served by public systems and their families. Second, the Center has contributed to the development of new models of community-based systems of care (Stroul & Friedman, 1986), and the staff have served as consultants on systems of care to many state and local governments. third, in an effort to stimulate more rezearch on service delivery and system-of-care issues and to create a network of researchers interested in this complex topic, the Center has organized and conducted an annual national conference on system-of-care research in children's mental health. The fifth such conference was held on March 2–4, 1992, in Tampa, Florida.

By virtue of our involvement in these issues and our concern for their growth, in October, 1989, we were invited by Dr. Lewis Judd, the Director of NIMH, to organize a panel of experts for the purpose of preparing a set of recommendations for enhancing research on service delivery and system-of-care issues. The report resulting from this effort (Research and Training Center for Children's Mental Health, 1989) was used by the National Advisory Mental Health Council (NAMHC) in preparing the "National Plan for Research on Child and Adolescent Mental Disorders," submitted to Congress in 1990.

In our report to NAMHC we pointed out that research on service delivery and systems of care in mental health is a relatively new area, having a much briefer history than the longer established traditions of basic and clinical research. It should be pointed out in this regard that our advocacy for service delivery and system-of-care research is in no way intended to diminish the need for basic and clinical research. We agree with the NAMHC and with the Institute of Medicine, which in 1989 published a significant report on research in children's mental health, that increased funding is needed for research in each of the three major categories: basic, clinical, and service delivery.

Service Delivery and System-of-Care Research

Essentially, service delivery and system-of-care research seeks to address two fairly simple questions: How should service delivery systems be organized to provide cost-effective services, and should these service delivery systems be financed to provide such services? (Burns & Friedman, 1990). The problem is that although these questions are simple to ask, they are very complex to answer and typically involve complicated and often difficult-to-measure independent variables. The task of describing community-based systems of care, with all of the different policies, procedures, service components, resources, and public and private agencies, is enormously complex by itself. In addition, the task of relating structural and process variables within these service delivery systems to specific outcome measures further complicates the research. However, unless progress is made in understanding the impact of organizational and financing variables on such dependent measures as access to care, utilization of care, cost of care, and the outcome of care, the likelihood is that much of the gains that are made through basic and clinical research will never be adequately translated into meaningful changes affecting the lives of children and their families. Furthermore, the financial resources required to provide needed services will not be available.

Within the last 10–15 years, there have been at least four significant developments at a service and policy level that have converged to create an especially strong need for more and better research on systems of care (Research and Training Center for Children's Mental Health, 1989). First, the primary locus of treatment in the mental health field has moved from hospitals to community settings. This creates special challenges in understanding how to develop effective community-based systems of care. Second, within both the child and adult areas, public mental health systems have identified as their top priority the delivery of services to individuals with severe and persistent problems. Typically, these are individuals who require services from a variety of agencies other than just mental health (e.g., general health, child welfare, juvenile justice, special education, or rehabilitation), thereby creating a need to identify strategies for promoting effective interagency collaboration.

Third, the role of states in planning and administering mental health services has grown with the implementation of the Alcohol, Drug Abuse, and Mental Health Block Grant program in 1980. This provides a more centralized responsibility within states for policymaking and planning and has generated an increased need to determine how to develop effective service systems. Fourth, there has been a rapid escalation of costs for health care and social services in general, including mental health care. At the present time, this increased cost in the health and social service area has clearly contributed to the budgetary crisis experienced by many states and localities. This has led to the need for more research on such issues as approaches to cost containment, the impact of different reimbursement strategies on service delivery, and the cost-effectiveness of different treatment approaches.

Changes in the Service Delivery Paradigm

As great as the need is for more research on service delivery and system-of-care issues, it is important to place the need for research into the context of several significant changes in the service delivery paradigm. It should be noted that these changes can largely be attributed to the influence of the Child and Adolescent Service System Program (CASSP), a modest NIMH effort that has provided grants to states for enhancing their system capacity to serve children and their families and grants to three academically based centers to provide technical assistance and conduct research (Duchnowski & Friedman, 1990; Stroul & Friedman, 1986). Recently, CASSP has added a competitive grant program by which states could initiate research–demonstration efforts.

The first major shift in the field has been toward an emphasis on the need for community-based systems of care that include a wide range of services of varying degrees of intensity, strong partnerships between parents and professionals, multiagency collaboration, and competence in addressing the needs of culturally diverse populations (Stroul & Friedman, 1986). This shift is based on the belief that children with serious emotional disturbances and their families have multiple and varied needs and that in order to serve them effectively there must be a communitywide effort involving many different agencies and services. Although this emphasis does not take away from the need for effective service components, such as day treatment programs or group homes, it focuses on the interrelatedness of all parts of the system.

This shift toward a system-of-care emphasis and away from a focus on specific programs has several implications for research. First, it is important that a greater focus in research be on the whole community-based system of care as the unit of analysis rather than individual programs. It is important to determine, for example, how well a community is doing overall in serving children with emotional disturbances and their families in addition to determining how well a particular program that may serve a relatively small number of children is doing.

Although this calls for complicated research, there are encouraging signs that the very process of clearly identifying target populations and desired quantitative outcomes for systems of care can be an important step toward improving services and increasing knowledge about systems (Jordan & Hernandez, 1990). Significant system-of-care research projects in which the unit of analysis is the entire system are currently taking place, for example, within several communities in California (Rosenblatt & Attkisson, 1992; Rosenblatt, Attkisson, & Fernandez, 1992), at our own Center (Duchnowski, Johnson, Hall, Kutash, & Friedman, 1993), within a demonstration project targeted at military dependents from the Ft. Bragg area (Bickman, 1993; Heflinger et al., 1992), and within demonstration sites for a special initiative of the Robert Wood Johnson Foundation (Beachler, 1990; Cross, Gallon, Gardner, Adnopoz, & Saxe, 1993; England & Cole, 1992).

Second, it is important that research focused on particular treatment programs also incorporates a system-of-care perspective (Burns & Friedman, 1990; Friedman, 1989):

> To determine if a particular program is effective as a part of a system, for example, it is not sufficient to determine overall success rates or to simply compare two similar programs (e.g., Group Home A vs. Group Home B). It is also important to determine how the youngsters served in the particular program compare to those served in other components of the system of care, and to examine whether some of them might have been served in less restrictive components of the system of care. It is also important to place the program in the broader context of the community in which it is located and the service system of which it is a part. (Burns & Friedman, 1990 p. 90)

It may be, for example, that a day treatment program in a community with a high density of other high-quality services may appear to be effective. However, a system analysis may reveal that its success is related to the support it gets from other services, and the fact that the existence of so many other services allows it to be selective in accepting youngsters. Without this systems perspective, the results of a program evaluation may be deceptive.

It may also be, for example, that out of 100 consecutive admissions to a group home, 75% of the youngsters made good progress. From a systems perspective, however, it is important to determine how many of those youngsters really required the service to begin with or could have been served in a less restrictive service if it were available. From a community-based system-of-care perspective, that same group home program may be more valuable if it serves only children who have gone through intensive nonresidential services before being admitted even if its success rate is reduced to 40% than it is if it has a higher success rate but with youngsters who may not have needed such an expensive and restrictive service (Friedman, 1989).

A second major paradigm shift in the field has been toward an increased emphasis on individual treatment, using multiple services in a flexible way (Burchard & Clarke, 1990; Staff, 1988; VanDenBerg, 1990). Such efforts, supported by discretionary funds that can be used to "wrap" services around individual clients, have carried to a new extreme the notions of individualized care and multifaceted intervention. They may result in extra services in a youngster's home, school, or community on a daily basis. They involve building on strengths and needs in a number of life domains as much as they do addressing specific problem areas (Johnson & Friedman, 1991).

The evaluation of these highly individualized approaches creates a much more difficult research test than evaluating any unitary intervention that all youngsters receive in a standard way because the independent variable, the intervention, is now much more complex. In fact, if treatment integrity is defined as using the same intervention in a well-controlled manner with all subjects, then obviously individualized approaches are in conflict with the need to maintain treatment integrity. However, unless services are provided in a flexible and individualized manner, is it realistic to expect that they will be effective when used with populations of youngsters with serious and multiple needs and problems?

A review article on treatment of antisocial behavior and conduct disorders in youngsters, published in *Psychological Bulletin,* illustrates this dilemma (Kazdin, 1987). The author reviewed studies that looked at different treatment approaches, specifically including parent training, family systems intervention, skill building, and a less clear category called community intervention. Based on this review, the author concluded that there was no empirical support for the effectiveness of these interventions with antisocial behavior and conduct disorders.

Such a conclusion was clearly justified by the findings. Also, it is not surprising that studies have focused on single interventions that are relatively simple to describe and define, given the greater ease with which such studies can be conducted. Is it not to be expected, however, that any single, unitary intervention is unlikely to have a great success rate with problems as serious and heterogeneous as conduct disorders?

It could be argued that the approach to research that emphasizes unidimensional interventions for the most serious problems is becoming outdated in light of new developments in service delivery. What is needed is research that studies intensive, comprehensive, and flexible interventions that are individualized but still can be described sufficiently to permit research to be done instead of testing. It may be with such approaches that the integrity of the intervention rests more with describing the process of conducting an assessment and translating the assessment into an individualized intervention than it does with using the same intervention with all people.

Conclusion

In summary, this chapter has addressed the issue of service delivery and system-of-care research in children's mental health. This type of research is of growing importance if the knowledge being gained through clinical research is to be put to full use and if the range of services needed to address complex problems are to be available and accessible. Particularly as financial resources to address problems of children and families diminish at the same time as the prevalence and seriousness of such problems increases (Friedman, 1992), the need for research on how to develop cost-effective systems of care becomes even greater.

Adequate progress in service delivery and system-of-care research clearly requires the active participation of psychologists. However, it must be recognized that this research is always complicated, often involves factors in communities that are beyond the direct control of the research, and stretches typical approaches to research to incorporate new concepts of systems of care and individualized treatment.

Service systems change in response to many factors, only some of which have to do with research findings (Behar, 1989). Typically, policymakers and administrators within systems do not have the time to wait until a sound empirical base is present to guide the direction of change. Most frequently, service systems seek to change in response to clinical and epidemiological changes in the nature and prevalence of problems presented by children and their families and in response to the need to improve cost-effectiveness of services.

Psychologists have much to contribute to the process of change. They have much to contribute both to the research that is needed to guide the change before it happens and to study the change after it has happened. Given that the service system represents the basic context in which clinical psychologists will function, it is hoped that at a minimum the professional training of psychologists will adequately prepare them to understand the legal, organizational, and financial complexities of community-based systems of care. This would represent an important improvement in professional training that would enhance the preparation of clinical psychologists, whether they work in the public or private sector. Given the need for an improved knowledge base for the development and modification of community-based systems of care, it is further hoped that professional training will go a step further and prepare psychologists to respond to the opportunity and challenge to make a significant research contribution to the service delivery and system-of-care field as well.

References

Behar, L. (1989). The forces impacting on public policy. In P. Greenbaum, R. Friedman, A. Duchnowski, K. Kutash, & S. Silver (Eds.), *Children's mental health services and policy: Building a research base: Confer-*

ence proceedings (pp. 91–92). Tampa: Florida Mental Health Institute, University of South Florida.

Burchard, J. D., & Clarke, R. T. (1990). The role of individualized care in a service delivery system for children and adolescents with severely maladjusted behavior. *The Journal of Mental Health Administration, 17*, 48–60.

Burns, B. J., & Friedman, R. M. (1990). Examining the research base for child mental health services and policy. *The Journal of Mental Health Administration, 17*, 87–98.

Duchnowski, A. J., & Friedman, R. M. (1990). Children's mental health: Challenges for the nineties. *The Journal of Mental Health Administration, 17*, 3–12.

Friedman, R. M. (1989). Service system research: Implications of a systems perspective. In P. Greenbaum, R. Friedman, A. Duchnowski, K. Kutash, & S. Silver (Eds.), *Children's mental health services and policy: Building a research base* (pp. 1–6). Tampa: Florida Mental Health Institute, University of South Florida.

Friedman, R. M. (1992). Mental health and substance abuse services for adolescents: Clinical and service system issues. *Administration and Policy in Mental Health, 19*(3), 159–178.

Institute of Medicine. (1989). *Research on children and adolescents with mental, behavioral, and developmental disorders*. Washington, DC: National Academy of Sciences.

Johnson, M. K., & Friedman, R. M. (1991). Strength-based assessment. *Update, 7*, 10–13.

Jordan, D. D., & Hernandez, M. (1990). The Ventura Planning Model: A proposal for mental health reform. *The Journal of Mental Health Administration, 17*, 26–47.

Kazdin, A. E. (1987). Treatment of antisocial behavior in children: Current status and future directions. *Psychological Bulletin, 102*, 187–203.

National Advisory Mental Health Council. (1990). *National Plan for Research on Child and Adolescent Mental Disorders*. Rockville, MD: U.S. Department of Health and Human Services, National Institute of Mental Health.

Research and Training Center for Children's Mental Health. (1989). *Report to NIMH on service system research*. Unpublished manuscript, University of South Florida, Florida Mental Health Institute, Tampa.

Stroul, B. A., & Friedman, R. M. (1986). *A system of care for severely emotionally disturbed children and youth*. Washington, DC: Georgetown University Child Development Center.

Staff. (1988, Summer). Individualizing services. *Update, 3*(2), 10–12.

VanDenBerg, J. (1990). The Alaska Youth Initiative: An experiment in individualized treatment and education. In A. Algarin, R. M. Friedman, A. J. Duchnowski, K. M. Kutash, S. E. Silver, & M. K. Johnson (Eds.), *Children's mental health services and policy: Building a research base: 2nd annual conference proceedings* (pp. 59–72). Tampa: Florida Mental Health Institute, University of South Florida.

CHAPTER

25

Public Mental Health Systems and Research: Can This Relationship Survive?

Michael F. Hogan
Ohio Department of Mental Health

Introduction

Mental health services—especially those for individuals with the most serious, long-term conditions—are still struggling to recover from societal neglect as well as the failed public policies of deinstitutionalization and total institutionalization. There are many signs that this recovery is well underway, including improvements in the level of mental health services. There has been a substantial expansion of access to care in the past generation, illustrated by the growth in outpatient services. From 1969 to 1983, the number of outpatient psychiatric admissions in the United States grew from 1.1 million to 2.7 million (Witkin, Atay, Fell, & Manderscheid, 1987).

Although access to care was facilitated by expanded insurance coverage, public mental health systems remained the foundation of service delivery. In 1987, the state mental health authorities (SMHAs) expended over $9 billion to provide care (Lutterman & Hogan, 1990). Due to Congress's historic reluctance to take responsibility for these state-supported efforts, the SMHAs remain a crucial underpinning of mental health care.

States have labored to maintain and improve the quality of their mental health programs, benefiting in particular from the conceptual approach labeled "community support." This concept of care is predicated on an understanding of serious mental illness as a frequently long-term problem of uncertain course. Adjustment and recovery are facilitated by integrated medical, psychological, social, and rehabilitative services delivered over time and across settings. As Morrissey and Goldman (1984) have noted, this approach is a radical departure from earlier mental health reform strategies that emphasized short-term treatment and focused on a single locus of care (e.g., the asylum, the psychiatric hospital, or the mental health center).

Although the community support concept may be considered a product of social reform, it also has its roots in research findings. In particular, the work of Stein and Test (1980) provided an empirical foundation for the new approach. It is, of course, completely uncertain whether the chicken of public policy or the egg of research findings came first. Nonetheless, this issue has new meaning as public mental health systems strive to adapt and develop in the 1990s.

Although issues related to the availability and quality of services remain prominent, there are a range of new issues and populations requiring attention. The co-occurrence of mental illness and chemical dependency is newly recognized as a major problem. Deteriorating systems of low-income housing, social supports, and affordable health care have an urgent impact on individuals with mental illness. The role of research in facilitating system improvement is uncertain. Can well-designed studies co-exist with the turbulent environment of public agencies? Can data provide "feed-forward" (as opposed to feedback) on the crucial problems that lie ahead, or is research necessarily reactive? Recent advances in both service delivery and services research may seem to hold out the prospect of a favorable union. What are the issues involved in achieving the promise of this marriage?

State Mental Health Agencies as a Locus for Research

It may appear that the culture of the typical state agency is incompatible with the culture required to support research activities. State agency time perspectives are frequently short, driven both by annual budget cycles and the short tenure of SMHA leadership. As of 1990, the median tenure of state directors and commissioners was only 2.2 years (National Association of State Mental Health Program Directors, 1990). More time is required to conceive and conduct research, particularly when controlled studies are involved.

State agencies may also appear dominated by political and bureaucratic considerations, given the brief tenure of leadership and the relative infrequency of commissioners trained at the masters or doctoral level. As of December 1990, only 16 commissioners had either of these degrees (National Association of State Mental Health Program Directors, 1990).

The environment of state mental health systems is also complex and turbulent. Although SMHA systems evolve gradually over a long period of time (Wolf, 1990), they are complex open systems. The Connecticut Department of Mental Health is not unrepresentative. A system administered through five regions and 23 catchment areas includes nine state facilities and 512 community-based programs administered by a total of 130 not-for-profit agencies or general hospitals. The boundaries of the system are also highly permeable. Many individuals receive care simultaneously in the public, nonprofit, and private sectors (e.g., from a state case manager, a community rehabilitation agency, and a private therapist). Others move through different sectors of care as their condition changes. Is such a complex system too "messy" to conduct rigorous research?

Finally, the supports and rewards for research in the SMHA are limited. Leadership changes, marginal salaries, and poor connections with academia are chronic problems. The SMHA is unlikely to be able to support a cadre of researchers, so peer support is limited. Budget pressures and the pressing priorities of unmet needs mean that equipment and logistical support may be hard to come by.

State Agency Research Efforts

Despite these problems, many SMHAs are actively engaged in research, both via direct management of research projects and through funding to academic or independent investigators. A survey of the states and territories (National Association of State Mental Health Program Directors, 1988) showed that 33 of the states were conducting or funding services research. Sixty percent of the states had employees conducting research directly, half had employees collaborating on research with colleges or universities, and 19 states awarded contracts or grants to higher education to complete research. This is clearly a substantial level of effort, and one that belies the impression that SMHAs are not in a position to conduct research.

The levels of investment and activity indicated by the states in the 1988 survey are also substantial. The total reported research budget of the states from all sources was $70.3 million, of which $18.8 million was focused on services research. These funds supported a total of 457 research projects. Also, despite the possible view of SMHAs as unable to support research staffing, the states reported a total of 218 professional staff engaged in research activities (National Association of State Mental Health Program Directors, 1988).

In addition to this significant breadth of state agency research involvement, the length and depth of the research efforts in a number of states is impressive. In states like New York, Ohio, Pennsylvania, and Connecticut, substantial investments in research have been made for many years. One prototypic approach has been state support of academic research institutes with a tripartite service, teaching, and research mission. Additionally, however, a number of the larger states have conducted or supported their own research efforts over many years.

Recent Developments Encouraging SMHA Research Efforts

Several developments within the past few years have increased the support for state agency research efforts and the profile of these activities. The general visibility of public mental health services research efforts received a major boost when a substantial research and evaluation component was made a crucial part of the Robert Wood Johnson Foundation initiatives. The first and most significant of the foundation's efforts involved a 5-year program to improve the quality of care of seriously mentally ill people in nine major American cities. The evaluation program is a substantial collaboration among a number of institutions and investigators, which considers five groups of interrelated studies: site-level analysis, community care study, housing studies, financing studies, and disability and vocational rehabilitation studies (Goldman et al., 1990). Although not an SMHA effort, this research project addresses issues in and crucial to states and involves many researchers who are collaborators in SMHA research endeavors.

A second set of positive influences emerges from the National Institute of Mental Health (NIMH), and begins with the Public–Academic Liaison (PAL) Program for research (National Institute on Mental Health, 1988). The PAL approach was promoted by former NIMH director Dr. Lewis Judd as a cross-cutting theme: Psychiatric research and services would both be improved by a higher level of collaboration between public mental health programming and academic institutions. Although few research grants have specifically been funded as PAL projects, there appears to be broad agreement that the announcement is stimulating increased levels of collaboration.

Another factor shaped by NIMH was the opportunity to increase services research provided indirectly by the passage of the 1988 reauthorization of the Alcohol, Drug Abuse, and Mental Health Block Grant. In the reauthorization of this legislation, a 5%–15% set-aside was created for data collection and research activities. The mental health share of this set-aside (which was agreed to be capped at 5%) amounted to about $20 million annually. In consultation with state representatives, NIMH developed a program for these funds that included activities such as development of SMHA data systems for both reporting and research purposes, funding of a national entity to work with the states on research and data collection, grants to the states for enhancing SMHA research capacity, and studies of high-priority areas such as substance abuse co-morbidity and children's mental health. Thus, the set-aside provided both funding support and encouragement of SMHA research endeavors.

Finally, NIMH undertook a range of activities to improve and expand its support of services research. These included convening advisory panels to develop a plan of research to improve care of individuals with serious mental illness and to enhance the NIMH National Reporting Program (sources of federal data on mental health care). Additionally, the Institute revised its approach to Community Support Program (CSP) demonstration grants, converting the program to a research demonstration project approach targeted specifically at SMHAs. The intersection of support for data system enhancement, CSP research, and SMHA research capacity enhancement clearly emphasized new possibilities for state agency research.

State Mental Health Research Priorities

These new possibilities have caused state agencies to reassess their interest in and ability to carry out such research efforts. Although many states are involved in research, the range of effort varies greatly. This is partly because the obstacles to SMHA research are substantial. Therefore, the level of state commitment and the relative priorities of the states are uncertain and variable.

As a way to catalyze state agency interest in services research and to promote dialogue among SMHA leaders and academic researchers, NIMH has sponsored several conferences to bring these groups together. In September, 1990, NIMH supported a "New England PAL conference," bringing together commissioners and/or their senior staff involved in research with academics having similar interests. At one level, the meeting provided an opportunity to discuss current research projects. At another, it occasioned a discussion of the "fit" between SMHA policy and research. A review of some of the critical issues discussed at the conferences provides some insight into these questions—at least for one region of the country.

Some context on the New England SMHAs is useful as background for this discussion. First, the New England states are relatively small and compact, with well-regarded mental health systems. In the recent national rankings of the states, four states ranked numbers 1–4 (i.e., Vermont, New Hampshire, Rhode Island, and Connecticut), whereas Maine was ranked 11th and Massachusetts 16th (Torrey, Erdman, Wolfe, & Flynn, 1990). New England states have moved aggressively to develop systems of community care, building on the community support concept. Additionally, the level of investment in mental health care is better than national norms. In 1990, the average New England state was spending $65 per capita on mental health care, although the national average was only $48 (Lutterman, Hollen, & Hogan, 1993). Thus, the New England mental health systems tend to be of manageable scale, relatively well funded, and have relatively coherent policy directions.

The New England SMHAs also tend to have well-developed relationships with higher education programs involved in mental health research. Higher education is also well developed in this region, and most of the states have long-standing collaborative SMHA–university research relationships. Thus, New England provides a favorable climate for considering mental health services research efforts.

A number of research projects discussed at the meeting reflected a model or prototypic approach to services research: SMHA and university researchers collaborating on well-designed studies of current clinical or policy problems. Topics included the use of clozapine (Bunney, 1990); comorbidity of substance abuse and mental illness (Fox, Drake, Teague, Noordsy, & Bartels, 1990); assessment of outcomes in a mobile demonstration program (Romeo, Detrick, McCarthy, Wagner, & Steipock, 1990); and research and strategic systems development (Hogan & Essock, 1990).

In addition, other generic problems discussed included challenges in blending research and service, the differing cultures of SMHAs and academia, and challenges for the future. A broad consensus about SMHA services research priorities emerged from discussions at this meeting. These priorities are suggested as a template for discussion of services research.

Sound SMHA Policy and Management as a Foundation

It appears to be no accident that services research appears to do better in states with well-developed service programs. Because such research engages in description and evaluation of programs and systems, it follows that a well-conceptualized and organized setting will be more conducive to research activity. It also seems logical that the potential problems associated with the instability and turbulence of SMHA environments may be ameliorated when sounder management structures and better designed systems are in place. This also implies that a degree of policy clarity and organizational integrity may be a prerequisite to initiating SMHA research. Put simply, long-term thinking may not be that productive when the ship of state is taking on water heavily.

Substantive SMHA–University Collaboration

Although a description of issues in state–university collaboration is beyond the scope of this chapter, they have been reviewed in other contexts (e.g., Bloom, 1989). However, one theme from the New England conference is that substantial and long-term public–university collaborations—particularly where policy goals are shared—create a setting in which shared services research activities are enhanced. An example illustrates this point.

In New Hampshire, the SMHA (Department of Health and Human Services) and Dartmouth Medical School collaborate in a variety of ways, including in the management of New Hampshire Hospital, the state psychiatric hospital. In the context of this relationship, the New Hampshire Psychiatric Research Center was established as a joint endeavor to conduct and stimulate services and clinical research activities. The project has a shared mission (which is inherent in the joint venture) and benefits from the presence of clinical and research resources. Given these factors, coupled with access to public policy issues and programs, a variety of well-designed and relevant services research projects have been initiated.

Policy-Relevant Issues at the Cutting Edge of Service Delivery

A final critical theme that emerged from discussion at the New England meeting is that SMHAs have the most to gain from services research that tackles urgent clinical and policy issues. These problems are vexing for states, require action based on limited knowledge, and are immediate. Although it may be thought that the orientation of research is of necessity more long-term and "academic," many of these problems would benefit from careful inquiry. Approaches to such problems that are thoughtfully designed are arguably more likely to work well than are hastily assembled, ad hoc solutions.

Thus, states at the New England meeting presented a range of challenging clinical and systems issues that were being addressed through well-structured studies. Such issues included how to introduce clozapine (a novel and expensive new treatment) in a system when demand far exceeds resources, how to assess the quality and impact of various case management strategies, and how to address the addiction problems that bedevil many people with serious mental illness.

Conclusion

This brief review of services research issues of concern to state mental health programs yields a number of conclusions about the importance of such efforts and the priorities of states. Although there are many apparent obstacles to supporting or conducting research in SMHAs, the states together support or conduct many services research projects—indeed more than those now supported by NIMH.

Clearly, research benefits from public–academic collaboration—the NIMH PAL for research initiatives is based on sound reasoning and experience. However, collaborative research into mental health services is most likely to be fruitful when the state agency has a well-defined policy mission and a reasonable degree of organizational stability and competence. Collaborative state–university research endeavors that are linked to policy goals are particularly likely to serve as a productive context for services research.

Finally, the New England experience suggests that current vexing problems in service delivery may be the highest priority for services research. Such approaches as rigorously evaluated pilot projects, exploratory studies, and experimental analysis of new treatment strategies can offer much for both clinicians and policymakers. If these approaches are utilized, research perspectives can help provide guidance to practical problems while adding to the knowledge base in mental health care.

References

Bloom, J. D. (Ed.). (1989). *State–university collaboration: The Oregon experience.* San Francisco: Jossey-Bass.

Bunney, S. B. (1990, September). *The clozapine story: Problems and promises.* Paper presented at the New England State Mental Health Services Research Conference, New Haven, CT.

Fox, T. S., Drake, R. E., Teague, G. B., Noordsy, D. L., & Bartels, S. J. (1990, September). *Dual diagnosis substance abuse and mental illness service systems and research.* Paper presented at the New England State Mental Health Services Research Conference, New Haven, CT.

Goldman, H. H., Lehman, A. F., Morrissey, J. P., Newman, S. J., Frank, R. G., & Steinwachs, D. M. (1990). Design for the national evaluation of the Robert Wood Johnson Foundation program on chronic mental illness. *Hospital and Community Psychiatry, 41,* 1217–1221. 1990.

Hogan, M. F., & Essock, S. (1990, September). *Research and strategic systems development: Conflict or complement?* Paper presented at the New England State Mental Health Services Research Conference, New Haven, CT.

Lutterman, T., Hollen, & Hogan, M. F. (1993). *Funding sources and expenditures of state mental health agencies: Revenue/expenditure study results, fiscal year 1990.* Alexandria, VA: National Association of State Mental Health Program Directors Research Institute.

Morrissey, J. P., & Goldman, H. H. (1984). Cycles of reform in the care of the chronically mentally ill. *Hospital and Community Psychiatry, 35,* 785–793.

National Association of State Mental Health Program Directors. (1988). *Study 87-597: Survey of state level research interests and capacity.* Alexandria, VA: Author.

National Association of State Mental Health Program Directors. (1990). *Study 89-629: Seniority of state mental health directors.* Alexandria, VA: Author.

National Institute of Mental Health. (1988). *Announcement: Public–academic liaison (PAL) for research on serious mental disorders.* Washington, DC: Author.

Romeo, T., Detrick, A., McCarthy, D. J., Wagner, R., & Steipock, V. (1990, September). *Assessing outcomes in Rhode Island's mobile treatment team demonstration program.* Paper presented at the New England state mental health services research conference, New Haven, CT.

Stein, L. I., & Test, M. A. (1980). Alternatives to mental hospital treatment. *Archives of General Psychiatry, 37,* 392–397.

Torrey, E. F., Erdman, K., Wolfe, S. M., & Flynn, L. M. (1990). *Care of the seriously mentally ill: A rating of state programs.* Washington, DC: Public Citizen Health Research Group/National Alliance for the Mentally Ill.

Witkin, M. J., Atay, J. E., Fell, A. S., & Manderscheid, R. W. (1987). Specialty mental health system characteristics. In R. W. Manderscheid & S. A. Barrett (Eds.), *Mental health, United States, 1987* (pp. 14–27). Washington, DC: U.S. Government Printing Office.

Wolf, J. (1990). Organization of state mental health systems. In C. G. Hudson & A. J. Cox (Eds.), *Dimensions of state mental health policy* (pp. 84–96) New York: Praeger.

Conclusion

CHAPTER

26

Current Progress and Future Directions

Paul Wohlford
Center for Mental Health Services

Hector F. Myers
University of California, Los Angeles

Joanne E. Callan
American Psychological Association

In early 1988, when we and our many colleagues began the series of conferences and books leading to the present volume, we were concerned primarily with improving clinical training for public mental health service. We still are. Through the processes described in chapters 1 through 6, however, we came to realize that, in order to significantly improve clinical training, the improvement of services for each of the underserved priority populations must be the first focus of the change process. The Linkages Conference recommendations summarized this by stating that quality clinical training should be driven by quality services (see Appendix A of this volume). We also reflected this recommendation by placing services before training in this book's title.

Improving public mental health services is a major national concern and challenge. The reform movement to address this is already underway—to move from hospital-based treatment services to community-based treatment/rehabilitation services—as described in chapters 7 through 12. The central theme of this book is that professionals in clinical training and public mental health services should network with each other and with consumers to form working, collaborative relationships and address these problems together. Chapter 13 presents a conceptual model for collaboration between the public mental health system and universities, and chapters 14 through 19 present several examples of how such collaboration is actually occurring.

The unique, important role of the consumer in this reform movement, which is discussed in chapter 12, is summarized later in this chapter in a discussion of the concept of consumer-assisted reform of mental health services and training. In order to facilitate reform of these complex interactive systems, both consumers and training programs must be involved.

If consumer-assisted reforms of mental health services and training are to succeed within the larger context of national health-care reform, they will have to be cost-effective. To ensure this efficiency, interventions must have a sound scientific basis in the latest research evidence showing which mental health services work and which do not work. Clinical training programs must continually stay up-to-date in order to conduct both pre-service and in-service training based on the best

The opinions expressed in this chapter are those of the authors and do not necessarily reflect the official policy or position of the American Psychological Association, the Center for Mental Health Services, or UCLA.

research evidence. Chapters 20 through 25 elaborate these points. Thus, an equally important component of the mission to improve clinical training is to incorporate the latest and most relevant clinical research and services research into the training. Therefore, improving clinical training, our initial objective, is an essential part of a whole dynamic process, portrayed in Figure 1 of chapter 20 and Figures 1 through 4 of this chapter, and also reflected in this book's title, *Serving the Seriously Mental Ill: Public–Academic Linkages in Services, Research, and Training.*

The central theme of this book is that, based on the consumers' need for quality public mental health services, a new or renewed initiative is needed to forge effective public–academic collaboration for improving psychological service, research, and training. This final chapter is organized in three parts related to this central theme. The first part covers the critical review and synthesis of key conceptual issues in public–academic linkages for clinical training, the second covers the review of current progress in support of this new initiative, and the third part covers future directions in professional training that make use of the preceding recommendations for projecting a new clinical training process model to address our country's mental health needs.

Key Conceptual Issues in Public–Academic Linkages for Clinical Training

Mental Health and National Health-Care Reform

Now paying about 40% of the total health costs, the public has a major stake in national health care. Its stake in mental health care is even greater, because it pays for about 60% of certain mental health costs (Hall, chapter 22, this volume). Unserved and underserved mentally ill people are likely to be among the 37 million Americans who now have no health insurance and among the millions more who have the type of health insurance that excludes or severely limits mental health services. Thus, their care often depends on public resources. Services for mentally ill people will continue to be a public responsibility for the foreseeable future, as discussed in chapter 7. For these and other reasons, mental health services will probably be included under the plan for national health-care reform.[1]

The most interesting question, therefore, becomes, How will quality mental health services be included in the national health-care reform plan? Criteria that have emerged from the preceding chapters regarding basic minimum provisions of mental health services are pertinent to this query.

Consumer needs. Mental health services must be responsive to various consumer needs, including those of recognized unserved and underserved groups such as seriously mentally ill adults, seriously disturbed children and adolescents, elderly and ethnic minorities with mental disorders, mentally ill individuals in rural areas, dually diagnosed individuals (with both mental and substance abuse disorders), homeless mentally ill individuals, mentally ill individuals in prisons, and others. Services will need to be tailored to meet the needs of each of these different groups, and services will need to be provided by adequately trained personnel.

Quality services. Consumers and family members must be involved in monitoring the quality and relevance of services at every level, including the scientific evidence on which the services are based. Community-based treatment and psychosocial rehabilitation approaches, as described in chapter 8 by Blanch, and in Appendix A by Leon, Callan, Johnson, Magrab, & Myers, are examples of services that are particularly responsive to consumers and their families.

Competent service providers and competent service systems. To ensure quality services for the various priority populations, there must be correspondingly differentiated groups of competent service providers (Sechrest & Scott, chapter 21) who are working in competent service systems (Manderscheid & Wohlford, chapter 20).

Science-based services. In order to provide efficient, cost-effective, quality services to ensure reasonable costs, providers should be trained to be clinically competent (Sechrest & Scott, chapter 21) in effective service delivery systems (Manderscheid & Wohlford, chapter 20), using methods

[1] Before this volume went to press, President Clinton appointed his wife, Hillary Rodham Clinton, to head the Task Force on National Health Care Reform, and Tipper Gore to head the Panel on Mental Health. Although the Task Force report had not yet been released to the public, a "White House Advisor confirms [the] commitment . . . [that President Clinton's] health-care plan [will] cover [the] cost of [treating] mental illness" (NAMI, 1993, p. 1).

that are based on the best research evidence (Friedman, chapter 24; Hogan, chapter 25). In order to be implemented effectively, the array of recommendations noted from recent conferences will require support at national, state, and local levels by the widest possible constituency including consumers, families, providers, administrators, and academics.

Ethnic minority psychologists. As discussed by Myers in chapter 5, by the year 2000 at least one third of our national population will consist of people of color. Regrettably, only 6–10% of psychology faculty, students, and service providers are of ethnic minority descent. A tremendous gap exists between the large number of ethnic minorities with mental disorders and the small number of mental health professionals who are members of ethnic minority groups (Wohlford, 1992). Hammond and Yung (1993) attribute the low utilization of outpatient mental health services by ethnic minorities at least in part to the lack of ethnic minority providers. This lack of providers is an obvious and important reason why ethnic minority populations are grossly underserved.

In spite of various special programs and conferences over the past several decades to address this deficit, the situation has not improved significantly. Piecemeal solutions have been inadequate to address the problem, even though many of them have been well designed and relevant to the special needs of ethnic minorities. A more comprehensive approach is required that recognizes that all parts of the educational system are interrelated. For example, although minority recruitment is contingent on having minority faculty as role models and effective scientist–professionals, one cannot recruit sufficient minority faculty because the educational pipeline has a limited supply of such talent.

Thus, a bold new approach is needed that recognizes the scope and interrelatedness of the problem. In order to increase the number of well-trained ethnic minority psychology service providers, one must simultaneously address recruitment of ethnic minorities into each level of the educational pipeline, including high school, undergraduate, graduate, postdoctoral, and faculty. One such new approach is outlined later in the section of this chapter called "Future Directions."

Major Structural Changes in Services and Training

Small incremental changes in mental health services and training have resulted in some truly excellent, state-of-the-art service systems and training programs responsive to public service needs. What is needed now are changes that would rapidly bring about many more service systems and training programs to address the critical needs within public mental health services. Not only is such change desirable from a social policy and humanitarian perspective, it is also necessary from an economic viewpoint. In order to include mental health in any national health-care reform without also creating overwhelming costs, concurrent structural reform in the delivery of mental health services and training will have to take place. In short, the current slow evolution of improved services and training must be replaced by a more revolutionary redesign of mental health service delivery and training.

Although the immediate imperative for revolutionizing mental health services and training comes largely in response to economic pressures, the relevance and effectiveness of future services, especially for underserved groups, will rely on the professional and institutional expertise that has been unutilized or underutilized, especially in the last decade.

Such a reform movement is likely to pose unique problems and challenges to academic training programs in professional psychology. Doctoral programs whose primary mission is to train professionals for service (e.g., the professional schools of psychology preparing for the PsyD and other programs that emphasize the application of psychological knowledge to service) and hospital or clinic-based internships are likely to find service-based clinical training to be congruent with their mission. However, university programs committed to training scholar–clinicians may find emphasis on service more difficult to incorporate. Such programs have as their primary mission the creation and dissemination of new knowledge, so their primary goal is the training of clinical scholars and scientists and not the training of service providers for the public sector. As Albee (1970) observed, the traditional interpretation of the scientist–practitioner model has tended to bifurcate science and practice into separate domains. Consequently, a major challenge to the reform movement's success is to reconcile such basic differences.

Fortunately, one way to achieve such reconciliation already exists. Improving the quality of clinical services requires the application of sound scientific methodology and principles both in the development and evaluation of clinical services for priority populations and in professional training. According to Hoshmond and Polkinghorne (1992), the training of professional psychologists requires a more complete integration of science and practice than is the case at present. They urge redefining the science–practice relationship by placing "emphasis on broadened choices of research methods, the development of reflective skills, and better linkage between teaching in the domains of research and practice" (p. 55). They argue that professional education should emphasize more action research, in which discovery and theory testing occur in the context of practice. This type of scientific activity "definitely requires collaboration among researchers, practitioners, and the public" (from Tyler, Pergament, and Gatz, 1983, in Hoshmond and Polkinghorne, 1992, p. 60).

In conclusion, science–practitioner training programs in psychology will play a requisite role in the public–academic linkage initiative, but only if faculty actively involve themselves in community-based service programs through research and evaluation. In the past, these components of public service programs have often been either absent or woefully inadequate. Because available research on priority populations—especially ethnic minorities and elderly with mental disorders, and dually diagnosed individuals—is so limited, substantial need exists for training more clinical scientists to conduct clinical research on the provision of appropriate services to these populations.

Current Progress in Support of Public–Academic Linkages for Clinical Training

Consumer-Assisted Reform of Mental Health Service and Training

As described by Frese in chapter 12, the consumer has the unique role in the reform of mental health services. The 1990 Linkages Conference summarized this in the recommendation that quality services should be consumer-driven. Since then, the need to clarify the emphasis on consumer-oriented services, to soften the rhetoric but retain the message, has become more apparent. For instance, Pallak (1990) has called for "client outcome orientation in research, program planning, and service delivery" (p. 1237). We have concluded that there should be consumer-assisted reform of mental health service and training.

Although the consumer movement in mental health is a rather recent phenomenon, it is quite complex. Primary consumers, who are former (or current) patients or clients, must be distinguished from secondary consumers who are the family members of the patients or clients. Since 1979, family members have been organized into the National Alliance for the Mentally Ill (NAMI), which has grown into a powerful national organization with state and local affiliates.

From its inception, NAMI has been dedicated to improving services, providing support and education to families, and to eradicating mental illness through research. During its first 12 years, NAMI had its greatest success in advocating for increased funding for research.

Starting in 1992, however, under the leadership of Dale L. Johnson as President of the Board of Directors, NAMI has placed increased emphasis on advocacy for improved services and improved clinical training of service providers. (Please see chapter 3 in this volume for other NAMI activities.) Since 1988, Victoria Conn has chaired the NAMI Committee on Curriculum and Training and has worked tirelessly to advocate for reform in all mental health professional educational programs, including psychology. Conn observes that family members (spouses, siblings, parents, and children) of seriously mentally ill people are themselves at risk for various disorders and "that psychologists are ideal professionals to intervene in these situations. Yet in most professional programs, psychologists are not trained to work in preventive ways with these populations" (V. Conn, personal communication, May 5, 1993). Lefley (1989) has reviewed the literature on family burdens, and Marsh (1992) calls understanding the phenomenological reality of these families' multitudinous stresses an essential parameter of professional practice. Yet, as Conn points out, training programs have largely ignored the service needs of family members, who have been largely left to fend for themselves.

In the mid-1980s, primary consumers, who are or have been seriously mentally ill adults, formed national organizations, including the National Mental Health Consumers Association, for which Frederick Frese, author of chapter 12, has served as president from 1992 to 1993; the National Alliance of Mental Patients; the National Depressive and Manic Depressive Association; Project Share, a self-help and advocacy resource exchange; and the National Association for Rights Protection and Advocacy.

Besides the above-noted consumer groups that focus mainly on seriously mentally ill adults, consumer groups for other priority populations deserve mention. Families of seriously emotionally disturbed children and adolescents have organized into the Federation of Families for Children's Mental Health. For mentally ill people in rural areas, there is the National Association for Rural Mental Health. The closest advocacy organization for the elderly with mental disorders is the American Association of Retired Persons. There is no comparable national advocacy or consumer organization for ethnic minorities with mental disorders.

If elderly, ethnic minority, and rural consumers and their advocates were to organize and demand special mental health service programs like the Community Support Program (CSP) for seriously mentally ill adults and the Child and Adolescent Service System Program (CASSP) for children, it would be easier to tailor clinical training programs that embody these principles.

The diversity of the consumer organizations reflects the diverse views held by consumers who only recently have begun to gain confidence as individual proponents and to organize themselves into formal groups that speak out publicly about their concerns. As Frese eloquently observes (chapter 12), he and other consumers had to overcome all too pervasive stigmas, including those expressed by professionals. Organizational development involving diverse participants has been neither quick nor easy. Some consumers are very angry and seek greater rights or retribution from institutions in which they feel they were abused. Regrettably, alleged abuses of patients in mental institutions have been real. This has been recognized by the creation of Center for Mental Health Services' (CMHS) Protection and Advocacy Program, which provided grant support to establish protection and advocacy offices in each state.

Other consumers, however, have no overwhelming grievances, and many of them are motivated to help their peers. Many such individuals seek to provide more meaningful services and various supportive approaches, including self-help groups. CMHS and state mental health authorities have actively assisted such consumer self-help groups. These efforts have recently blossomed to include consumer participation at high levels of state and federal policy-making panels.

Consumers have a critical role in all state mental health advisory groups that are mandated under the state mental health block grant provisions of PL 99-660 and PL 102-321. State mental health advisory committees, including consumers, must review all state mental health plans, as discussed in chapter 7 and Appendix C. Some states have fulfilled both the letter and the spirit of this requirement by having active networks of local advisory mental health committees, again with consumer participation, that inform the state advisory committees.

Elevating the role of the consumer to ensure a major voice and influence in improving the quality of services is also a feature of Total Quality Management (TQM), which includes:

- Quality—Providers must conform to standards of practice while also meeting the individual needs of mental health consumers.

- Recognition of consumers as customers.

- Empowerment—Only when as consumers gain a greater voice in, or control over, their treatment will they be able to take greater charge of their lives and responsibility for their behavior.

- Quality improvement teams—To develop competent providers, such teams must include trainers, providers, consumers, and family members (Rago & Reid, 1991).

In summary, one goal of TQM is continuous monitoring and evaluation of the treatment process with the consumers' view recognized as essential to the success of the process.

In addition to the obvious and fundamental roles of consumers in improving the quality of services, consumers have much potential to contribute to education and training programs (Frese, chapter 12, this volume). Perhaps the consumer's most important contribution is to help students to appreciate patients' underlying sensitivities and humanity, regardless of how psychotic they may be at any given moment (New York State Office of Mental Health, 1993). Consumers or former patients can be invaluable in helping professionals or professionals-in-training gain a better understanding of mental illness, recovery, and good clinical practice (Blanch, Fisher, Tucker, Walsh, & Chessman, 1993). A major goal of consumer-assisted reform of mental health services and training would be to have consumers participate in both service programs and training programs for undergraduate and graduate students.

How could this goal be achieved? For some years, Carling (1990) has welcomed consumers into his community psychology courses at the University of Vermont, not only as students, but also as instructors, as research assistants in a number of studies, and as key advisors in curriculum development. The Boston University Center for Psychiatric Rehabilitation also helps consumers attend college in a special supported-learning approach (Unger, Anthony, Sciarappa, & Rogers, 1991; Walsh, Sharac, Danley, & Unger, 1991). Also, professional training programs should reach out to consumers who have potential for assuming a training role.

Consumer-organized self-help groups may be one source of individuals who are interested in forging effective partnerships with mental health professionals. For example, in a survey of 104 self-help groups of former mental patients, Emerick (1990) found that the majority were moderately supportive groups in which partnerships with professionals could occur. Certainly, this seems to be a fertile area for applied psychological research to discover ways of effectively working with consumer groups and, in turn, developing a cadre of consumer trainers.

The small subset of consumers who are also mental health professionals may play a pivotal role in translating consumers' concerns to other mental health professionals and in assuming leadership in the consumer groups. Special training support for this objective, perhaps modeled after the CMHS/NIMH Minority Fellowship Program—a Consumer Fellowship Program—could greatly expand the number of consumer–professionals.

Impact of Federal Reorganization and Support

The 1992 Alcohol, Drug Abuse, and Mental Health Administration (ADAMHA) Reorganization law (PL 102-321) should have a positive impact on clinical training for several reasons. First, it reunites clinical training with the major mental health services organization, CMHS, which should facilitate conjoint programming of clinical training with CASSP, CSP, and homeless programs. Second, it places clinical training in the same division as the state block grant program with its provisions for state mental health planning. Providing well-trained personnel is a fundamental requirement for obtaining quality services. Third, it places clinical training and state human resource development (HRD) in the same administrative branch, which facilitates the integration of clinical training preservice programs with HRD in-service programs. Finally, it places clinical training within the same organization that is responsible for service data systems, facilitating possible improvement in training data systems.

Federal Support for Preparation of Clinical Providers

In the past two decades, public mental health administrators have complained, both in anecdotal and formal reports, that many professionals they hired were not prepared to perform necessary services in the public sector. This situation frequently required staff retraining or on-the-job training.

In 1981, Congress required that preservice clinical training programs focus on one or more underserved priority populations. Also, mental health trainees who received federal support were required to pay it back, in a period equal to their period of support, through service to the priority populations in public settings.

From 1980 to 1993, however, the NIMH/CMHS[2] mental health clinical training budget plummeted from about $70 million to $3 million. In this same period, the proportion of trainees supported by NIMH/CMHS correspondingly plummeted from about one fifth of the new mental health professional graduates to less than 2% of graduates between 1986 and 1992, and to less than 1% of graduates in 1993.

Ironically, these massive reductions in support came just at the time when clinical training programs in psychology and other disciplines were actually targeting the priority populations more effectively, when 93% of the graduates receiving support actually completed their payback service obligation, and when 80% of those who completed their payback service were remaining with either the public or private, nonprofit sector (CMHS, 1993a).

Federal Support for Clinical Training Programs Involved in Public–Academic Linkages

From 1988 to 1993, institutional training grants in psychology accounted for about 40% to 45% of the total grants for all disciplines. With intense competition, only 14% to 26% of the applications were funded, and those funded had to be judged either excellent or outstanding on all criteria. Since 1989, a program's demonstration of public–academic linkages has been elevated to be a primary review criterion. Usually, funded programs

[2] Since CMHS was created, it has had responsibility for mental health clinical training that previously was that of NIMH.

demonstrated active collaborations with one or more local public mental health facilities and provided documentation of support from the appropriate state mental health program (e.g., from the CASSP director for a seriously emotionally disturbed child program or from the CSP director for an adult program).

CMHS/NIMH has supported 65 psychology programs meeting these criteria during the period from 1988 to 1993. These programs are listed in Appendix D of this volume along with priority population(s), program type (general or minority student), program purpose (doctoral, internship, or postdoctoral), and whether the program was multidisciplinary. Most grants addressed the priority population of children with mental disorders, and the other grants are distributed across the other four priority populations. About half the grants supported ethnic minority professional training, and the other half supported general professional training. About half of the grants were awarded to doctoral programs and the other half to internships and postdoctoral programs.

Special Initiatives for Ethnic Minority Students

Given the poor record of training ethnic minority mental health professionals, CMHS/NIMH developed two special initiatives for supporting clinical training of ethnic minority students. One is a separate type of institutional grant for the professional mental health training of ethnic minority and disadvantaged students. This type of grant has trained hundreds of minority students in the past several years. It requires that a training program have an appropriate pool of minority students from which to draw, appropriate faculty, curriculum, and field experiences or practica that further the objectives of the ethnic minority training program.

The second special initiative is the Minority Fellowship Program (MFP) for clinical training. Since 1974, the American Psychological Association (APA) has been one of four mental health professional organizations that has been receiving support in the form of a special institutional training grant from CMHS/NIMH for the graduate study of minority students selected in national competition. These students may attend graduate programs anywhere in the country. In recent years, the APA/MFP program has supported 25–35 students per year.

Evaluation of Public–Academic Linkages for Clinical Training

As a goal, fostering effective public–academic linkages for services and training is fraught with many obstacles. To achieve this goal, formal means of evaluating training programs with regard to level of collaboration must be identified. Clearly, plans must note general criteria of quality, but other criteria such as those reflecting state and local needs must also be taken into account—for example, size (i.e., large state vs. small state), relative affluence (i.e., affluent state vs. poor state), geography (i.e., rural vs. urban state), and the population's percentages of ethnic minorities and age distribution in the population. Each of these factors is likely to influence the focus of service and training programs, as well as the relative ease or difficulty faced in trying to establish new collaborative service and training relationships.

New strategies must be used by training programs to overcome institutional and disciplinary barriers and to forge collaborative mental health service and training networks for the seriously mentally ill. As noted by Davis (chapter 13), efforts must ensure positive outcomes for all parties. Initiatives in North Carolina, Ohio, Cincinnati, Maryland, Vermont, and Colorado, as described in chapters 14 through 19, illustrate how these strategies can be implemented. In each case, training has been built on state-of-the-art services, that is, community-based treatment/rehabilitation, as contrasted with hospital-based treatment programs. Great care was taken to define and assign meaningful roles for all stakeholders, including consumers and their families, mental health administrators and providers, and academics and trainers. Recognition was given to the unique contributions of each mental health discipline in the context of collaborative multidisciplinary teams.

In each of the above programs, collaboration was initiated by interested and committed individuals from both the public and private sectors, although different structures were used among them to accomplish the goal. A specific structure (e.g., consortia for training, networks for service and training, etc.) depends on the unique characteristics of the groups, disciplines and institutions involved, stated goals and objectives, and available resources. Establishing specific collaborative arrangements for services and training is easier for some institutions and settings than for others. For example, collaborative service arrangements are easier to implement in communities with already established, even though loosely integrated, service networks. Similarly, collaborative training programs will be easier to implement in hospitals and community mental health facilities in which such teams already exist and are already part of the clinical experience.

Specific follow-up activities to the 1990 Linkages Conference have been generated as well. A month after the conference, Andrea Blanch, CSP Director in New York, invited all clinical training grantees in New York to participate in new state outpatient programs focusing on public–academic linkages for clinical training. Also, as presented in chapter 19, Carl Zimet and Courtenay Harding of the University of Colorado followed up on the conference by reaching out to several public mental health agencies in Denver to initiate a new postdoctoral program. The resulting consortium of several public agencies in Denver and the University of Colorado made plans to support four postdoctoral fellows for the year 1993–1994.

Finally, psychology may be able to learn something from psychiatry. In 1986, Talbott and Robinowitz presented 10 model programs of state–university collaboration, in which psychiatry departments collaborated with state mental health authorities. From 1989 to 1993, Pew Charitable Trusts supported the State/University Collaboration Project to develop and strengthen collaborative relationships between state mental health programs and university departments of psychiatry. The project's goal—to improve services to seriously mentally ill individuals—was designed to expand and improve psychiatric training, thereby strengthening recruitment and retention of psychiatrists in the public mental health sector. The project had three primary functions: First, a central project office at American Psychiatric Association coordinated other activities and served as an information clearinghouse; second, regional meetings brought together state and university representatives to inform each other about the project and to start or renew collaboration; and third, state–university teams in 41 states sought and received individual consultation from expert consultation teams. As a result of the project, there are at least 25 new training collaborations, 18 new service collaborations, and 11 new research collaborations. Ten formal collaborative agreements have been signed, and joint boards, faculty/staff meetings, and leadership meetings have been established at 14 sites (C. Robinowitz, personal communication, May 17, 1993). The creation of collaborative relationships has succeeded in directly influencing care to seriously mentally ill people by increasing the number of psychiatrists in the public sector. Early results of the project were presented in 12 articles on state–university collaboration in *Hospital and Community Psychiatry* (January, 1991). Proposals are being made to continue this project and to expand it to other disciplines, including psychology.

As stated earlier, the successes of the psychology programs presented in chapters 14–19 should be capitalized on and expanded systematically. The funding of an office at APA would certainly facilitate the implementation of many of the recommendations made by the Linkages Conference and presented in Appendix A.

Future Directions for Clinical Training

In order to plan policy directions in clinical training and human resource development, CMHS sponsored the National Conference, "Building a Competent Mental Health Workforce for the 21st Century," held in Washington, D.C., February 9–10, 1993. Conference participants included mental health providers, consumers, trainers in six mental health disciplines (psychology, psychiatry, psychiatric nursing, social work, marriage and family therapy, and counseling), students, and administrators at federal, state, and local levels. As recommended earlier (see Figure 4, chapter 1), this conference was, in many respects, a multidisciplinary version of the December 1990 Linkages Conference. Not surprisingly, the Linkages Conference recommendations are highly congruent with the main recommendation from the February 1993 conference, which is that

> the public mental health system and the academic community need to establish and maintain an interactive process to address pressing training needs.
> The two major systems in place to provide the education, training, and development of mental health care providers are the degree-granting academic institutions and the service delivery systems in hospitals and communities. These two complex worlds must establish and maintain collaborative working relationships so a continuous, numerically sufficient, and clinically competent workforce will be developed and sustained. (CMHS, 1993b, p. 6)

An Interactive Model of Mental Health Services, Research, and Training

As discussed in chapter 20, the mental health field has historically had the three primary functions

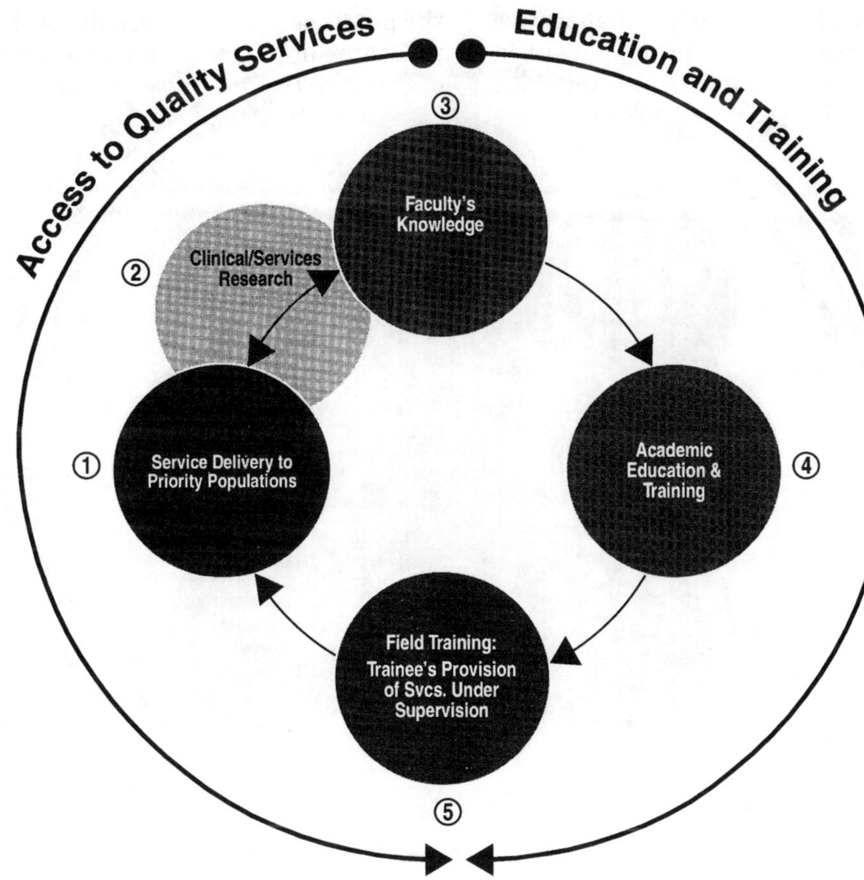

Figure 1. Interactive model to improve mental health services, research, and training: Basic functions.

of services, research, and training. These functions are basically interdependent in fundamentally important ways that generally are not recognized, even today. An interactive model describing these functions was introduced in chapter 20. The main purpose of the presentation of this model is to show the interdependence of the parts of the system and the necessity for cooperation between these parts in order to improve mental health services.

The interactive model: Basic functions. Ideally, the latest scientific advances in mental health research would be conveyed directly from the clinical researcher to the service provider, (e.g., in scholarly journals or professional meetings). More commonly, however, clinical research knowledge is translated and transferred to the service providers via clinical training programs, as discussed in chapter 20. A clinical training program with expert faculty usually serves as an intermediary between the clinical research scientist and the service provider, either in preservice training or in-service training. In Figure 1, the process begins with providing quality services to priority populations, then conveying clinical and service research knowledge to the faculty, who then share knowledge with students in academic education and training, and help students apply what they have learned by providing actual services to actual clients while under supervision in field training sites such as internships. After training is finished, the new provider goes on to practice as a credentialed professional for priority populations, thus completing the circle.

The interactive model: The general model. Recommendations from the Linkages Conference (Appendix A) were analyzed for each of the priority populations. This analysis helped identify several critical issues in clinical training that would enhance quality psychological services for each of the priority populations. Frequent recurrences of critical issues were then noted across the priority populations, making possible a general model that describes the clinical training process (see Figure 2).

The interactive model attempts to represent graphically several fundamental propositions that undergird the central thesis that quality clinical

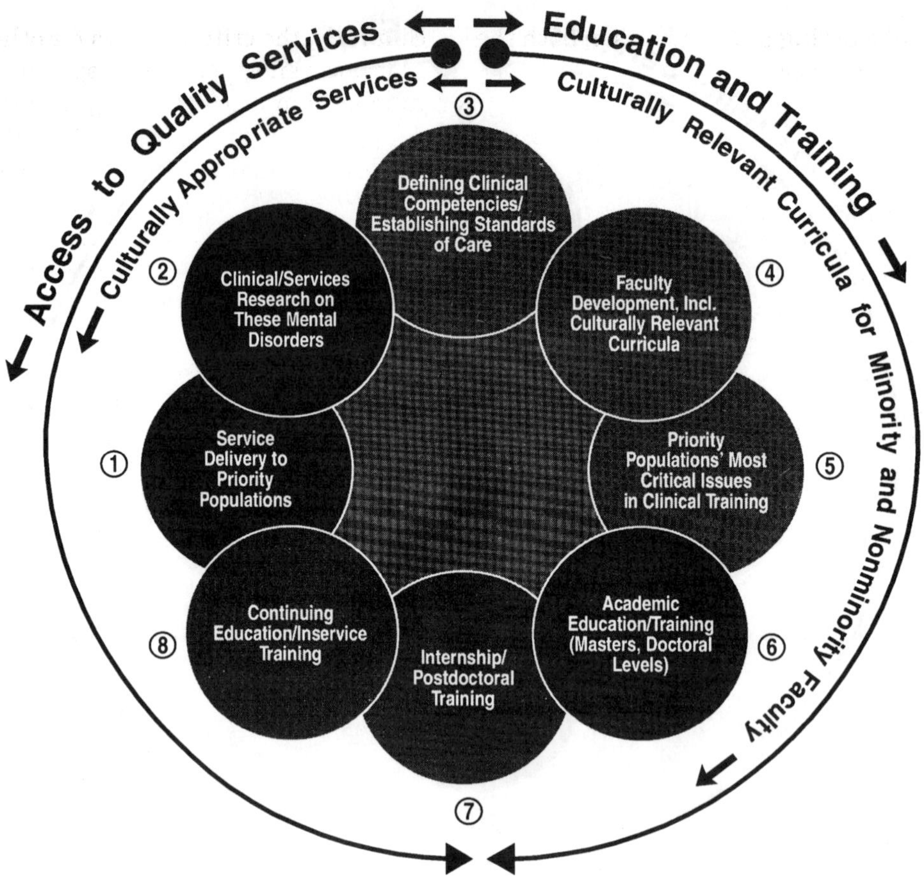

Figure 2. Interactive model to improve mental health services, research, and training: The general model.

training is services based and vice versa: Quality services plus education and training, although discriminable, form one continuous process, as represented by the large circle in Figure 2.

Clinical services, research, and training are intrinsically linked (as represented by the interlocking, numbered, small circles on the perimeter of the priority population circle):

1. Ideally, clinical training starts with quality services provided to the priority populations.

2. Clinical training programs are informed, again ideally, by the best and latest scientific research about what works and what does not work with a particular mental disorder.

3. Defining clinical competencies and establishing standards of care is of fundamental importance to the integration of all other processes. Clinical competencies may be derived from standards of care, and the education and training curricula may be derived from those clinical competencies. Also, defining clinical competencies is crucial for differentiating among several levels of services and training, namely, paraprofessional, associate, bachelors, masters, preinternship, postinternship, and postdoctoral. Note that, in Figure 2, competencies and standards occupy the key position between services and training.

4. Culturally appropriate services constitute one component of all quality services; similarly, culturally relevant curricula used by both minority and nonminority faculty constitute one component of all training programs. A critical issue for all priority populations is faculty development for culturally relevant curricula.

5. The priority population's most critical remaining issue is discussed below.

6. Academic education and training, at both the masters and the doctoral level for some priority populations, is at the heart of the training.

7. Internship and postdoctoral training is the central component that bridges academic training (on the right) and services (on the left).

8. Finally, continuing education and inservice training should be more systematically used to

upgrade skills of existing practitioners in both the private and public sectors.

The interactive model for specific priority populations. For seriously mentally ill adults (see Figure 3), the most critical issues include two areas specific to seriously mentally ill adults in slot number 5: psychopharmacology as a treatment modality of importance to seriously mentally ill adults, and all other priority populations, especially children, the elderly, and ethnic minorities; and psychosocial rehabilitation, behavioral and cognitive systems, consumer consultation, and family collaboration as they pertain to seriously mentally ill adults. For seriously mentally ill adults, three other cross-cutting issues are critical: the definition of clinical competencies and the establishment of standards of care; the development of faculty for culturally relevant curricula; and the availability of academic education and training, including masters and doctoral levels. Similarly, the critical issues for other priority populations reflect both the specific issues in slot number 5 and cross-cutting issues.

For each priority population, the emphasis of the model may be articulated somewhat differently but still follows the general model:

For children with serious emotional disturbances (see Figure 4), the most critical issues are refining training guidelines for children's psychological services and defining clinical competencies and establishing standards of care.

For ethnic minorities with disorders, the most critical issues include minority student recruitment and retention, faculty development for culturally relevant curricula, defining clinical competencies, and psychopharmacology.

For elderly with mental disorders, the four most critical issues are (a) the creation of an APA interdirectorate/public policy mechanism for the elderly, (b) services financing, (c) professional competencies and standards of care, and (d) funding for higher education.

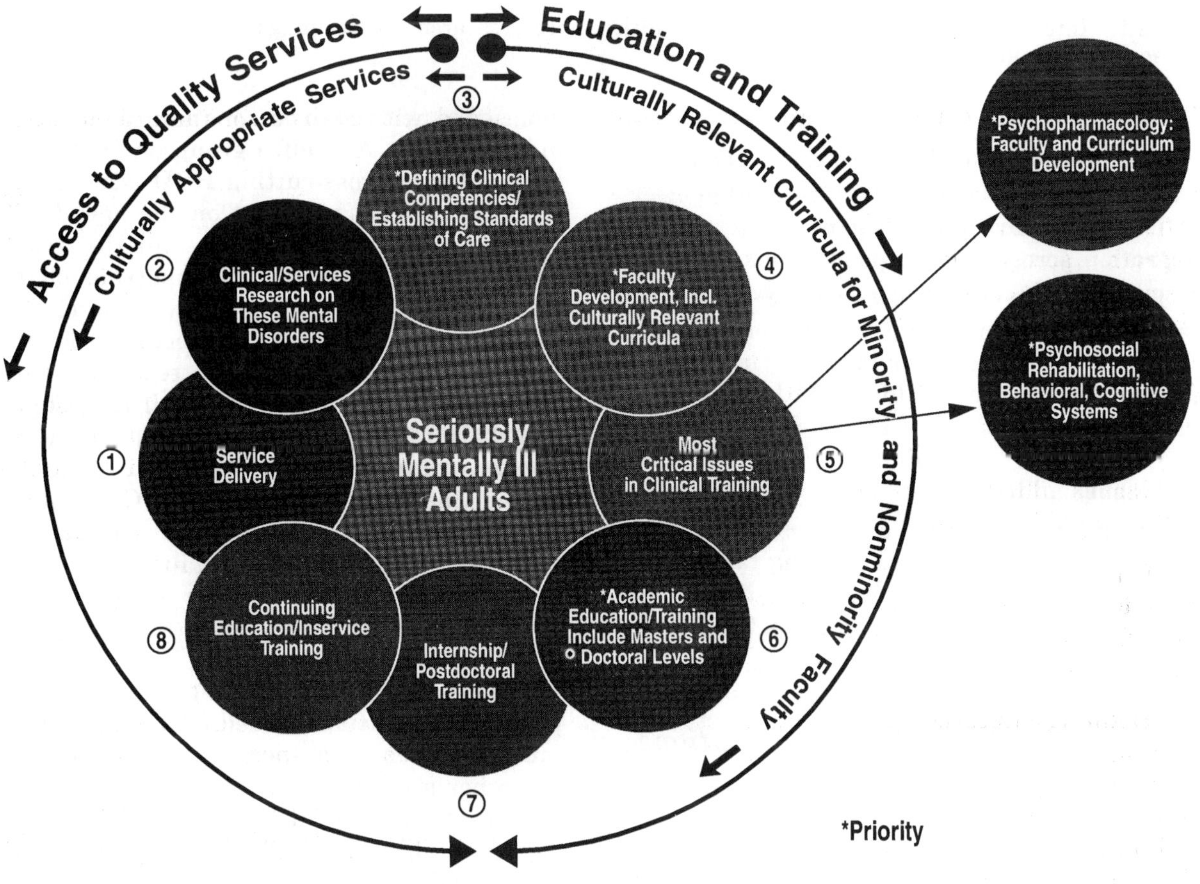

Figure 3. Interactive model to improve mental health services, research, and training for seriously mentally ill adults.

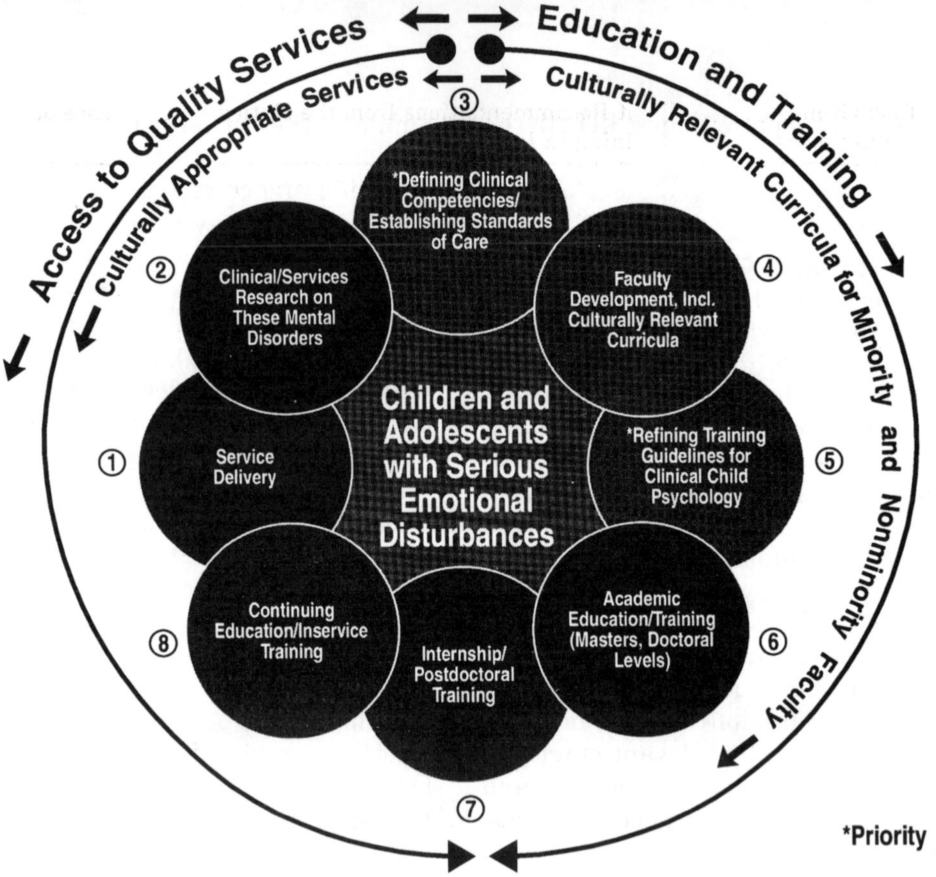

Figure 4. Interactive model to improve mental health services, research, and training for children and adolescents with serious emotional disturbances.

Features of the interactive model.

• The interactive model was inductively derived from the needs of each priority population.

• The interactive model is general and permits integration across priority populations.

• The interactive model can be a grid to see if a significant training or service component is adequately addressed. For instance, in planning the 1992 Conference on Elderly With Mental Disorders, it was possible to ask such questions as Are issues concerning minorities addressed? Are rural issues addressed?

• The interactive model can be used to plan for future activities, such as organizing task groups based on the critical issues just cited, to implement recommendations from the Linkages Conference.

Task Groups to Help Implement Linkages Conference Recommendations

In 1991–1992, informal task groups[3] were organized around the 11 priorities or critical issues mentioned, with chairpersons and 15–20 members in each group. A twelfth group on HRD was set up to address cross-cutting HRD issues and any other issues that were not on the agenda of the other task groups. Table 1 presents the structure, priority populations, and chairpersons of the 12 task groups. Each task group was matched with the most appropriate APA directorate for implementing those particular recommendations, which is also shown in Table 1. All 12 task groups had their initial meetings in at the APA Convention in Washington, DC, in August, 1992, and their second meetings at the APA Convention in Toronto, Ontario, Canada, in August, 1993. Reports of all 12 task groups, including its membership, specific purpose, progress at initial meeting, and plans for future activities were prepared and circulated to all members.

Table 1 also lists the task groups according to priority population served. Although six task groups addressed a specific priority population, the other six cut across all priority populations. In order to implement the recommendations efficiently, duplication of effort with current APA task forces was avoided where possible. For example, regarding the psychopharmacology task group, APA commissioned a Task Force on Psychophar-

[3] We chose the somewhat unusual term informal advisory task group to clarify that our activities were neither an official APA Task Force nor an official CMHS/NIMH Advisory Committee.

Table 1. CMHS Task Groups to Implement Recommendations from the National Conference on Public–Academic Linkages for Clinical Training in Psychology

Task group	Chairpersons
APA Education Directorate	
Defining Clinical Competencies and Establishing Standards of Care	Child[a]—Lenore Behar Adult[b]—Lee Sechrest Elderly[c]—Margaret Hastings
Seriously Mentally Ill	Adult—Robert Coursey Andrea Blanch Marianne Farkas Dale Johnson Harriet Lefley
Refining Clinical Training Guidelines for Children's Psychological Services	Child—Michael Roberts Robert Friedman
Masters Level Services and Training	All—Larry Alferink Arthur Horne
Comorbidity/Substance Abuse	All—Holly Hills Robert Zucker
Human Resources Development	All—Rodney Hammond Sara Sparrow
APA Practice Directorate	
Psychopharmacology Training	All—Antonio Puente Elsie Golu
Rural Services and Training	Rural[e]—Scotty Hargrove Ruben Echemendia
Older Adults With Mental Disorders	Elderly—Deborah King Linda Teri
APA Public Interest Directorate	
Faculty Development/Culturally Relevant Curriculum	Minority[d]—Hector Myers Bernadette Gray-Little
Minority Student Recruitment/ Retention	Minority—Richard Suinn Linda Berg-Cross
APA Science Directorate	
Clinical/Services Research	Child—Sandra Russ Adult—Timothy Kuehnel Elderly—M. Lawton Powell Minority—Samuel Turner

[a] Children with serious emotional disturbances;
[b] adults with serious mental illness;
[c] elderly with mental disorders;
[d] ethnic minorities with mental disorders
[e] individuals with mental disorders living in rural areas

macology in 1990. Because the agenda of the APA task force had already been established, we decided to dovetail our task group activities with those of the APA Task Force to make use of the latter's best efforts. This pattern parallels that for task groups on minority recruitment, masters level services and training, rural services and training, and clinical and services research.

Task group activities: Some examples. Several of the task groups have taken or are taking concrete action. The Task Group on Refining Clinical Training Guidelines for Children's Psychological Services, with the support of APA Division 12 (Section 1), Division 29, and the University of Kansas, held its second meeting (a writing conference) at the University of Kansas in May, 1993. Based on existing training guidelines for academic training, predoctoral internships, and postdoctoral training (Magrab & Wohlford, 1990), it consolidated and updated them based on community-based systems of care principles (see chapter 2).

The task groups on ethnic minority recruitment and on faculty development have proposed establishing an APA blue ribbon panel to set ethnic minority goals for the year 2000. This proposal was endorsed by the APA Committee on Ethnic Minority Affairs in March 1993 and will be forwarded through the APA governance process. As discussed earlier in this chapter, a fresh, bold approach is needed in order to significantly increase the number of ethnic minority professional psychologists. The proposal will set increased goals for ethnic minority recruitment for the year 2000 at all levels of the educational pipeline—high school, undergraduate, graduate, postdoctoral, and faculty—in order to significantly increase the number of ethnic minority professional psychologists. These goals, if reached, would significantly improve the current status quo. By setting specific goals that are publicly stated and well publicized, the chance of attaining these objectives will be enhanced.

The main recommendations from the task groups on rural services and training and Substance Abuse/Comorbidity are to hold national conferences on clinical training issues on these topics, because the important issues have not been previously addressed.

Both the task groups on clinical competencies and research divided into subgroups according to priority populations: seriously mentally ill adults, and so on. After meeting as subgroups, they plan to reconvene as a whole group to identify overarching issues. As a result of the creation of the APA Task Force on Standards for Psychological Interventions in August, 1993, the task group on clinical research will merge with the respective priority population task groups.

In summary, all 12 task groups have engaged critical issues that should be addressed if clinical training is to progress. Given the fiscal constraints and the programmatic need to make progress in all disciplines, it is likely that new initiatives will be multidisciplinary in approach. For example, if there is a national conference on rural services and training, it would be a multidisciplinary conference not limited to psychology. During their first meetings in 1992, most of the task groups seemed to be moving in the multidisciplinary direction.

Conclusion

In this book, a case is made for consumer-assisted reform of mental health services and training, in which clinical training is reorganized in order to pay more focused attention to the needs of priority populations of seriously mentally ill adults, seriously emotionally disturbed children, elderly and ethnic minorities with mental disorders, mentally ill in rural communities, and dually diagnosed. Because these populations are likely to be served in the public sector, providing services in public mental health settings should be incorporated into the preclinical and practicum training of psychological service professionals. Such integration can be most effectively accomplished through mutually beneficial collaboration between academic institutions and public sector agencies.

If mental health becomes a part of national health-care reform, the issues that have emerged from the preceding chapters in this book will be critical to the reform process. This would include the recognition of consumer needs, assurance of quality services, training of competent service providers and competent service systems, cost-effective quality of services that are science-based, and recognition and correction of shortages of ethnic minority providers. Special attention in the proposed service–research–training model should be given to the active participation of primary (patients) and secondary (family members) consumers in service delivery decisions and in the training of professionals. In addition, the premise that services provided should be based on the best available scientific evidence, and that service programs must demonstrate their effectiveness using sound scientific methods, is reaffirmed.

The editors and contributors to this volume hope that the ideas articulated herein will stimulate greater creativity and innovative thinking in the pursuit of effective treatment approaches to serving these targeted populations. We also hope to encourage a spirit of collaboration among the training and service institutions in mental health in order to ensure that new providers are adequately trained to meet the needs of their clients in the public mental health sector. We are hopeful that the new health care reform proposals will incorporate many of the principles and ideas presented in this volume, and in doing so, stimulate the fundamental structural changes in the mental health care services and training systems that have been long overdue.

References

Albee, G. W. (1970). The uncertain future of clinical psychology. *American Psychologist, 25,* 1071–1080.

Blanch, A., Fisher, D., Tucker, W., Walsh, D., & Chessman, J. (1993). Consumer–practitioners and psychiatrists share insights into recovery and coping. *Disability Studies Quarterly, 13,* 17–20.

Carling, P. J. (1990). Strategic attempts of a psychology department to promote community integration: The University of Vermont experience. In D. L. Johnson (Ed.), *Service needs of the seriously mentally ill: Training implications for psychology* (pp. 129–134). Washington, D.C.: American Psychological Association.

CMHS (1993a). *Report to the United States Congress: Evaluation of the mental health clinical training program payback requirement.* Rockville, MD: DHHS, CMHS.

CMHS (1993b). *Workforce training and development for mental health systems.* Rockville, MD: DHHS, CMHS.

Emerick, R. D. (1990). Self-help groups for former patients: Relations with mental health professionals. *Hospital and Community Psychiatry, 41,* 401–407.

Hammond, W. R., & Yung, B. (1993). Minority student recruitment and retention practices among schools of professional psychology: A national survey and analysis. *Professional Psychology: Research and Practice, 24,* 3–12.

Hoshmond, L. T., & Polkinghorne, D. E. (1992). Redefining the science–practice relationship and professional training. *American Psychologist, 47,* 55–66.

Lefley, H. P. (1989). Family burden and family stigma in major mental illness. *American Psychologist, 44,* 556–560.

Magrab, P. R., & Wohlford, P. (Eds.). (1990). Improving psychological services for children and adolescents with severe mental disorders: Clinical training in psychology. Washington, DC: American Psychological Association.

Marsh, D. T. (1992). Working with families of people with serious mental illness. In L. Vandecreek, S. Knapp, & T. L. Jackson (Eds.), *Innovations in clinical practice: A source book.* (Vol. 11, pp. 389–402). Sarasota, FL: Professional Resource Press.

NAMI (1993). Clinton health care plan to cover cost of mental illness. *NAMI Advocate, 14*(3), 1.

New York State Office of Mental Health (1993). *The role of psychology in the public mental health system: A two-day meeting of psychologists and mental health service recipients.* Albany, NY: Author.

Pallak, M. S. (1990). Community-based care for the mentally ill: Client outcome orientation in research, program planning, and service delivery. *American Psychologist, 45,* 1237.

Rago, W. V., & Reid, W. H. (1991). Total quality management strategies in mental health systems. *Journal of Mental Health Administration, 18,* 253–263.

Talbott, J. A., & Robinowitz, C. B. (Eds.). (1986). *Working together: State-university collaboration in mental health.* Washington, DC: American Psychiatric Press.

Tyler, F. B., Pergament, K. I., & Gatz, M. (1983). The resource collaborator: A model for interactions involving psychologists. *American Psychologist, 38,* 388–398.

Unger, K. V., Anthony, W. A., Sciarappa, K., & Rogers, E. S. (1991). A supported education program for young adults with long-term mental illness. *Hospital and Community Psychiatry, 42,* 838–842.

Walsh, D., Sharac, J., Danley, K. S., & Unger, K. (1991). The campus support project: An innovative supported education program model. *Innovations and Research: Clinical Services, Community Support, and Rehabilitation,* 1991, 1, 15–21.

Wohlford, P. (1992). Patterns of NIMH support of clinical training for ethnic minorities. *The Clinical Psychologist, 45,* 13–21.

Appendixes

APPENDIX

A

Policy Recommendations From the National Conference on Implementing Public–Academic Linkages for Clinical Training in Psychology

Executive Summary

Recommendations to Congress

Shortages of well-trained personnel are one of the major reasons why millions of seriously mentally ill Americans do not receive adequate services. A primary goal of clinical training in psychology is to improve the quality and quantity of psychology personnel who provide services for the Center for Mental Health Services (CMHS)[1]/National Institute of Mental Health (NIMH) underserved priority populations of seriously mentally ill adults and children, adolescents, elderly, ethnic minorities, and rural populations with mental disorders. CMHS/NIMH's present institutional clinical training programs addressing severe mental disorders and training ethnic minority students are excellent. Since the congressionally mandated payback was instituted in 1981, more than 5,400 trainees have completed their payback obligation in public mental health service.

However, the 20%–25% cuts in the funding of CMHS/NIMH training in 1987, 1989, and 1992 have undermined and destabilized clinical training efforts to improve clinical services for underserved priority populations. Therefore, every effort should be made to restore the fiscal year 1993 NIMH clinical training program at least to its 1986 level of $20 million in order to provide more adequate funding of the present institutional clinical training grants with payback to attract new professionals to careers in public mental health and to provide support for new initiatives for multidisciplinary clinical training to meet the mental health services objectives of the 1990s and beyond as recommended in recent conferences.

Additional Funding Needed for New Initiatives

1. CMHS/NIMH should support a new grant for public–academic linkages for clinical training that would support partnerships between university and state and community service system programs; state and community service personnel

This report was prepared by Gloria R. Leon, Joanne E. Callan, Dale L. Johnson, Phyllis R. Magrab, and Hector F. Myers.

[1] References originally made to the National Institute of Mental Health (NIMH) now apply to the new Center for Mental Health Services (CMHS), part of the Substance Abuse and Mental Health Services Administration (SAMHSA) which, after October 1, 1992, has responsibility for the mental health clinical training program under Public Law (PL) 102-321, the Alcohol, Drug Abuse, and Mental Health Administration (ADAMHA) Reorganization Act.

needs, as presented in the state mental health plan under PL 99-660, and obligations for trainees in preservice training, in-service training, and continuing education; and high-quality, research-based university mental health training programs.

2. CMHS/NIMH should take the lead to increase programs to develop ethnic minority faculty and students. The major obstacle is the unacceptably limited pool of ethnic minority student and faculty candidates. Thus, significant new program efforts, like the Minority Access to Research Careers program for research training, must be used to enlarge the pools of ethnic minority candidates at each level, from undergraduate students, graduate students, and postdoctoral trainees to faculty.

3. CMHS/NIMH should improve programs for faculty development with the stipulation that such new faculty development awards be more flexible than the present Individual Faculty Scholar Awards. Specifically, new faculty development grants should permit short-term and long-term training; they should be given as institutional training grants and should encourage exchange of academic faculty and state and local staff.

4. CMHS/NIMH should provide leadership by supporting new Regional Centers of Excellence for Clinical Services, Training, and Research as a major means of enhancing curriculum and faculty development. Focusing on one or more priority populations and enlisting state and local service agencies, these multidisciplinary centers should represent a true partnership between the public and academic sectors. Each center should have as its foundation excellent service delivery and clinical and services research components and should be a continuing education resource to other service providers in the community. The model is mental retardation's university-affiliated facilities.

5. CMHS/NIMH services and clinical research grants that are appropriate should have clinical training as a required component of significant scope; the training component would be a supplement and receive separate review.

6. CMHS/NIMH should systematically improve services and clinical training for the elderly, ethnic minorities, and rural populations with mental disorders, just as it now does for seriously mentally ill adults and children through the Community Support Program (CSP) and Children and Adolescent Service System Program (CASSP).

Recommendations to the CMHS/NIMH

The Conference's recommendations to CMHS/NIMH are in two parts: recommendations calling for increased funding, and recommendations that do not require significantly increased funding.

I. Recommendations calling for increased funding:

1. CMHS/NIMH should continue to expand the present institutional clinical training grant, which is severely underfunded at present, and

2. CMHS/NIMH should take the lead in support of six new initiatives for clinical training to meet the mental health services objectives of the 1990s and beyond, in the preceding recommendations to Congress.

II. Recommendations that do not require significantly increased funding. CMHS/NIMH should carry out the following eight clinical training initiatives within current levels of funding:

1. To strengthen public–academic linkages for clinical training, CMHS/NIMH should exercise a leadership role to bring together other federal agencies, state agencies, community organizations, and consumer and advocacy groups to improve services and clinical training for priority populations (i.e., seriously mentally ill adults and children, elderly, ethnic minorities, and rural populations with mental disorders). To do this, CMHS/NIMH should promote collaborative funding for clinical training from multiple sources: federal (e.g., CMHS/NIMH's CASSP, CSP, human resource development, clinical training, and research), state and local foundations and universities. CMHS/NIMH's role is to provide catalytic incentives for such broad-based funding.

2. CMHS/NIMH should recognize and reward those programs that have made noteworthy achievements in minority mental health training, producing substantial numbers of graduates, making substantial improvements in their curriculum, and/or developing model programs. One type of reward would be 5-year grants instead of 3-year grants.

3. CMHS/NIMH and the American Psychological Association (APA) should jointly sponsor a national conference on predoctoral internships and postdoctoral training focused on public–academic linkages for the CMHS/NIMH priority populations.

4. CMHS/NIMH should conduct a systematic study, like the congressionally mandated 1987 study of personnel for aging, to assess the numbers and kinds of trained mental health personnel, including but not limited to psychologists, needed to render quality services to those with serious mental disorders in the years 2000 and 2020.

5. It is extremely important for CMHS/NIMH to evaluate the impact and effectiveness of both current clinical training programs and the proposed clinical training initiatives on service delivery systems, client outcomes, and students and, especially, which models trained significant numbers of ethnic minority psychologists.

6. CMHS/NIMH should establish effective mechanisms for the sharing of information with all participants in the services–clinical training–research network, including, but not limited to, (a) publishing case examples describing a variety of successful public–academic linkages programs, and (b) supporting the participation of psychologists in multidisciplinary network of faculty, providers, consumers, and families.

7. CMHS/NIMH should vigorously support collaboration in interface areas among clinical training, services, and clinical and services research on priority populations by encouraging clinical training as part of all appropriate public–academic liaison research, clinical research, and services research grants and by encouraging clinical research as part of all appropriate clinical training grants (e.g., awarding supplements for dissertation research on priority populations).

8. CMHS/NIMH should reestablish standing committees to review clinical training grant applications. These committees should be multidisciplinary and expert to review applications for training to work with specific priority populations.

Recommendations to APA

The Conference's recommendations to APA are in four parts:

I. Recommendations for APA to advocate to Congress for increased funds for the present clinical training program and six new initiatives for clinical training in the preceding recommendations to Congress. This is the single most important recommendation for APA's action.

II. Recommendations for APA to advocate to CMHS/NIMH to carry out eight initiatives within the current level of funding for clinical training in the preceeding recommendations to CMHS/NIMH.

III. Recommendations for APA to carry out directly:

1. APA should promote, through an effective coalition of the Education, Practice, Public Interest, and Science Directorates, the clinical training goals regarding exposure, experience, and expertise for services to the priority populations of adults, children, elderly, ethnic minorities, and rural populations with serious mental disorders (see the Policy Recommendations that follow).

- APA, CMHS/NIMH, universities, internships and postdoctoral training institutions, state and local agencies, and consumers should collaborate to define and enhance the education and training experiences to better prepare students for working with priority populations. Task forces comprised of representatives from these groups should be developed to carry out these efforts.
- APA accreditation criteria for doctoral and internship programs should be responsive to the needs of the priority populations and, especially, their cultural diversity. The accreditation criteria should be reviewed by the above task forces, which should recommend changes as needed.

2. APA should increase efforts to recruit minority students for careers in psychology, including students in high school and college. APA, state, and university efforts must be increased and coordinated to provide enhanced funding; foundations should be approached for training grants.

3. APA should organize a national conference on predoctoral internships and postdoctoral training focused on public–academic linkages for the CMHS/NIMH priority populations.

4. The issue of masters-level training as an appropriate entry point for psychologists working in the public sector is complex; APA should organize a national conference to examine the ramifications of changing the entry level to accommodate the needs for greater service provision in the public sector.

5. APA should initiate evaluation research on the effectiveness of priority population-focused

doctoral, internship, and postdoctoral training on service delivery systems and client outcomes. It is important to include participation by federal, state, and professional groups.

6. APA should clarify the issue of practicing within the limits of one's training and experience and promote continuing education for both enhancing skills and reinforcing the ethical responsibility for practicing within one's area of competence. For example, one should not practice with children if one has not had adequate training and supervision in working with children nor should one practice with ethnic minorities if one has not had adequate training and supervision in working with ethnic minorities.

IV. Recommendations for APA to advocate to state and state-level agencies or organizations:

7. To provide better job opportunities in the public sector, APA and its Practice Directorate should (a) address concerns of psychologists employed within the public mental health system, including salary, benefits, career path, and status; and (b) lobby state legislatures to make them more aware of mental health service needs and to increase funding to meet these needs.

8. APA should exert national leadership to promote improved standards at the state and local levels:

- Continuing education requirements for state license renewal should provide incentives to meet the service needs of one or more of the priority populations. The aim is to upgrade the skills of professional staff in the public mental health system as well as those working in academic, community, and private practice settings.

- State and local agencies should support the retraining of current public sector psychologists who lack training in key areas related to priority populations. If these psychologists are now providing services to these populations, they should be supervised until they receive training.

Overview

Important themes of the National Conference on Implementing Public–Academic Linkages for Clinical Training in Psychology were (a) clinical training should be driven by service needs; (b) the academic and public sector professional communities should establish collaborative partnerships; and (c) all parties should recognize the important contributions that can be made by community, state, and federal personnel through their continued collaboration in the development and implementation of all phases of public–academic linkages. It is imperative that federal and state funding provide incentives to develop stronger and more effective linkages between academic training programs, internship and postdoctoral training programs, and service delivery facilities, to improve the quality of clinical training.

The Conference recommended that, in addition to the current priority populations targeted for improved psychological services and training, priorities should also include those with substance abuse problems (particularly the dually diagnosed with both mental disorders and substance abuse disorders), the families and children of those suffering from these difficulties,[2] as well as people suffering from acquired immunodeficiency syndrome (AIDS). Prevention was also an important concern.

Moreover, the whole mental health services–research–training system should be restructured because of significant gaps between science, clinical training, and clinical practice (i.e., the knowl-

[2] On the basis of NIMH's Epidemiologic Catchment Area (ECA) study, it is apparent that the single largest category of diagnosable behavior disorders is substance abuse and related disorders. It is also clear from a number of recent analyses of the ECA data set that comorbidity (i.e. dual diagnosis) is the rule rather than the exception for the more serious forms of mental disorder. It is vital to acknowledge the importance of dual diagnosis as a reality of serious behavioral disturbance, even though current administrative boundaries dictate that these problems are, to some degree, treated as if they were separate. From a policy standpoint as well as from an intervention perspective, it is important for the several institutes who have overlapping missions in this area to articulate more clearly ways they may help each other with clinical training, service delivery, and the implementation of public–academic linkages. It is vital that CMHS/NIMH, along with the Center for Substance Abuse Prevention and the Center for Substance Abuse Treatment (and perhaps also National Institute on Drug Abuse (NIDA) and National Institute on Alcoholism and Alcohol Abuse (NIAAA), insofar as these institutes are concerned with not just etiology but also the evaluation of service efficacy) move ahead in grappling with training issues pertaining to those with dual diagnosis and begin to plan a conference focusing on these issues. There are some important concerns in this area that are different from those regarding the singly diagnosed mentally ill. These include the general lack of awareness in the professional community of the knowledge base pertaining to substance abuse; the parallel lack of sophistication of substance abuse workers in diagnosing and treating the other diagnoses; comparative differences in standard levels of training in the substance abuse versus mental illness areas (i.e., the doctoral level is more common in the mental illness area), and so forth.

edge exists, but training programs are slow to teach it and professionals are even slower to use it because of outdated concepts and methods). This underlying set of systems problems should be addressed by translating the latest scientific knowledge about effective mental health services into current education and training curricula for use in the preservice training of new professionals and also for the continuing education of current professionals. The aim is to translate the latest scientific knowledge into practice. Part of this process would be to regularly update the description of priority populations.

In summary, the concept of "service-driven clinical training" recognizes that mental health services, research, and training are all parts of the same system (see chapters 20 and 26 for discussion of a model of services–research–training). The explicit intent of improving services and clinical training as a joint effort is to gain recognition that an effective systems intervention requires faculty to develop their knowledge, skills, and curricula to better educate the next generation of mental health practitioners.

Specific implementing strategies emanating from the four Conference work groups were generally complementary, with several groups focusing at times on somewhat different aspects of the same issue. There appeared to be significant consensus among the groups in recommending the collaboration principles and implementation strategies that follow below.

I. Services to Priority Populations

Principles

1. To ensure that clinical training is driven by services, there must be a continuous focus on enhancing the provision of public mental health services to priority populations by people from all levels of training: academic (masters, doctoral), predoctoral internship, postdoctoral training, continuing education, and faculty development. Public includes all levels of public or private nonprofit agencies (e.g., community mental health centers, state hospitals, state agencies, and federal agencies).

2. Service and training programs should be driven by consumers (i.e., they should be modified to make them more consumer-oriented). Service and training programs should provide choices for and empower consumers. Consumers should be assisted in acquiring self-advocacy and leadership skills.

3. Service and training programs should recognize the special needs of some populations (e.g., children, adolescents, the elderly, and families require special approaches); the common problem of people with dual diagnoses requires the augmentation of traditional approaches with those more relevant to this population's needs.

4. Service and training programs at all levels (e.g., faculty, students) should appreciate their probable need for general and specific consultation regarding ethnic group issues. Both service and training programs should move beyond mere "cultural awareness" to dealing with attitudes, norms, and behavior that promote genuine cultural competencies for providing services to relevant ethnic groups.

Implementation

CMHS/NIMH

1. CMHS/NIMH should continue to support clinical training for students with payback requirements to provide services to priority populations.

2. CMHS/NIMH should exercise a leadership role with other federal agencies to bring state agencies, community organizations, advocacy groups, and other relevant parties together to improve services and clinical training for the elderly and ethnic minorities with mental disorders, just as CMHS/NIMH does for seriously mentally ill adults and children through the CSP and CASSP programs. Also, CMHS/NIMH should take the initiative to address the critical interface issues among services, clinical training, and research for all priority populations.

3. CMHS/NIMH should establish an effective mechanism for the sharing of information with all participants in the services–clinical training–research network.

4. If additional funds were available, CMHS/NIMH should support Regional Centers of Excellence for Clinical Services, Training, and Research, described more fully in Section V, Curriculum Development.

5. If additional funds were available, CMHS/NIMH should provide seed money to faculty to establish and implement linkage activities for clinical training, services, and research.

6. If additional funds were available, CMHS/NIMH should create a Staff College or other training entity jointly sponsored by National Association of State Mental Health Program Directors (NASMHPD), National Alliance for the Mentally Ill (NAMI), and APA as well as other professional organizations and consumer organizations to update and train state commissioners, clinical directors, chief psychologists, and academic and internship faculty in the latest and most effective treatment models. The Staff College would employ psychologists and others with expertise in conceptualizing and developing treatment models and would present workshops to develop training materials and course outlines.

APA

1. APA should advocate more effectively with Congress to increase CMHS/NIMH clinical training funds to support the above new initiatives.

2. To provide better posttraining job opportunities in the public sector, APA, and especially the Practice Directorate, should (a) address concerns of psychologists employed within the public mental health system, including salary, benefits, career path, and status; and (b) lobby state legislatures to make them more aware of service provision needs and encourage legislators to increase funding to meet these needs.

States

1. State-level task forces with representatives from public service agencies and graduate programs as well as liaisons from CMHS/NIMH, APA, minority professional organizations, and state professional organizations should be organized to advocate for and develop more effective service provisions.

2. Salary levels of public sector psychologists need to be increased to induce more professionals to work in settings serving priority populations.

3. State agencies need to take a leadership role in meeting with state higher education departments to set a training direction that can be worked out in collaboration with university departments and community-based organizations.

4. State agencies should require that all relevant mental health staff, including psychologists, receive in-service training on the latest and soundest approaches for the priority populations, including psychosocial and community interventions and cultural competence regarding ethnic group issues. (See Staff College recommendation, CMHS/NIMH, no. 6, above.)

Universities[3]

1. Universities and public agencies at state and local levels should establish new joint appointments for psychologists by expanding and strengthening existing appointments, especially with respect to clinical and services research.

2. Universities should recruit students with specific interests in working with priority populations, including ethnic minority populations and those who have language skills for doing so. One way to conduct such student recruitment effectively is to intensively recruit existing service personnel who currently work with the priority populations.

Furthermore, all training programs should be encouraged to incorporate within their didactic and practica components opportunities for all students to confront their assumptions about diverse groups and to acquire insights about those assumptions. The objective for each student is to learn to work effectively with diverse groups, including developing a network of colleagues and resources for examining and, hopefully, resolving diversity-related issues.

II. Academic Issues

Principles

1. Psychology students/trainees who seek professional mental health service careers may reasonably expect to attain the following levels of competence in providing services to the priority

[3] The term *university* or *universities* in this document refers to institutions with masters or doctoral programs, both PhD and PsyD, whether located in universities or professional schools of psychology.

populations of seriously mentally ill adults; children and adolescents, elderly, and minorities with mental disorders; mentally ill individuals in rural areas; and the dually diagnosed.

- *Exposure.* All students who seek professional mental health service careers should have a minimum core foundation in knowledge and experiential contact with several, if not all of the six priority populations, as noted above.

- *Experience.* All students should receive additional knowledge and supervised experience to attain at least minimal competence to work with minorities and one or more other priority populations. In the case of minorities, for all students, minority content should be mainstreamed throughout all the courses and practica, including courses in psychopathology, evaluation, and intervention. In the case of the other priority populations, students may be expected to select one or more, according to their service and clinical research interests.

- *Expertise.* A limited number of students who plan to focus their careers on a priority population specialty should attain an *advanced level of competence* in clinical and administrative services and/or clinical research with this population. These students will do their dissertation research and postdoctoral training with this population.

2. Academic leadership should encourage collaborative partnerships with public mental health service agencies at the state and local levels and on multidisciplinary efforts in research and clinical training.

3. The issue of masters-level training as an appropriate entry point for psychologists working in the public sector is complex, with implications regarding quality of training in non-APA-accredited schools, licensure, supervisory relationships, and professional identity. APA, with CMHS/NIMH support and the participation of the Council of Applied Masters Programs in Psychology (CAMPP), the Council of University Directors of Clinical Psychology (CUDCP), the National Council of Schools of Professional Psychology (NCSPP), the Association of Psychology Internship Centers (APIC), NASMHPD, NAMI, and so forth, should fund a future conference to examine the ramifications of changing the entry level for the professional psychologist from the doctoral level (the APA position) to the masters level. Such a conference should describe appropriate roles masters-level psychologists may play in providing service to priority populations that doctoral psychologists will not fill in the foreseeable future.

4. Increased efforts should be made to recruit minority faculty and students. CMHS/NIMH and state and university funding sources must be increased and coordinated to provide enhanced funding to recruit and educate minority students so they can seek careers in psychology in the public sector. Because the major obstacle is the unacceptably limited pool of minority student and faculty candidates, significant new efforts must be made to enlarge the pools of minority candidates at each level, from undergraduate students to faculty.

Implementation

CMHS/NIMH

1. If additional funds were made available by Congress, CMHS/NIMH should support more programs with a strong training focus on the priority populations, which have the above-noted goals of exposure, experience, and expertise.

2. Current institutional clinical training grants and new initiatives recommended here must be enhanced by overcoming current barriers such as instability of funding, how resources are distributed, and "turf" issues. If annual funding by Congress were increased and stabilized, then the period of clinical training grants should be increased from 3 years to 5 years to enhance the programs' stability.

States

1. See the preceeding CMHS/NIMH recommendation no. 4.

APA

1. APA should more effectively advocate with Congress to increase CMHS/NIMH clinical training funds to support the above new initiatives. The funding cuts of 20%–25% in 1987, 1989, and 1992 have undermined and destabilized clinical training efforts to improve clinical services for underserved priority populations.

2. APA should promote, through an effective coalition of the Education, Practice, Public Interest, and Science Directorates, the above-stated goals regarding exposure, experience, and expertise in the priority populations.

Universities

1. Universities should have as a goal the development of curricular and training models that enable graduates to produce innovative service system designs for treatment and research on priority populations.

2. Both faculty and students of university child clinical and school psychology programs should participate in the CASSP program demonstration training and service delivery projects; faculty and students of clinical and counseling programs working with seriously mentally ill adults should participate with the CSP program and local NAMI chapters.

3. To increase student training in community settings serving seriously mentally ill adults and other priority populations, supervised clinical training in community facilities including those serving priority populations should occur at the preinternship level as part of the practicum placements to which students are assigned. These community placements are key components in developing the exposure-experience-expertise levels of competence in the priority populations made available as options to students. Faculty should work with public agencies (including private nonprofit) at the state and local levels to expand and strengthen these student options by actively engaging their own research, supervising students where desirable or necessary, and serving as informed services advocates for the state mental health plan under P.L. 102-321. There should be (a) increased assignments of preinternship practicum placements in such facilities supervised by licensed staff psychologists; (b) enhanced roles of community staff in university programs; (c) enhanced roles of university faculty in community settings, including direct supervision of practicum students where necessary or feasible; and (d) systematic development of clinical research opportunities in community settings.

4. University training should include an introduction to the theory, research, and practice of consumer advocacy and self-help as they pertain to these priority populations.

5. Universities should consider state employees and community paraprofessional workers as a potential pool of graduate students, with provisions and incentives for their continuing to work in state agencies after completing their academic training (discussed more fully under Section VII).

6. See the preceeding CMHS/NIMH recommendation no. 4.

III. Internship and Postdoctoral Issues

Principles

1. A critical interface between academic training and the public sector is the internship and postdoctoral training, most of which occurs in public or private nonprofit mental health service agencies.

2. The formal predoctoral internship should remain a 1-year requirement. However, a variety of postdoctoral fellowships should be developed for training focusing on priority populations: 1–2 years for clinical service and administrative training and 2–3 years for combined clinical service and research training.

3. Stronger linkages should be developed between university, internship, and postdoctoral facilities to ensure that this training focuses on the actual needs of priority populations, high-quality services, and continuity of training experiences for the students.

4. Internships in which children and adolescents receive services should develop a conceptual, holistic knowledge base that centers on families and their needs within the community context, as well as focuses on the needs of individual children.

Implementation

CMHS/NIMH

1. CMHS/NIMH should continue to fund internships and postdoctoral training, however, if more funds were available, CMHS/NIMH should support such programs more extensively and in collaboration with state agencies, as described else-

where. Stipends should be specifically targeted for work in the public sector, with a required payback.

2. A separate conference should be held, sponsored by CMHS/NIMH, APA, APIC, CUDCP, NCSPP, NAMI, and so forth to develop guidelines for predoctoral internships and postdoctoral fellowships focused on academic–public linkages, with mental health consumers, community-level agencies, and state agencies an integral part of this conference. The conference should seek to define and specify the content of internship and postdoctoral training and should define minimal standards needed to make these experiences more distinct and relevant to studying and serving the needs of priority populations.

3. It is extremely important to evaluate the impact and effectiveness of the above-recommended postdoctoral training procedures on service delivery systems, client outcomes, and students. This evaluation should be funded by CMHS/NIMH with the participation of APIC, APA, CUDCP, NCSPP, NASMHPD, NAMI, and consumer groups.

APA

1. APA should advocate more effectively with Congress to increase CMHS/NIMH clinical training funds to support the above new initiatives.

2. APA should review accreditation standards for internships in order to make changes to enhance the public–academic linkages initiative.

Internship Training Institutions

1. Internships should be encouraged to follow a consortium model that includes training in state and community facilities. Personnel from these agencies would then have more impact on training than they currently do, and students would have opportunities to work in a variety of settings under multidisciplinary supervision. Release time should be made available for state supervisors of those interns who may be in sites that do not have in-house licensed professionals. Public sector supervisors should be appointed as adjunct professors at the participating university and should also give lectures and serve on committees relevant to the trainee.

IV. Faculty Development

Principles

1. It is imperative to have faculty with specialization in the priority populations. Training and research funds are needed for generating and communicating knowledge about services to these populations.

Implementation

CMHS/NIMH

1. If additional funds were available, CMHS/NIMH and state agencies should provide new institutional grants for faculty development in each priority population, to enable academic and public sector personnel to enhance their expertise. Grants for sabbatical leaves, summer salaries, and part-time salaries to tenured and nontenured faculty for practicum and service as well as for research activities in the public sector are examples of such support. Stipends should also be established for faculty to take continuing education courses on public mental health issues and to support teaching by public sector professionals within universities. Grants should be multidisciplinary and should be part of Regional Centers of Excellence for Clinical Services, Training and Research discussed under V. Curriculum Development. These grants should include cost-sharing of stipends with other university or public agencies and mandatory payback.

APA

1. APA should advocate with Congress more effectively to increase CMHS/NIMH clinical training funds to support the above new initiatives.

2. See I. Services for Priority Populations, APA, principle no. 2.

Universities

1. Academic personnel may need training in collaborative skills to be effective consultants to public sector professionals. Faculty consciousness may have to be raised regarding public–academic linkages and serving priority populations through formal courses and applied experiences. A specific

means of raising faculty consciousness is given next.

2. Consultation and collaboration with family groups such as NAMI and consumer groups is important in developing faculty awareness about the specific issues of concern to people with mental illness and their families. This consultation is also important in planning the necessary training for faculty to provide appropriate services to the priority populations. The concept of pro bono work should be promoted.

3. Minority faculty should not be assigned all of the minority roles with regard to service and administration within their departments, as this is a hindrance to their retention, promotion, and tenure. Universities need to develop a reward system to encourage all faculty to pursue minority-relevant activities and should recognize the contribution of these activities to the educational mission in considering standards for promotion and tenure.

V. Curriculum Development

Principles

1. In psychology, faculty development and curriculum development must go hand in hand. Curriculum development follows faculty development or occurs at the same time but never occurs apart from faculty development. That is, the world's best curriculum would not be used if the responsible faculty are not ready to teach it.

2. Collaborative efforts need to be directed at developing innovative and high-quality curricula that will better address the needs of priority populations. These efforts must focus on the content of curricula as well as establishing new structures to develop, guide, and support continuing collaboration. (See I. Services to Priority Populations, CMHS/NIMH, no. 6.)

3. Course work, research, and practicum training for graduate students related to public sector activities should not be at the expense of increasing the time to attain the doctorate. All students should be exposed to some didactic, research, and applied work with priority populations. Curricular planning should focus on the development of a specialized public–academic linkage predoctoral track supported by stipends from various sources. Other course work and requirements should be adjusted accordingly to avoid delay in program completion.

4. A multidisciplinary curriculum is advantageous. University, community, and state agency personnel as well as consumers and families should be included in its development, as well as representatives from all mental health disciplines.

Implementation

CMHS/NIMH

1. If more funds were available, CMHS/NIMH should support Regional Centers of Excellence for Clinical Services, Training and Research as the major means of enhancing curriculum development and faculty development. Focusing on one or more priority populations, these centers can represent a true partnership between the public and academic sectors with possible labor exchanges between the two for the establishment of joint summer institutes, course development, teaching, and supervision of clinical services, preventive services, and research. Attention can be provided to public policy issues and the development of leadership skills, and support can be given for research consistent with the primary objectives of the center, ultimately including evaluation research. Each center should have as its foundation an excellent service delivery component and an excellent clinical and services research component and should be a resource to other service providers in the community.

2. CMHS/NIMH should publish case examples describing a variety of successful public–academic linkage programs with a range of populations from across the country.

APA and State Licensing Boards

1. APA should advocate more effectively with Congress to increase CMHS/NIMH clinical training funds to support the above new initiatives.

2. APA accreditation criteria should reflect attention to curricular content responsive to the above needs, as should state licensing examinations in their test items and skills evaluation.

Universities

1. Universities, state agencies, community agencies, consumer groups, and professional organizations should work together to define and enhance the content of predoctoral courses and practicum experiences to better prepare students for working with the seriously mentally ill and other underserved populations. Task forces comprised of representatives from these groups should be developed to carry out this work.

2. The core curriculum should include the basic content as well as an expanded focus on community support systems, social networks, primary prevention, advocacy, psychosocial rehabilitation models and techniques, psychoeducational approaches with patients and families, culturally responsive services, and case management. Attention to appropriate sequencing of classes prior to internships with priority populations should be encouraged.

3. Practicum training should also occur in nontraditional training environments such as nursing homes, homeless shelters, criminal justice systems, and work settings.

4. Personal sensitivity regarding issues such as cultural diversity and mental illness needs to be made an integral part of training for both faculty and students. This goal can be achieved in part through exposure to consumers and their families and through participant group methods, such as role reversal and so forth.

VI. Research

Principles

1. Collaborative research between universities and state and local public agencies should be increased to build a greater knowledge base regarding priority populations and to ensure a greater involvement of universities with the public system.

Implementation

CMHS/NIMH

1. CMHS/NIMH should fund collaborative and public–academic liaison research on priority populations, particularly research that is applied, innovative, and outcome oriented. These grants should include support for the development of faculty and public sector staff and student stipends. The emphasis is on collaboration with federal support providing incentive for state and local agencies to work in concert with the universities for services and clinical research.

2. CMHS/NIMH should provide incentive grants for collaborative research among university, community, and state personnel on priority populations with job sharing relevant to each party's interests. Job sharing could involve university and state personnel or university and community personnel, each being paid for time spent working in the others' facility. The specific financial arrangements would be arranged by the particular institutions.

3. All appropriate CMHS/NIMH services and clinical research grants should have clinical training as a required component of significant scope. If additional funds were available, the clinical training component could be a supplement to the research grants.

4. CMHS/NIMH announcements for clinical training in psychology should include special incentives for research with priority populations (e.g., supplemental awards for dissertation research related to the priority populations).

APA

1. APA should advocate with Congress more effectively to increase CMHS/NIMH clinical training funds to support the above new initiatives.

VII. Continuing Education and In-Service Training

Principles

1. University, state, and community personnel should be involved jointly in education and training activities for faculty, students, and psychologists in public settings at all levels: community, state, and federal (including the Veterans Administration, the Indian Health Service, etc.). These joint training activities will have an additional benefit by providing role models for students, ulti-

mately enhancing the recruitment of students to work in the public sector.

2. Grants should be funded jointly to academic and public sector facilities, so all can have an equal opportunity for input in the distribution of funds.

3. Specialty areas of training should be addressed through continuing education in addition to predoctoral or postdoctoral programs.

4. Consumer empowerment in continuing education and in-service training should be fostered through attention to the agendas of consumer groups. Following the agriculture-extension model at land-grant universities, the needs of consumer groups should be one of the forces driving the education and training of mental health professionals.

Implementation

CMHS/NIMH and Other Federal Agencies

1. CMHS/NIMH, other federal agencies, and states should co-fund training grants for continuing education and in-service activities as well as pre- and postdoctoral training. State higher education departments, university faculty, and service providers can work together to develop the content for training.

2. For in-service training and continuing education, CMHS/NIMH should also support short-term (a few weeks) intensive training courses, such as summer institutes, that use actual work in excellent programs as the training model.

APA

1. APA should work with other national organizations such as NASMHPD and minority mental health professional organizations to approach foundations for educational training grants.

2. See Executive Summary, Recommendations for APA to carry out directly, no. 6.

States

1. State license renewal should be contingent on meeting continuing education requirements focused on the needs of one or more of the priority populations. This requirement will upgrade the skills of professional staff in the public mental health system as well as those working in academic, community, and private practice settings.

2. State agencies should support the retraining of current public sector psychologists who lack training in key areas related to priority populations. If these psychologists are now providing services to these populations, they should be supervised until they receive training.

Bibliography

Callan, J. E., Johnson, D. L., Leon, G. R., Magrab, P. R., & Myers, H. F. (1990, December). *Improving clinical training in psychology: Consolidated recommendations from conferences on seriously mentally ill adults: Children and adolescents, elderly, and ethnic minorities with mental disorders.* Paper presented at the National Conference on Implementing Public–Academic Linkages for Clinical Training in Psychology, Georgetown University Child Development Center, Washington, DC.

Johnson, D. L. (Ed.). (1990). *Service needs of the seriously mentally ill: Training implications for psychology.* Washington, DC: American Psychological Association.

Knight, B. G., Teri, L., Santos, J. F., & Wohlford, P. (Eds.). (1993). *Applying geropsychology to services for older adults: Implications for training and practice.* Unpublished manuscript.

Magrab, P. R., & Wohlford, P. (Eds.). (1990). *Improving psychological services for children and adolescents with severe mental disorders: Clinical training in psychology.* Washington, DC: American Psychological Association.

Myers, H. F., Wohlford, P., Guzman, L. P., Echemendia, R. J. (Eds.). (1991). *Ethnic minority perspectives on clinical training and services in psychology.* Washington, DC: American Psychological Association.

Santos, J. F., & VandenBos, G. R. (1982). *Psychology and the older adult: Challenges for training in the 1980s.* Washington, DC: American Psychological Association.

Zarit, J. M., Zarit, S. H., Frazer, D. W., Hartman-Stein, P., Knight, R., & Teri, L. (1990). Training in Clinical Geropsychology: Report of the Division 20 Education Subcommittee on Clinical Practice and Training. *Adult Development and Aging News, 18,* 3–6.

APPENDIX

B

National Conference on Implementing Public–Academic Linkages for Clinical Training in Psychology: Participants List

Norman Abeles, PhD
Director of Clinical Training
Department of Psychology
129 Psychology Research Bldg.
Michigan State University
East Lansing, MI 48824

Robert E. Anderson, PhD
S. Dakota Division of Alcohol & Drug Abuse
Kneip Building
700 Governors Drive
Pierre, SD 57501-2291

Bernard S. Arons, MD
Director, Center for Mental Health Services
5600 Fishers Lane, Rom 15-105
Rockville, MD 20857

Ralph Barocas, PhD
Director of Clinical Training
Professor of Psychology
Department of Psychology
George Mason University
Fairfax, VA 22030

Cynthia G. Baum, PhD
Assistant Executive Director, Education Directorate
American Psychological Association
750 First Street, NE
Washington, DC 20002-4242

Lenore Behar, PhD
Special Assistant for Child & Family Services
Division of Mental Health/Mental Retardation
Room #523, Alberemorle Bldg.
325 N. Salisbury Street
Raleigh, NC 27603

Linda Berg-Cross, PhD
Director, Clinical Psychology Program
Psychology Department
Howard University
Washington, DC 20059

Andrea Blanch, PhD
Director of Community Support Programs
New York State Office of Mental Health
44 Holland Avenue
Albany, NY 12229

Bruce Bongar, PhD
Professor of Psychology
Department of Clinical Psychology
Pacific Graduate School of Psychology
431 Burgess Drive
Menlo Park, CA 94025

Stuart Broad, JD
Division Administrator, Human Resource Development Division
National Association of State Mental Health Program Directors
1101 King Street, Suite 160
Alexandria, VA 22314

Mary Rose Brogan, PhD
Director of Psychological Services
Connecticut Valley Hospital
P.O. Box 351
Eastern Drive
Middletown, CT 06457

John Burchard, PhD
Professor of Psychology
Psychology Department
University of Vermont
177 Killarney Drive
Burlington, VT 05401

Carol Bush, PhD
Chief, Nursing Education Program
Center for Mental Health Services
Rockwall II, Room 501
5600 Fishers Lane
Rockville, MD 20857

Mardi Carter, PhD
Director, Division of Human Resources
Department of Mental Health
1101 Robert E. Lee Building
239 North Lamar Street
Jackson, MS 39201

Jean Lau Chin, EdD
Executive Director
South Cove Community Health Center
885 Washington Street
Boston, MA 02111

Sandra Christenson, PhD
Assistant Professor of Psychology
University of Minnesota
School Psychology Program
N-548 Elliott Hall, 75 E. River Road
Minneapolis, MN 55455

Anna Marie Ciofarri, PhD
Director of Higher Education Initiative
Center for Community Change
Trinity College
208 Colchester Avenue
Burlington, VT 05401

Lemuel Clark, MD
Chief, Human Resources Planning
and Development Branch
Center for Mental Health Services
Rockwall II, Room 501
5600 Fishers Lane
Rockville, MD 20857

Rod Copeland, PhD
Director, Division of Mental Health
Department of Mental Health & Mental Retardation
103 South Main Street
Waterbury, VT 05676

Robert D. Coursey, PhD
Associate Professor of Psychology
Department of Psychology
University of Maryland
College Park, MD 20742

Jan L. Culbertson, PhD
Associate Professor of Pediatrics
Director of Child Neuropsychology
University of Oklahoma Health Sciences Center
Child Study Center, 1100 N.E. 13th Street
Oklahoma City, OK 73117

Dorynne Czechowica, MD
Associate Director for Medical
and Professional Affairs
National Institute on Drug Abuse Room 10-A-12
5600 Fishers Lane
Rockville, MD 20857

King E. Davis, PhD
Commissioner
Department of Mental Health, Mental Retardation
and Substance Abuse Services
P.O. Box 1797
Richmond, VA 23214

Peg Dawson, PhD
President, National Association
of School Psychologists
1 Marshall Road
Brentwood, NH 03044

Barry Edelstein, PhD
Chair and Professor of Psychology
Department of Psychology
West Virginia University
Morgantown, WV 26506-6040

Anita Ellis, PhD
Superintendent
Blue Hill Hospital
51 Coventry Street
Hanford, CT 06106

Raymond D. Fowler, PhD
Chief Executive Officer
American Psychological Association
750 First Street, NE
Washington, DC 20002-4242

Frederick J. Frese, PhD
Director of Psychology
Western Reserve Psychiatric Hospital
1756 Sagamore Rd.
Northfield, OH 44067

Bruce R. Fretz, PhD
Professor of Psychology
Department of Psychology
University of Maryland
College Park, MD 20742

Robert M. Friedman, PhD
Professor and Chair
Florida Mental Health Institute
University of South Florida
13301 Bruce B. Boulevard
Tampa, FL 33612

Barbara J. Friesen, PhD
Director, Research & Training Center on
Family Support & Children's Mental Health
Regional Research Institute
Portland State University, P.O. Box 751
Portland, OR 97207-0751

Ellen Gerrity, PhD
National Institute of Mental Health
5600 Fishers Lane, Room 18C25
Rockville, MD 20857

Elsie Go Lu, PhD
Deputy Director
Los Angeles County
Department of Mental Health
505 S. Virgil Avenue
Los Angeles, CA 90020

Bernadette Gray-Little, PhD
Chair and Professor of Clinical Psychology
Department of Psychology
University of North Carolina
Davie Hall, CB #3270
Chapel Hill, NC 27599

L. Philip Guzman, PhD
Executive Director
Child Guidance Center of Greater Bridgeport
1081 Iranistan Avenue
Bridgeport, CT 06604

W. Rodney Hammond, PhD
Assistant Dean
Wright State University
School of Professional Psychology
110 Health Sciences Building
Dayton, OH 45435

Jerome H. Hanley, PhD
Director, Division of Children,
Adolescents, & Their Families
S. Carolina Department of Mental Health
P.O. Box 485, 2414 Bull St., # 304
Columbia, SC 29202

David S. Hargrove, PhD
Chair and Professor of Psychology
Department of Psychology
301 Peabody Hall
University of Mississippi
University, MS 38677

Robert P. Hawkins, PhD
Professor of Psychology
Coordinator of Child Clinical Training
Department of Psychology
West Virginia University
Morgantown, WV 26506-6040

David T. Hellkamp, PhD
Professor of Psychology
Department of Psychology
Xavier University
Cincinnati, OH 45207

Simon Holliday
Chief, DC Health Planning
and Development
1660 L Street, NW
Washington, DC 20036

Dale L. Johnson, PhD
Professor of Psychology
Department of Psychology
University of Houston
Houston, TX 77204-5341

Margaret Johnson, MA
Consultant
Child Development Center
Georgetown University
2233 Wisconsin Avenue, NW, Suite 215
Washington, DC 20007

James Jones, PhD
Director, Affirmative Action &
Minority Fellowship Programs
American Psychological Association
750 First Street, NE
Washington, DC 20002-4242

Ellen B. Kagen, MSW
Washington Business Group on Health
777 North Capitol Street, Suite 800
Washington, DC 20002

Thomas J. Kenny, PhD
Professor & Director of Pediatric Psychology
University of Maryland School of Medicine
W. P. Carter Center
630 West Fayette Street
Baltimore, MD 21201

Christopher Keys, PhD
Director of Clinical Training
Department of Psychology
University of Illinois at Chicago
Box 4348
Chicago, IL 60680

Darrell G. Kirch, MD
Acting Deputy Director
Division of Clinical Treatment & Research
National Institute of Mental Health, Room 18-C-26
5600 Fishers Lane
Rockville, MD 20857

Eric Kohatsu
(student representative)
6700 Belcrest Road, #1126
Hyattsville, MD 20782

Jessica L. Kohout, PhD
Director, Office of Demographics,
Employment, and Educational Research
American Psychological Association
750 First Street, NE
Washington, DC 20002-4242

Nadine M. Lambert, EdD
Professor of Education
School of Education
University of California
Berkeley, CA 94720

Harriet P. Lefley, PhD
Professor of Psychiatry
Department of Psychiatry, D-29
University of Miami, School of Medicine
P.O. Box 016960
Miami, FL 33101

Gloria Leon, PhD
Professor of Psychology
Department of Psychology
University of Minnesota
Elliott Hall, 75 E. River Rd.
Minneapolis, MN 55455

Rebecca Levine
Personnel Coordinator
Department of Surgery
Georgetown University
3800 Reservoir Road, NW
Washington, DC 20007

Maury Lieberman, MSW
Division of Program Development,
Special Populations and Projects
Center for Mental Health Services
5600 Fishers Lane, Room 7-C-02
Rockville, MD 20857

Lewis P. Lipsitt, PhD
Professor of Psychology & Medical Science
Department of Psychology
Brown University
Providence, RI 02912

Raymond P. Lorion, PhD
Professor & Director
Clinical/Community Psychology
Department of Psychology
University of Maryland
College Park, MD 20742

Helene Lycaki, PhD
Director of Psychology & Psychology
Internship Training
Lafayette Clinic
951 East Lafayette
Detroit, MI 48207

Gary Macbeth, MSW
Director, Child & Adolescent Mental Health Service
Virginia Department of Mental Health, Mental
Retardation & Substance Abuse Services
P.O. Box 1797
Richmond, VA 23214

Phyllis R. Magrab, PhD
Director, Child Development Center and
Child and Adolescent Service System Program
Technical Assistance Center
Georgetown University
3800 Reservoir Road, NW
Washington, DC 20007

Ronald W. Manderscheid, PhD
Acting Director, Division of
State & Community Systems Development
Center for Mental Health Services
Rockwall II, Room 501
5600 Fishers Lane
Rockville, MD 20857

Elizabeth McCauley, PhD
Professor of Psychiatry & Behavioral Science
University of Washington
Children's Hospital & Medical Center
P.O. Box C-5371
Seattle, WA 98105

Jahi-Anabwile McCurtis
Division of Addiction Services
Indiana Department of Mental Health
117 East Washington Street
Indianapolis, IN 46204

Susan Moses
Staff Writer, *Monitor*
American Psychological Association
750 First Street, NE
Washington, DC 20002-4242

Hector F. Myers, PhD
Professor of Psychology
Department of Psychology
UCLA
405 Hilgard Avenue
Los Angeles, CA 90024

Paul D. Nelson, PhD
Deputy Executive, Education Directorate
American Psychological Association
750 First Street, NE
Washington, DC 20002-4242

Patricia O'Connor, PhD
Professor of Psychology
Department of Psychology
Russell Sage College
Troy, NY 12180

Donald R. Peterson, PhD
Professor of Psychology
School of Professional Psychology
Busch Campus, Rutgers University
P.O. Box 819
Piscataway, NJ 08855-0819

Sheila A. Pires
Human Service Collaborative
2262 Hall Place, NW
Suite 204
Washington, DC 20007

Ruth R. Pitlick
Director
State/University Collaboration Project
American Psychiatric Association
1400 K Street, NW
Washington, DC 20005

Lisa Porche-Burke, PhD
Provost
California School of Professional Psychology
1000 South Fremont
Alhambra, CA 91803-1360

Jean C. Ramage, PhD
Dean
College of Education & Psychology
James Madison University
Harrisonburg, VA 22807

Juanita Yvonne Reaves, PhD
Chief, Planning and Evaluation Division
Center for Mental Health Services/SE
Campus—Behavioral Studies Bldg.
2700 Martin Luther King Jr. Ave., SE
Washington, DC 20032

Jill N. Reich, PhD
Professor and Chairman
Department of Psychology
Loyola University
6525 North Sheridan Road
Chicago, IL 60626

Todd R. Risley, PhD
Director, Division of Mental Health & Developmental Disabilities
State of Alaska
P.O. Box H-04
Juneau, AK 99811

Michael C. Roberts, PhD
Professor of Psychology
Department of Psychology
University of Kansas
Lawrence, KS 66045

Sandra W. Russ, PhD
Assistant Provost
Professor of Psychology
Case Western Reserve University
Cleveland, OH 44106

Susan Salasin, PhD
Division of Program Development, Special Populations and Projects
Center for Mental Health Services
5600 Fishers Lane, Room 7-C-02
Rockville, MD 20857

Stanley R. Schneider, PhD
Associate Director, Research Training & Development
Division of Neuroscience & Behavioral Sciences
National Institute of Mental Health
5600 Fishers Lane
Rockville, MD 20857

Harry Schnibbe
Executive Director
National Association of State Mental Health Program Directors
1101 King Street, Suite 160
Alexandria, VA 22314

Lee Sechrest, PhD
Professor of Psychology
Department of Psychology
312 Psychology Building
University of Arizona
Tucson, AZ 85721

Steven L. Seitz
Public Health Analyst
Center for Substance Abuse Prevention,
Substance Abuse & Mental Health Services Administration, Rockwall II
5600 Fishers Lane
Rockville, MD 20857

Milton F. Shore, PhD
1370 Lamberton Drive
Silver Spring, MD 20902

Mary Lynn Skutley
Manager, Editorial Development
APA Books
American Psychological Association
750 First Street, NE
Washington, DC 20002-4242

Douglas K. Snyder, PhD
Professor of Clinical Psychology
Department of Psychology
Texas A & M University
College Station, TX 77843-4235

Andrea Solarz, PhD
Assistant Director, Science Policy
Public Policy Office
American Psychological Association
750 First Street, NE
Washington, DC 20002-4242

Sara S. Sparrow, PhD
Professor of Psychology
Yale Child Study Center
230 South Frontage Road
P.O. Box 3333
New Haven, CT 06510

Tony Speier, PhD
Director of Community Services
Department of Health & Hospitals
Division of Mental Health
P.O. Box 4049, Bin #12
Baton Rouge, LA 70821

Charles Spielberger, PhD
Professor of Psychology
Department of Psychology
University of South Florida
Tampa, FL 33620

James Stockdill, LLD
Deputy Director
Department of Health & Mental Hygiene
201 West Preston Street
Baltimore, MD 21201

Martha Storandt, PhD
Professor of Psychology
Department of Psychology
Washington University
St. Louis, MO 63130

Carole Stovall, PhD
(student representative)
2950 Van Ness Street, NW
#615
Washington, DC 20008

James P. Stratoudakis, PhD
Director, Office of Mental Health Services
Fairfax–Falls Church Community Services Board
3340 Woodburn Road
Annandale, VA 22003

George Stricker, PhD
Professor of Psychology
The Derner Institute
Adelphi University
Garden City, NY 11530

Kenley R. Wade, MM
Administrator & Children and Adolescent Service Systems Program Project Director
Bureau of Child & Adolescent Services
Department of Mental Health/Developmental Disabilities
401 Stratton Building
Springfield, IL 62706

Stanley E. Weinstein, PhD
Workforce Management Specialist
Department of Health & Mental Hygiene
Mental Hygiene Administration-4th Floor
201 West Preston Street
Baltimore, MD 21201-2399

Richard Weise, MA
Research Psychologist
Mood Anxiety & Personality Disorders Research Branch
National Institute of Mental Health, Room 10-C-24
5600 Fishers Lane
Rockville, MD 20857

Bryant L. Welch, JD, PhD
Consultant & Senior Advisor
Practice/Administration
American Psychological Association
750 First Street, NE
Washington, DC 20002-4242

R. Douglas Whitman, PhD
Professor & Director of Clinical Training
Department of Psychology
Wayne State University
71 W. Warren Avenue
Detroit, MI 48202

Rosemary A. Wilson, PhD
Director of Psychology Education
Spring Grove Hospital
Wade Avenue
Catonsville, MD 21228

Paul Wohlford, PhD
Chief, Psychology Education Program
Center for Mental Health Services
Rockwall II, Room 501
5600 Fishers Lane
Rockville, MD 20857

Betty Yung, PhD
Grant Specialist
School of Professional Psychology
110 Health Sciences Building
Dayton, OH 45435

Carl N. Zimet, PhD
Professor of Clinical Psychology
Director, Division of Clinical Psychology
University of Colorado Health Sciences Center
Box C-256, 4300 East 9th Avenue
Denver, CO 80262

Robert A. Zucker, PhD
Professor & Co-Director of Clinical Training
Department of Psychology
Michigan State University
East Lansing, MI 48824-1117

APPENDIX

C

State Mental Health Planning

Mental health planning has re-emerged as a priority under the law titled the State Comprehensive Mental Health Plan Act of 1986, Public Law 99-660 (PL 99-660). This law required states to plan and implement a comprehensive community-based system of care for seriously mentally ill individuals as a condition for receiving alcohol, drug abuse, and mental health block grant funds.

PL 99-660 has been an expression of the values of those who would advocate for the increasing delivery of mental health services to the seriously mentally ill outside of institutions, and against the structures of present state mental health systems that have been mainly institutionally oriented, PL 99-660 argued for a community support oriented systems reform and redesign with the attendant reallocation and addition of new resources.

In brief, the original legislation required the achievement of a total case management system by 1992. There was also a request for the states to set other service delivery targets that were to be achieved. In 1990, Congress strengthened the state planning law, through the amendment PL 101-639, which has required an additional separate plan for child and adolescent services with formal service requirements. The 1992 law on mental health, PL 102-321, which has subsumed the preceding laws on state mental health planning and specifically made the State Mental Health Block Grant, totaling $278 million in 1993, partly contingent on meeting the state planning requirements.

Stratoudakis, Tomes, Wohlford, and Stockdill in chapter 7 of this volume describe the context of PL 99-660's potential for building linkages for the training of psychologists as part of the mental health service delivery workforce. The issue of needing trained personnel to meet service goals in the state mental health plans is discussed in a particularly relevant document sponsored by the National Institute of Mental Health (NIMH) and titled "Planning for the Mental Health Workforce Under Public Law 99-660: A Manual for Planners to Provide Community-Based Services for Persons with Serious Mental Illness."[1]

Executive Summary

The first annual report to Congress, as required by the Mental Health Amendments of 1990 (PL 101-639), which amended PL 99-660, reported Fiscal Year 1990 activities. It was prepared in 1991 and released by DHHS in 1992. It is based on an analysis of three reviews of state submissions by panels of outside experts and NIMH officials. This report describes NIMH activity related to PL 99-660; reviews the status of the implementation of the mental health plans by the states (following the criteria established by the Act); describes the extent of participation of the State planning councils; describes coordinated services for children and adults; assesses the extent to which State and local public and private resources have been

This appendix is based on excerpts from *Fiscal Year 1990 Report to Congress on Activities Under PL 99-660, Title V: State and State Comprehensive Mental Health Services Plan Act of 1986* U.S. Department of Health and Human Services, Public Health Services, Alcohol, Drug Abuse, and Mental Health Administration (ADAMHA), National Institute of Mental Health (NIMH), February, 1992. It also presents excerpts from the 1992 law (PL 102-321) that has subsumed the earlier state planning requirements as part of the state block grant provisions for mental health services. Thanks to Maury Lieberman who contributed to the prefatory paragraphs.

[1] Published by the Western Interstate Commission for Higher Education, Boulder, CO, April, 1990.

utilized; and discusses quantitative measures of improvement of services provided under the plan.

Overview

The planning process moved States toward the provision of community-based services for the severely mentally ill. The process responded to the differences among States; some States devised a way to plan while others moved to an explicit blueprint for action. No State was completely static; no State has failed to move in some respect.

NIMH provided guidance and support to states and organized and conducted a plan review process. Guidance and support have taken two forms: 1) disbursement of planning funds to each state for 2 years to aid in the development of plans; and 2) provision of technical assistance through reports and manuals, advisory mechanisms and conferences. The plan review process involved three separate reviews of state submissions.

Development and implementation of comprehensive mental health plans for community-based services for the severely mentally ill occurred in states with dramatically different structural, population and policy realities. State plans and implementation progress reflect that diversity, and states responded to the planning requirements of PL 99-660 in distinctive ways, as described below.

Requirements Under PL 99-660

A. An organized community-based system of care for the severely mentally ill: States were expected to define their ideal future system, analyze the current situation, design change strategies, and organize and carry out a planning process. State responses to this requirement were unique and varied. Some states had already engaged in planning; others had already committed themselves to a community-based system. Still others confronted these issues for the first time.

B. Quantitative targets to be achieved in implementing such a system: States were required to define the populations to be served (both adults and children), provide a rationale for those definitions, estimate numbers in particular categories, explain service needs, set quantitative targets and devise tracking and management information systems. State variation in response to this requirement reflected both the technical complexity of these issues as well as the diversity of experience among the states.

C. Services to be provided to the severely mentally ill that would enable them to gain access to mental health services: States were asked to identify the services provided to enable individuals to gain access and to describe services available and accessible to protect client rights. For many States, this requirement prompted attention to a consumer and family orientation.

D. Provide rehabilitation services, employment services, housing services, medical and dental care, and other support services to allow the severely mentally ill to function outside of inpatient institutions: States were required to show evidence of the involvement of other State agencies in the planning process and the potential of funding for these services. While some States could describe their existing relationships with other service providers within the State, others were required to foster new relationships with service providers at both the state and local levels. Developing these relationships proved to be challenging.

E. Activities that reduce the rate of hospitalization: States proposed and are in the process of implementing activities to reduce and measure the rate of hospitalization. . . .Some states encountered difficulties.

F. Case management services: States described their case management philosophies and approaches and defined the roles and functions of the case managers. They were expected to indicate efforts to tailor services tc different populations within the state. Various models of case management were used by different States. . . . The scope of eligibility for case management services also varied. States faced staffing issues (particularly caseload size) and problems of interagency collaborations (especially between community mental health centers and hospitals).

G. Programs of outreach and services to the severely mentally ill who are homeless: States were asked to describe the location of the homeless mentally ill populations, their service needs, and to devise outreach activities and methods of ensuring accessibility to services. It was challenging for many States to assess the severity of the problem, understand its dimensions, and locate the major populations.

H. Consultation with representatives of employees of State institutions and nursing homes: States were expected to describe mechanisms that they used to obtain input from employees of state institutions and long term care facilities. States used a variety of methods.

Other Plan Requirements (Under PL 101-639)

A. The extent of participation of the state mental health planning councils: Many States already had formal advisory groups in place when the planning process began, either because of past Federal activity or because of prior State activity. [This requirement] necessitated some shifting of membership and focus in those States; other jurisdictions put advisory mechanisms into place for the first time.

B. Coordinated services for children and adults conducted under the plans: Coordination for purposes of P.L. 99-660 involves relationships between various State agencies, between State and Federal agencies, between State and local agencies, and between public and private entities. The emphasis in many States on the development of the case manager is evidence of the importance given to this issue; the case manager is often the participant within the system with the ability to link fragmented services together. Many States face special problems involving coordinated services for children. A number of States built coordinated activity around grants received through the Child and Adolescent Service Systems Project (CASSP) and the Community Support Program (CSP).

C. Utilization of state and local public and private resources in the enhancement and delivery of designated services: Despite tight budgets and major fiscal limitations, funds for community-based services are increasing in many States due to reallocation of funds from hospital budgets to community facilities and some increase in legislative support for these initiatives. Medicaid funds have been crucial financing mechanisms in many states.

D. Quantitative measurement of the improvement in services projected and achieved under the plan: Although States are moving toward the ability to develop quantitative measures of improvement in services, few States have been able to develop information systems that define services and specify indicators of performance measures that would allow for them to develop such measures.

Conclusion

The implementation of PL 99-660 has taken place within a context characterized by variable conditions, resources, and experiences within the states. However, despite the differences, a number of common elements can be discerned. This summary section of the report analyzes the context as well as the achievements and shared problems among the states. It also discusses the issues faced by both the states and NIMH for the future.

A. The Context of Implementation

The development and implementation of comprehensive mental health plans for community-based services for the severely mentally ill has occurred in States with dramatically different structural, population and policy realities. For some States, the implementation involved activities centered around the State capitol; for others, close relationships with strong county or other local jurisdictions were required. Some States could build their planning and implementation efforts on programs and relationships that were already in place. These involved previous hospital rate reductions; relationships with CMHCS; attention to court orders or consent decrees; use of Federal programs; State mandated planning efforts; and State statutory definitions of populations and programs. For other States, however, the Federal mandates served as the first time response to these issues.

States also varied in the attributes of the populations that are to be served. Demographic patterns of age distribution, cultural and racial diversity as well as rural–urban variances created different realities for states.

Other contextual attributes contributed to this variability. Some States had a tradition of active consumer, family member, and advocacy activity. Others did not. Some State mental health agencies were organized as free-standing autonomous bureaucracies; others were located within the confines of broader departmental structures. And during the past few years, some States have experienced more severe economic downturns than others.

Given these characteristics, it is not surprising that the implementation of PL 99-660 took different forms around the U.S. NIMH's activities within this program were devised to respond to this diversity. While focusing on the common themes for compliance, the technical assistance efforts sponsored by NIMH were developed to assist states to work on these issues within the context of their own realities. The three review processes that were undertaken not only had a compliance review function but also emphasized the need for feedback to the States on their progress. Within the bounds of limited staff and dependence on review of documents, the State variability and needs were respected.

B. Achievements

Despite the variety around the U.S., when viewed as a national program, certain common patterns were found in the development and implementation of the State efforts. There are a number of common positive elements:

1. The planning process that was put in place around the country was able to move States along the path to the provision of community-based services for the severely mentally ill. The process had the ability to respond to the differences among States; some States devised a plan to plan while others were able to move to an explicit blueprint for action. No State . . . has failed to move in some respect.

2. The creation of the State planning councils provided the structure for a mechanism that could be used in the future . . . [for] involvement of key stakeholders.

3. The involvement of consumers in a variety of roles within the system was emphasized. Consumer representation on the council was important to empowerment as was consumer participation in various service delivery mechanisms.

4. The planning process set a system of incentives in motion to create linkages between State mental health agencies, other State human service agencies, local level providers and governments, and the private sector.

5. There was increased attention to the role of the case manager within the service delivery system, sometimes as a centerpiece for [a variety of] system changes.

6. Despite real fiscal problems in many States, the process provided a way for States to think about packaging and reallocating existing fiscal resources.

7. States were able to use limited resources to develop model programs or demonstrations of new methods to provide services.

8. Overall, States indicated an ability to move toward decentralization in their service delivery systems . . . to CMHCs as well as local governments or regional units of State agencies.

C. Problems

At the same time, States also shared some common problems as they moved to implement PL 99-660:

1. Most States found it difficult to develop linkages between hospital-based programs and community-based systems.

2. The problems of children and adolescents have not been addressed by many States.

3. States are apprehensive about the budget situation . . . with limited or declining State and Federal resources.

4. Data issues plagued many States: definitional problems, collection obstacles, or utilization obstacles.

5. Efforts to focus on client outcomes were less than successful . . . both because of the data system questions as well as for service systems to focus on input and process issues.

6. Human resource development problems were common. Existing staff often had limited specialized training or experience with the severely mentally ill. Staff shortages were common, particularly to deal with special populations.

7. Interagency relationships were extremely difficult to develop. Competing priorities, reward systems and bureaucratic locations worked against close linkages.

8. State agencies were concerned about the lack of control they would have in the determination of service quality and character when decentralization occurred.

D. State-Anticipated Problems for Complete Implementation

States anticipate a variety of problems in the achievement of full implementation of plans.

These include funding issues, human resources questions, characteristics of the service delivery system, characteristics of the political context, the pace and demands of change, responses to the present implementation deadline, specific service problems, and data systems and administration procedures.

E. CMHS/NIMH Future Activities and Issues

Four issues face CMHS/NIMH as the agency responsible for the implementation of PL 99-660.

1. Monitoring and review: Viewed over several years, it is apparent that the feedback received by States through the review process organized by CMHS/NIMH had an impact on the way that the responses to the legislation were crafted. While this process was useful to many States during the planning phase, it has real limitations when the agency is asked to monitor the actual implementation of plans, not the plans themselves. Unlike the planning process, which does produce a document that can be assessed, implementation assessment requires contextual data and observation. Exclusive reliance on documents and paper submissions does not provide the type of information that can be gleaned when reviewers are actually in a State for a site visit or when there is an opportunity to discuss issues directly with State officials.

2. Quantitive measurement: The variability among States and the technical complexity involved in devising data systems make this a challenging requirement.

3. Technical assistance: As Appendix 4 indicates, a number of areas of technical assistance are recommended for some states.

4. Responsibilities related to additional plan requirements: With the amendment of PL 99-660 by PL 101-639 . . . [the States] must now apply all of the original PL 99-660 requirements to specify development of a community-based mental health services plan for children.

State-Anticipated Problems for Complete Implementation Funding

- Additional funding needed to continue present system
- Facing [mental health program] cuts due to revenue shortfalls
- Lack of legislative appropriation to fund parts of proposed or present system

Characteristics of the Service Delivery System

- Difficult interagency coordination, especially for children
- Autonomy of community mental health centers—their relationship to state level divisions
- Fixing local accountability for service delivery

Specific Service Problems

- Case management: hard to achieve full implementation
- Diminishing affordable housing
- Racial and ethnic service gaps
- Shortages of specialized service

Characteristics of the Political Context

- Political opposition in the transition from the current system to client-oriented systems of care
- Community resistance and need for public education
- Austerity and uncertainty
- Lack of support from counties and key system stakeholders

Human Resources

- Recruitment problems: unavailability of qualified mental health professionals (including rural areas and special populations)
- Hiring freezes affecting key positions

- Redeploying the work force presently in institutions
- High turnover rates (e.g., of case managers) which severely inhibit continuity of services and deplete training efforts
- Lack of materials for training and support [at all levels, local, State, and Federal]

Deadlines

- Complete implementation cannot be achieved in 2 to 3 years—5 to 8 years is more realistic given the complexity of the issues

Excerpts from State Mental Health Planning Provisions of the 1992 ADAMHA Reorganization Act, PL 102-321, July 10, 1992[2]

SEC. 1911. Formula Grants to States. (a) In General—For the purpose described in subsection (b), the Secretary, acting through the Director of the Center for Mental Health Services, shall make an allotment each fiscal year for each state. . . . The Secretary shall make a grant to the state of the allotment made for the state for the fiscal year if the state submits to the Secretary an application.

(b) Purpose of Grants—A funding agreement for a grant under subsection (a) is that the state involved will expend the grant only for the purpose of (1) carrying out the plan submitted . . . by the state for the fiscal year involved; (2) evaluating programs and services carried out under the plan; and (3) planning, administration, and educational activities related to providing services under the plan.

SEC. 1912. State Plan for Comprehensive Community Mental Health Services for Certain Individuals. (a) In General—The Secretary may make a grant under section 1911 only if (1) the state involved submits to the Secretary a plan for providing comprehensive community mental health services to adults with a serious mental illness and to children with a serious emotional disturbance and (2) the plan meets the criteria specified.

(b) Criteria for Plan—With respect to the provision of comprehensive community mental health services to individuals who are either adults with a serious mental illness or children with a serious emotional disturbance, the criteria referred to in subsection (a) regarding a plan are as follows:

(1) The plan provides for the establishment and implementation of an organized community-based system of care for such individuals.

(2) The plan contains quantitative targets to be achieved in the implementation of such system, including the numbers of such individuals residing in the areas to be served under such system.

(3) The plan describes available services, available treatment options, and available resources (including federal, state, and local public services and resources, and to the extent practicable, private services and resources) to be provided such individuals.

(4) The plan describes health and mental health services, rehabilitation services, employment services, housing services, educational services, medical and dental care, and other support services to be provided to such individuals.

(5) The plan describes the financial resources and staffing necessary to implement the requirements of such plan, including programs to train individuals as providers of mental health services, and the plan emphasizes training of providers of emergency health services regarding mental health.

(6) The plan provides for activities to reduce the rate of hospitalization of such individuals.

(7) The plan requires the provision of case management services to each such individual in the state who receives substantial amounts of public funds or services.

(8) The plan provides for the establishment and implementation of a program of outreach to, and services for, such individuals who are homeless.

(9) In the case of children with a serious emotional disturbance, the plan

> **(A) subject to subparagraph (B), provides for a system of integrated social services, educational services, juvenile services,**

[2] Unlike the preceding 1990 Report to Congress, this is an excerpt from a different document, namely, the 1992 ADAMHA Reorganization Act, PL 102-321, pp. 58–61. It is extremely relevant because, with its mandated definitions of serious mental illness, standardized methods, and quantitative targets, it lays the foundation for an accountability structure for the future. This accountability structure will be of critical importance if mental health will be included under national health-care reform, as discussed in chapter 26.

and substance abuse services that, together with health and mental health services, will be provided in order for such children to receive care appropriate for their multiple needs.

(10) The plan describes the manner in which mental health services will be provided to individuals residing in rural areas.

(11) The plan contains an estimate of the incidence and prevalence in the state of serious mental illness among adults and serious emotional disturbance among children.

(12) The plan contains a description of the manner in which the state intends to expend the grant under section 1911 for the fiscal year involved to carry out the provisions of the plan required in paragraphs (1) through (11).

(d) Requirement of Implementation of Plan—If the Secretary determines that a state has not completely implemented the plan, the Secretary shall reduce the amount of the allotment under section 1911 for the state for the fiscal year involved by an amount equal to 10% of the amount for the state for the fiscal year.

APPENDIX

D

Public–Academic Linkages in Clinical Training Programs in Psychology Supported by CMHS/NIMH, 1988–1993

ALABAMA

Carl Clements, PhD[Cgd]
University of Alabama
Department of Psychology
Tuscaloosa, AL 34548-0348

CALIFORNIA

Hector F. Myers, PhD[Cmdp]
UCLA, Department of Psychology
405 Hilgard Avenue
Los Angeles, CA 90024-1563

Gary W. Small, MD[Egipx]
UCLA, Department of Psychiatry
760 Westwood Plaza
Los Angeles, CA 90024-1759

Russell L. Boxley, PhD[Smd]
California School of Professional Psychology
1000 S. Fremont Avenue
Alhambra, CA 91803-1360

Margaret J. Gatz, PhD[Egd]
University of South California
Department of Psychology
Los Angeles, CA 90089-1061

Irvin H. Hart, PhD[Sgi]
Camarillo State Hospital, Box A
Camarillo, CA 93011

Jean Holroyd, PhD[Cmi]
UCLA Neuropsychology Institute
760 Westwood Blvd., Room C8-532
Los Angeles, CA 90024-1563

Stephanie Pearson, PhD[Smi]
Didi Hirsch Community Mental Health Center
4760 S. Sepulveda Blvd.
Culver City, CA 90230

May Tung, PhD[SCMmi]
Richmond Area Multi-Services, Inc.
3626 Balboa Street
San Francisco, CA 94121

Priority Population Served
- S = Seriously mentally ill adults
- C = Children and adolescents with serious emotional disturbances
- E = Elderly with mental disorders
- R = Mentally ill in rural areas
- M = Minorities: ethnic, with mental disorders

Type of Program
- g = General professional training programs
- m = Professional training for ethnic minority and disadvantaged students
- d = Doctoral program
- p = Postdoctoral
- i = Internship program
- x = Multidisciplinary
- c = Counseling psychology
- s = School psychology

Note: All programs are clinical psychology programs, unless noted as counseling or school psychology.

Larry W. Thompson, PhD[Egp]
Veterans Administration Medical Center
3801 Miranda Avenue
Palo Alto, CA 94304

COLORADO

Candace M. Fleming, PhD[Cmi]
University of Colorado Health Science
4200 E. 9th Avenue
Denver, CO 80262

Kenneth Purcell, PhD[Cgdmd]
University of Denver
Department of Psychology
Denver, CO 80208

Scott B. Hamilton, PhD[Cmdc]
Colorado State University
Department of Psychology
Fort Collins, CO 80523

CONNECTICUT

William Sledge, MD[Sgix]
Connecticut Mental Health Center
34 Park Street, Room 137
New Haven, CT 06519

Thomas R. Lipscomb, PhD[Cgi]
Child and Family Services, Inc.
1680 Albany Avenue
Hartford, CT 06105

Mary F. Sink, PhD[Sgip]
Danbury Hospital
24 Hospital Avenue
Danbury, CT 06810

Sara S. Sparrow, PhD[Cgip]
Yale Child Study Center
P.O. Box 3333
New Haven, CT 06520

DISTRICT OF COLUMBIA

James M. Jones, PhD[1md]
American Psychological Association
750 First Street, NE
Washington, DC 20002-4242

Linda Berg-Cross, PhD[CMmd]
Howard University
Department of Psychology
Washington, DC 20059

Lee Crump, PhD[Mmip]
Howard University Hospital
Department of Psychiatry
2401 Georgia Avenue, NW
Washington, DC 20060

FLORIDA

Albert J. Duchnowski, PhD[Cgix]
University of South Florida
Florida Mental Health Institute
13301 Bruce B. Downs Blvd.
Tampa, FL 33612

GEORGIA

Rex L. Forehand, PhD[Cgd]
University of Georgia
Department of Psychology
Athens, GA 30602

HAWAII

Stephen N. Haynes, PhD[SMmd]
University of Hawaii
Department of Psychology
Honolulu, HI 96822

ILLINOIS

Sheila C. Ribordy, PhD[CMmd]
DePaul University
Department of Psychology
2219 N. Kenmore
Chicago, IL 60614-3504

Alexandria J. Rosen, PhD[Cgd]
University of Illinois
Department of Psychology
Chicago, IL 60680

MARYLAND

Robert D. Coursey, PhD[Sgdp]
University of Maryland
Department of Psychology
College Park, MD 20742

Bruce Fretz, PhD[Emdpc]
University of Maryland
Department of Psychology
College Park, MD 20742

[1] Dr. Jones directs APA's Minority Fellowship Program, which does not designate priority populations.

Thomas Kenny, PhD[Cmix]
University of Maryland
School of Medicine
630 West Fayette Street
Baltimore, MD 21201

Raymond Lorion, PhD[Mmd]
University of Maryland
Department of Psychology
College Park, MD 20742

MASSACHUSETTS

Herbert Joseph, PhD[CMmi]
Boston City Hospital
Department of Psychology
818 Harrison Avenue, Talbot 43
Boston, MA 02118

Leslie M. Brody, PhD[SCmd]
Boston University
Department of Psychology
Boston, MA 02215

Eugene J. D'Angelo, PhD[Cgi]
Judge Baker Children's Center
295 Longwood Avenue
Boston, MA 02215

Jessica Daniel, PhD[Cmpx]
Judge Baker Children's Center
295 Longwood Avenue
Boston, MA 02215

MICHIGAN

Robert Zucker, PhD[Cgd]
Michigan State University
Department of Psychology
East Lansing, MI 48824-1117

MINNESOTA

Richard Weinberg, PhD[Cgds]
University of Minnesota
Department of School Psychology
Minneapolis, MN 55455

MISSISSIPPI

David S. Hargrove, PhD[Rgd]
University of Mississippi
Department of Psychology
301 Peabody Hall
University, MS 38677

William Wagner, PhD[CMmd]
University of Southern Mississippi
Department of Psychology
Hattiesburg, MS 39406-5012

NEBRASKA

William Spaulding, PhD[Sgd]
University of Nebraska
Department of Psychology
Lincoln, NE 68588-0308

NEW YORK

Ian M. Evans, PhD[Cgd]
State University of New York-Binghamton
Department of Psychology
Binghamton, NY 13901

Carmen I. Vazquez, PhD[SMmi]
New York University—Bellevue Hospital
Room 20S-14
27th Street 1st Avenue
New York, NY 10016

Michael Raulin, PhD[Cgd]
State University of New York/Buffalo
Department of Psychology
Buffalo, NY 14260

Jefferey R. Bedell, PhD[Sgip]
Albert Einstein College of Medicine
Department of Psychiatry
1300 Morris Park Avenue
Bronx, NY 10461

Priority Population Served
- S = Seriously mentally ill adults
- C = Children and adolescents with serious emotional disturbances
- E = Elderly with mental disorders
- R = Mentally ill in rural areas
- M = Minorities: ethnic, with mental disorders

Type of Program
- g = General professional training programs
- m = Professional training for ethnic minority and disadvantaged students
- d = Doctoral program
- p = Postdoctoral
- i = Internship program
- x = Multidisciplinary
- c = Counseling psychology
- s = School psychology

Note: All programs are clinical psychology programs, unless noted as counseling or school psychology.

Anderson J. Franklin, PhD[CMmd]
City College of City University of New York
Department of Psychology
New York, NY 10031

Lawrence Lichenstein, PhD[Smi]
New York University Medical Center
Gouverneur Hospital
227 Madison Street, Room 306
New York, NY 10002

Robert H. Goldstein, PhD[Sgi]
University of Rochester Medical Center
Department of Psychiatry
300 Crittenden Boulevard
Rochester, NY 14642

Robert Pollard, PhD[CSmix]
University of Rochester
Department of Psychiatry
Medical Center
300 Crittenden Blvd.
Rochester, NY 14642-8409

Deborah A. King, PhD[Egpx]
University of Rochester
Medical Center
Department of Psychiatry
300 Crittenden Boulevard
Rochester, NY 14642

NORTH CAROLINA

Eric Schopler, PhD[Cgix]
University of North Carolina
CB# 7180 Medical School Wing E
Chapel Hill, NC 27599

Bernadette Gray-Little, PhD[CgdSgd]
University of North Carolina
Department of Psychology
Chapel Hill, NC 27599

NORTH DAKOTA

Jeffrey Holm, PhD[RCMmd]
University of North Dakota
Department of Psychology
Grand Forks, ND 58202

OHIO

Rodney I. Hammond, PhD[Cmd]
Wright State University
School of Professional Psychology
Dayton, OH 45435

OKLAHOMA

Kenneth Sanvold, PhD[Mmd]
Oklahoma State University
Department of Psychology
Stillwater, OK 74078

OREGON

Eric M. Johnson, PhD[Cgi]
Morrison Center
3355 SE Powell Boulevard
Portland, OR 97202

PENNSYLVANIA

Ruben Echenmendia, PhD[CMmd]
Pennsylvania State University
Department of Psychology
University Park, PA 16802

SOUTH CAROLINA

Robert V. Heckel, PhD[Cmd]
University of South Carolina
Department of Psychology
Columbia, SC 29208

Ronald Belter, PhD[Cgi]
Medical University of South Carolina
171 Ashley Avenue
Charleston, SC 29424-0742

TEXAS

John P. Vincent, PhD[Smd]
University of Houston
Department of Psychology
Houston, TX 77204-5341

Walter De Lange, PhD[Cgp]
Houston Child Guidance Center
3214 Austin Street
Houston, TX 77004

Freddy A. Paniagua, PhD[Cmix]
University of Texas Medical Branch
Department of Psychiatry &
Behavioral Science
Galveston, TX 77550

Deborah Tharinger, PhD[Cgds]
University of Texas
Department of School Psychology
Austin, TX 78712

UTAH

Michael Bertoch, PhD[Cmds]
Utah State University
Department of Psychology
Logan, UT 84332-2810

VIRGINIA

Thomas H. Ollendick, PhD[Cgd]
Virginia Polytech Institute
& State University
Department of Psychology
Blacksburg, VA 24060

Thomas F. Oltmanns, PhD[Smd]
University of Virginia
Department of Psychology
Charlottesville, VA 29903-2477

WASHINGTON

Linda Teri, PhD[Egipx]
University of Washington
Department of Psychiatry
Seattle, WA 98195

Eric Trupin, PhD[Cgi]
University of Washington
Department of Psychiatry
Seattle, WA 98195

Priority Population Served
- S = Seriously mentally ill adults
- C = Children and adolescents with serious emotional disturbances
- E = Elderly with mental disorders
- R = Mentally ill in rural areas
- M = Minorities: ethnic, with mental disorders

Type of Program
- g = General professional training programs
- m = Professional training for ethnic minority and disadvantaged students
- d = Doctoral program
- p = Postdoctoral
- i = Internship program
- x = Multidisciplinary
- c = Counseling psychology
- s = School psychology

Note: All programs are clinical psychology programs, unless noted as counseling or school psychology.

380B18 FM 1019
05/04/98 30805 SELB
ICI INFORMATION CONSERVATION, INC.